How to Read a Paper

How to Read a Paper

The Basics of Evidence-Based Healthcare

SEVENTH EDITION

Trisha Greenhalgh
Professor of Primary Care Health Sciences
University of Oxford
Oxford, UK

Paul Dijkstra
Director of Medical Education and Consultant Sport and Exercise Medicine Physician
Aspetar Orthopaedic and Sports Medicine Hospital
Doha, Qatar
Nuffield Department of Orthopaedics, Rheumatology and Musculoskeletal Sciences
University of Oxford
Oxford, UK

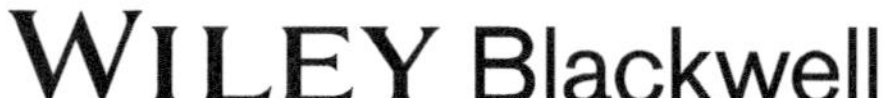

This edition first published 2025

Edition History
John Wiley & Sons Ltd (4e, 2010; 5e, 2014; 6e, 2019)

Registered Offices
John Wiley & Sons, Inc., 111 River Street, Hoboken, NJ 07030, USA
John Wiley & Sons Ltd, The Atrium, Southern Gate, Chichester, West Sussex, PO19 8SQ, UK

For details of our global editorial offices, customer services, and more information about Wiley products visit us at www.wiley.com.

Wiley also publishes its books in a variety of electronic formats and by print-on-demand. Some content that appears in standard print versions of this book may not be available in other formats.

Library of Congress Cataloging-in-Publication Data Applied for

Paperback ISBN: 9781394206902

Cover Design: Wiley

Set in 9.5/12pt Minion by Straive, Pondicherry, India

SKY10090925_111424

In November 1995, Trisha's friend Ruth Holland, book reviews editor of the *British Medical Journal*, suggested that she write a book to demystify the important but often inaccessible subject of evidence-based medicine. She provided invaluable comments on the original draft of the manuscript but was tragically killed in a train crash on 8th August 1996. This book is dedicated to her memory.

Contents

Foreword to the first edition by Professor Sir David Weatherall

Not surprisingly, the wide publicity given to what is now called *evidence-based* medicine has been greeted with mixed reactions by those who are involved in the provision of patient care. The bulk of the medical profession appears to be slightly hurt by the concept, suggesting as it does that until recently all medical practice was what Lewis Thomas has described as a frivolous and irresponsible kind of human experimentation, based on nothing but trial and error, and usually resulting in precisely that sequence. On the other hand, politicians and those who administrate our health services have greeted the notion with enormous glee. They had suspected all along that doctors were totally uncritical and now they had it on paper. Evidence-based medicine came as a gift from the gods because, at least as they perceived it, its implied efficiency must inevitably result in cost saving.

The concept of controlled clinical trials and evidence-based medicine is not new, however. It is recorded that Frederick II, Emperor of the Romans and King of Sicily and Jerusalem, who lived from 1192 to 1250 CE, and who was interested in the effects of exercise on digestion, took two knights and gave them identical meals. One was then sent out hunting and the other ordered to bed. At the end of several hours he killed both and examined the contents of their alimentary canals; digestion had proceeded further in the stomach of the sleeping knight. In the 17th century, Jan Baptista van Helmont, a physician and philosopher, became sceptical of the practice of blood-letting. Hence he proposed what was almost certainly the first clinical trial involving large numbers, randomisation and statistical analysis. This involved taking 200–500 poor people, dividing them into two groups by casting lots, and protecting one from phlebotomy while allowing the other to be treated with as much blood-letting as his colleagues thought appropriate. The number of funerals in each group would be used to assess the efficacy of blood-letting. History does not record why this splendid experiment was never carried out.

If modern scientific medicine can be said to have had a beginning, it was in Paris in the mid-19th century and where it had its roots in the work and teachings of Pierre Charles Alexandre Louis. Louis introduced statistical analysis to the evaluation of medical treatment and, incidentally, showed that blood-letting was a valueless form of treatment, although this did not change the habits of the physicians of the time, or for many years to come. Despite this pioneering work, few clinicians on either side of the Atlantic urged that trials of clinical outcome should be adopted, although the principles of numerically based experimental design were enunciated in the 1920s by the geneticist Ronald Fisher. The field only started to make a major impact on clinical practice after the Second World War following the seminal work of Sir Austin Bradford Hill and the British epidemiologists who followed him, notably Richard Doll and Archie Cochrane.

But although the idea of evidence-based medicine is not new, modern disciples like David Sackett and his colleagues are doing a great service to clinical practice, not just by popularising the idea, but by bringing home to clinicians the notion that it is not a dry academic subject but more a way of thinking that should permeate every aspect of medical practice. While much of it is based on mega-trials and meta-analyses, it should also be used to influence almost everything that a doctor does. After all, the medical profession has been brain-washed for years by examiners in medical schools and royal colleges to believe that there is only one way of examining a patient. Our bedside rituals could do with as much critical evaluation as our operations and drug regimes; the same goes for almost every aspect of doctoring. As clinical practice becomes busier, and time for reading and reflection becomes even more precious, the ability effectively to peruse the medical literature and, in the future, to become familiar with a knowledge of best practice from modern communication systems, will be essential skills for doctors. In this lively book, Trisha Greenhalgh provides an excellent approach to how to make best use of medical literature and the benefits of evidence-based medicine. It should have equal appeal for first year medical students and grey-haired consultants, and deserves to be read widely.

With increasing years, the privilege of being invited to write a foreword to a book by one's ex-students becomes less of a rarity. Trisha Greenhalgh was the kind of medical student who never let her teachers get away with a loose thought and this inquiring attitude seems to have flowered over the years; this is a splendid and timely book and I wish it all the success it deserves. After all, the concept of evidence-based medicine is nothing more than the state of mind that every clinical teacher hopes to develop in their students; Dr Greenhalgh's sceptical but constructive approach to medical literature suggests that such a happy outcome is possible at least once in the lifetime of a professor of medicine.

DJ Weatherall
Oxford
September 1996

Preface to the seventh edition

From Trisha

When I published the first edition of this book in 1996, I was a young physician in family medicine and a junior lecturer in a university; evidence-based medicine was still somewhat of an unknown quantity. It's now 2024, I am now approaching retirement (no longer practising clinical medicine but still working as a full-time professor) and evidence-based healthcare (no longer 'medicine' alone) is a major force in science and clinical practice. This seventh edition is co-written with new blood in the shape of Paul Dijkstra, a consultant physician and academic who has applied evidence-based healthcare in rigorous and imaginative ways in his own clinical field (sports medicine).

Back in 1995, when the idea for this book emerged, a handful of academics (including me) were already enthusiastic and had begun running 'training the trainers' courses to disseminate what we saw as a highly logical and systematic approach to clinical practice. Others – the majority of clinicians – were convinced that this was a passing fad that was of limited importance and would never catch on. I wrote *How to Read a Paper* for two reasons. First, students on my own courses were asking for a simple introduction to the principles presented in what was then known as 'Dave Sackett's big red book' (Sackett DL, Haynes RB, Guyatt GH, Tugwell P. *Clinical Epidemiology: A basic science for clinical medicine*. London: Little, Brown; 1991), an outstanding and inspirational volume that was already in its fourth reprint, but which some novices apparently found a hard read. Second, it was clear to me that many of the critics of evidence-based medicine did not really understand what they were dismissing and that until they did, serious debate on the clinical, pedagogical and even political place of evidence-based medicine as a discipline could not begin.

I am of course delighted that *How to Read a Paper* has become a standard reader in many medical and nursing schools, and that it so far been translated into over 20 languages, including French, German, Italian, Spanish, Portuguese, Chinese, Polish, Japanese, Czech and Russian. I am also delighted that what was initially dismissed as a fringe subject in academia has been well and truly mainstreamed in clinical service. In the UK, for example, it is now a contractual requirement for all doctors, nurses and pharmacists to practise (and for managers to manage) according to best research evidence.

In the 28 years since the first edition of this book was published, evidence-based medicine (and, more broadly, evidence-based healthcare) has waxed and waned in popularity. Hundreds of textbooks and tens of thousands of journal articles now offer different angles on the 'basics of EBM' covered briefly in the chapters that follow. An increasing number of these sources point out genuine limitations of evidence-based healthcare in certain contexts. Others look at evidence-based medicine and healthcare as a social movement – a 'bandwagon' that took off at a particular time (the 1990s) and place (North America) and spread quickly with all sorts of knock-on effects for particular interest groups.

It has been a delight working with Paul on this latest edition of what has become a classic introductory textbook. I think the new jointly authored text is more vibrant and varied than the previous single-author editions, and I hope you agree! As ever, we would welcome any feedback that will help make the text more accurate, readable and practical.

From Paul

When my wife Andrea and I bought our first copy of *How to Read a Paper* (at the time, I was a young sports medicine doctor and Andrea a masters student in experimental therapeutics at Oxford), I never thought I would one day have the privilege to co-author edition seven with Trisha Greenhalgh! While Andrea introduced Oxford and the Centre for Evidence-Based Medicine to me, Trisha opened my eyes to the new world (for me) of evidence-based healthcare: *How to Read a Paper* spotlighted shortcomings in my own undergraduate and early graduate training and changed how I practised sports medicine. The book inspired me to think and practice in a more 'evidence-based' way, to embrace patients' expertise more, to listen and question more, and to read healthcare (and other) papers more critically. Working with Trisha on the seventh edition (and to have had Trisha as one of my five DPhil in Evidence-Based Health Care mentors), was far more than an enlightening experience; it continues to be a joyous and humbling learning journey for which I'm eternally grateful! I am keen to share the lessons from this journey with you too.

When preparing this seventh edition, Trisha and I began with some formal reviews of the previous edition, and also a social media call for suggestions on how to improve it (including ones from students, who are the book's main target audience). They wanted a wider variety of chapters, updated examples and – the most significant suggestion perhaps – coverage of how the artificial intelligence (AI) revolution changes EBM and EBHC. After all, in these days of ChatGPT, maybe you don't need to read a paper at all, since your digital assistant could read it for you! We've included more examples of big data studies and other AI-supported research (see, in particular, Chapter 17). We added two more chapters, one on mechanistic evidence (Chapter 18) and another on papers reporting consensus exercises (Chapter 19).

Trisha Greenhalgh
Paul Dijkstra
September 2024

Preface to the first edition: do you need to read this book?

This book is intended for anyone, whether medically qualified or not, who wishes to find their way into the medical and healthcare literature, assess the scientific validity and practical relevance of the articles they find and, where appropriate, put the results into practice. These skills constitute the basics of evidence-based medicine (if you're thinking about what doctors do) or evidence-based healthcare (if you're looking at the care of patients more widely).

I hope this book will improve your confidence in reading and interpreting papers relating to clinical decision-making. I hope, in addition, to convey a further message, which is this. Many of the descriptions given by cynics of what evidence-based healthcare is (the glorification of things that can be measured without regard for the usefulness or accuracy of what is measured, the uncritical acceptance of published numerical data, the preparation of all-encompassing guidelines by self-appointed "experts" who are out of touch with real medicine, the debasement of clinical freedom through the imposition of rigid and dogmatic clinical protocols, and the over-reliance on simplistic, inappropriate, and often incorrect economic analyses), are actually criticisms of what the evidence-based healthcare movement is fighting against, rather than of what it represents.

Do not, however, think of me as an evangelist for the gospel according to evidence-based healthcare. I believe that the science of finding, evaluating and implementing the results of clinical research can, and often does, make patient care more objective, more logical, and more cost-effective. If I didn't believe that, I wouldn't spend so much of my time teaching it and trying, as a doctor, to practise it. Nevertheless, I believe that when applied in a vacuum (that is, in the absence of common sense and without regard to the individual circumstances and priorities of the person being offered treatment or to the complex nature of clinical practice and policymaking), 'evidence-based' decision-making is a reductionist process with a real potential for harm.

Finally, you should note that I am neither an epidemiologist nor a statistician, but a person who reads papers and who has developed a pragmatic (and at times unconventional) system for testing their merits. If you wish to pursue the epidemiological or statistical themes covered in this book, I would encourage you to move on to a more definitive text, references for which you will find at the end of each chapter.

Trisha Greenhalgh
November 1996

Acknowledgements

We are grateful to the people listed below for help and advice in preparing this book, though we take full responsibility for any inaccuracies.

To the people who, long ago, inspired and supported Trisha to write the first edition of *How to Read a Paper*, including Ruth Holland, Professor Sir Andy Haines, Professor Dave Sackett and Dr Anna Donald.

To people who have contributed ideas, references, feedback or suggestions to particular chapters for the current edition (those contributing to previous editions are mentioned in the text of the relevant chapter). We mention them in the relevant chapters. In sum, they are:

- Drs Jason Oke and Mohammed Farooq (chapter 5)
- Professor Mike Clarke (chapter 9)
- Professor Stavros Petrou (chapter 11)
- Dr Lennard Lee (chapter 15);
- Ms Yosra Mekki (chapter 17)

To the authors and publishers of articles who gave permission to reproduce figures or tables. Details are given in the text.

To various additional advisers and proofreaders who had direct input to this new edition or who advised Trisha on previous editions.

To the many readers, too numerous to mention individually, who took time to write in and point out ambiguities and typographical and factual errors in previous editions.

To our followers on social media who proposed numerous ideas and constructive criticisms. We are @trishgreenhalgh and @drpauldijkstra on X and can also be found on other platforms.

To our partners and families for their unfailing support for our academic work and writing. Shout out to Trisha's husband Dr Fraser Macfarlane and their sons Rob and Al Macfarlane. Our sons had not long been born when the first edition of this book was being written and are now pursuing their own scientific careers (Rob in marine biology, Al in medicine). Another shout out to Paul's wife Andrea Dijkstra and their daughters Elisabet and Anne – Elisabet pursuing doctoral studies in music at Guildhall School of Music and Drama in London and Anne well on her way to becoming an architect.

Chapter 1 **Why read papers at all?**

Does 'evidence-based medicine' simply mean 'reading papers in medical journals'?

Evidence-based medicine (EBM), which is part of the broader field of evidence-based healthcare (EBHC), is much more than just reading papers. According to what is still (more than 25 years after it was written) the most widely quoted definition, it is 'the conscientious, explicit and judicious use of current best evidence in making decisions about the care of individual patients' [1]. This definition is useful up to a point, but it misses out a very important aspect of the subject – and that is the use of mathematics. Even if you know almost nothing about EBHC, you probably know it talks a lot about numbers and ratios! A few years ago, Trisha and Anna Donald decided to be upfront about this in our own teaching, and proposed this alternative definition:

> *Evidence-based medicine is the use of mathematical estimates of the risk of benefit and harm, derived from high-quality research on population samples, to inform clinical decision-making in the diagnosis, investigation or management of individual patients.*

The defining feature of EBHC, then, is the use of *numbers* derived from research on *population samples* to inform decisions about *individuals*. This, of course, begs the question 'What is research?' – for which a reasonably accurate answer might be 'Focused, systematic enquiry aimed at generating new knowledge'. In later chapters, we explain how this definition can help you distinguish genuine research (which should inform your practice) from the poor-quality endeavours of well-meaning amateurs (which you should politely ignore). (As an aside, it has become fashionable to include qualitative research

How to Read a Paper: The Basics of Evidence-Based Healthcare, Seventh Edition.
Trisha Greenhalgh and Paul Dijkstra.

within EBHC, and we do cover this in chapter 12, but *most* people talking about EBM and EBHC are referring to research that generates *numbers*).

If you follow an evidence-based approach to clinical decision-making, therefore, all sorts of issues relating to your patients (or, if you work in public health medicine, issues relating to groups of people) will prompt you to ask questions about scientific evidence, seek answers to those questions in a systematic way and alter your practice accordingly.

You might ask questions, for example, about a patient's symptoms ('In a 34-year-old man with left-sided chest pain, what is the probability that there is a serious heart problem, and, if there is, will it show up on a resting ECG?'), about physical or diagnostic signs ('In an otherwise uncomplicated labour, does the presence of meconium [indicating fetal bowel movement] in the amniotic fluid indicate significant deterioration in the physiological state of the fetus?'), about the prognosis of an illness ('If a previously well two-year-old has a short fit associated with a high temperature, what is the chance that she will subsequently develop epilepsy?'), about therapy ('In patients with acute coronary syndrome [heart attack], are the risks associated with thrombolytic drugs [clot busters] outweighed by the benefits, whatever the patient's age, sex and ethnic origin?'), about cost-effectiveness ('Is the cost of this new anti-cancer drug justified, compared with other ways of spending limited healthcare resources?'), about patients' preferences ('In an 87-year-old woman with intermittent atrial fibrillation and a recent transient ischaemic attack, do the potential harms and inconvenience of thrombolytic therapy outweigh the risks of not taking it?') and about a host of other aspects of health and health services.

Professor Sackett, in the opening editorial of the very first issue of the journal *Evidence-Based Medicine*, summarised the essential steps in the emerging science of EBM [2]:

1. Convert our information needs into answerable questions (i.e. to formulate the problem).
2. Track down the best evidence with which to answer these questions – which may come from the clinical examination, the diagnostic laboratory, the published literature or other sources.
3. Appraise the evidence critically (i.e. weigh it up) to assess its validity (closeness to the truth) and usefulness (clinical applicability).
4. Implement the results of this appraisal in our clinical practice.
5. Evaluate our performance.

Hence, EBHC requires you not only to read papers but to read the *right* papers at the right time, and then to alter your behaviour (and, what is often more difficult, influence the behaviour of other people) in the light of what you have found. Sometimes, how-to-do-it courses in EBHC concentrate too heavily on the third of these five steps (critical appraisal) to the exclusion of all the others. Yet, if you have asked the wrong question or sought answers from the wrong sources, you might as well not read any papers at all. And all your training in search techniques and critical appraisal will go to waste if you do not put at least as much effort into implementing valid evidence and measuring progress towards your goals as you do into reading the paper. A few years ago, Trisha added three more stages to Sackett's five-stage model to incorporate the patient's perspective: the resulting eight stages, producing a *context-sensitive checklist for evidence-based practice*, which (like the other checklists in this book) is given in Appendix 1.

If we were to be pedantic about the title of this book, these broader aspects of EBHC should not even get a mention here. But we hope you understand that the book would be incomplete without the final section of this chapter (Before you start: formulate the problem), Chapter 2 (Searching the literature), and Chapter 16 (Applying evidence with patients). Chapters 3–15 describe step three of the EBHC process: critical appraisal; that is, what you should do when you actually have the paper in front of you. Chapter 20 deals with common criticisms of EBHC. The challenges of implementation are so complex that they needed a book of their own, *How to Implement Evidence-Based Healthcare* [3].

If you want to explore the subject of EBHC on the Internet, you could try the websites listed in Box 1.1 (these were the top suggestions when we asked our X [formerly Twitter] followers which ones they found most useful). If you're not ready for that yet, don't worry at this stage, but do put learning to use web-based resources on your to-do list. Don't worry either when you discover that there are over 1000 websites dedicated to EBM and EBHC; they all offer very similar material and you certainly don't need to visit them all.

Box 1.1 Web-based resources for evidence-based medicine

BMJ Evidence-Based Medicine Toolkit: a resource site maintained by this leading UK medical journal containing a wealth of resources and links for EBM, including links to critical appraisal checklists and statistical tools. https://bestpractice.bmj.com/info/toolkit

National Institute for Health and Care Excellence: this UK-based website, which is also popular outside the UK, links to evidence-based guidelines and topic reviews. www.nice.org.uk

The A–Z List of Evidence-Based Medicine Resources: A one-stop shop for various databases maintained by Dartmouth Libraries at Dartmouth College, Hanover, NH, USA, including PubMed, the Cochrane Database of Systematic Reviews and the Database of Abstracts of Reviews of Effectiveness (DARE): https://www.dartmouth.edu/library/biomed/guides/research/ebm-az-list.html

Why do people sometimes groan when you mention evidence-based healthcare?

Critics of EBHC might define it as 'the tendency of a group of young, confident and highly numerate medical academics to belittle the performance of experienced clinicians using a combination of epidemiological jargon and statistical sleight of hand' or 'the argument, usually presented with near-evangelistic zeal, that no health-related action should ever be taken by a doctor, a nurse, a purchaser of health services or a policymaker unless and until the results of several large and expensive research trials have appeared in print and approved by a committee of experts'.

Anyone who works face to face with patients knows how often it is necessary to seek new information before making a clinical decision. In general, we don't put a patient on a drug without evidence that it is likely to work. Apart from anything else, such off-licence use of medication is, strictly speaking, illegal. Surely we have all been practising EBHC for years?

Well, no, we haven't. There have been a number of surveys on the behaviour of doctors, nurses and related professionals and, while things seem to be improving, performance still falls short. It was estimated in the 1970s in the United States that only around 10–20% of all health technologies then available (i.e. drugs, procedures, operations, etc.) were evidence-based; that estimate improved to 21% in 1990. Studies of the interventions offered to consecutive series of patients suggested that 60–90% of clinical decisions, depending on the specialty, were 'evidence-based' [4]. But such studies had major methodological limitations (in particular, they were done in international centres of excellence and they did not take a particularly nuanced look at whether the patient would have been better off on a different drug or no drug at all).

Evidence-based decision-making is more common in some specialties than others. A large survey by an Australian team, for example, looked at 1000 patients treated for the 22 most commonly seen conditions in a primary-care setting. The researchers found that while 90% of patients received evidence-based care for coronary heart disease, only 13% did so for alcohol dependence [5]. Furthermore, the extent to which any individual practitioner provided evidence-based care varied in the sample from 32% of the time to 86% of the time. More recently, a review in *BMJ Evidence-Based Medicine* cited studies of the proportion of doctors' clinical decisions that were based on strong research evidence; the figure varied from 14% (in thoracic surgery) to 65% (in psychiatry); this paper also reported new data on primary healthcare, in which around 18% of decisions were based on 'patient-oriented high-quality evidence' [6].

The fashion to analyse what proportion of clinical decisions are evidence-based seems to have waned in recent years. But an online survey of UK general practitioners published by our team in 2020 showed that their knowledge of the quantitative benefits and harms of different treatments for long-term conditions such as diabetes or heart disease was very poor, and that most of them were aware that they were ignorant in this regard [7].

Let's take a look at the various approaches that health professionals use to reach their decisions in reality – all of which are examples of what EBHC *isn't*.

Decision-making by anecdote

When Trisha was a medical student, she occasionally joined the retinue of a distinguished professor as he made his daily ward rounds. On seeing a new patient, he would enquire about the patient's symptoms, turn to the massed ranks of juniors around the bed, and relate the story of a similar patient encountered a few years previously. 'Ah, yes. I remember we gave her such-and-such, and she was fine after that'. He was cynical, often rightly, about new drugs and technologies and his clinical acumen was second to none. Nevertheless, it had taken him 40 years to accumulate his expertise, and the largest medical textbook of all – the collection of cases that were outside his personal experience – was forever closed to him.

Anecdote (storytelling) has an important place in clinical practice [8]. Psychologists have shown that students acquire the skills of medicine, nursing and so on by memorising what was wrong with particular patients, and what happened to them, in the form of stories or 'illness scripts'. Stories about patients are the unit of analysis (i.e. the thing we study) in grand rounds and teaching sessions. Clinicians glean crucial information from patients' illness narratives; most crucially, perhaps, what being ill *means* to the patient. And experienced doctors and nurses rightly take account of the accumulated 'illness scripts' of all their previous patients when managing subsequent patients. But that doesn't mean simply doing the same for patient B as you did for patient A if your treatment worked, and doing precisely the opposite if it didn't!

The dangers of decision-making by anecdote are well illustrated by considering the risk–benefit ratio of drugs and medicines. When Trisha was in her first pregnancy, she developed severe vomiting and was given the anti-sickness drug prochlorperazine, and developed a very distressing neurological spasm. Two days later, she had recovered fully from this idiosyncratic reaction, but she never prescribed the drug since, even though the estimated prevalence of neurological reactions to prochlorperazine is only one in several thousand cases. Conversely, it is tempting to dismiss the possibility of rare but potentially serious adverse effects from familiar drugs, such as thrombosis on the contraceptive pill, when one has never encountered such problems in oneself or one's patients.

We clinicians would not be human if we ignored our personal clinical experiences, but we would be better to base our decisions on the collective experience of thousands of clinicians treating millions of patients, rather than on what we as individuals have seen and felt. Chapter 5 (Statistics for the non-statistician) describes some more objective methods, such as the number needed to treat, for deciding whether a particular drug (or other intervention) is likely to do a patient significant good or harm.

When the EBM movement was still in its infancy, Sackett emphasised that evidence-based practice was no threat to old-fashioned clinical experience or judgement [1]. The question of *how* clinicians can manage to be both 'evidence based' (i.e. systematically informing their decisions by research evidence) and 'narrative based' (i.e. embodying all the richness of their accumulated clinical anecdotes and treating each patient's problem as a unique illness story rather than as a 'case of X') is a difficult one to address philosophically, and beyond the scope of this book. The interested reader might like to look up two articles by Trisha on this topic [9, 10].

Decision-making by press cutting

Trisha qualified as a doctor back in 1983, when medical journals were mostly still in paper form. She used to keep a file of papers ripped out of her medical weeklies before binning the less interesting parts. If an article or editorial seemed to have something new to say, she consciously altered her clinical practice in line with its conclusions. One paper, for example, said that all children with suspected urinary tract infections should be sent for scans of the kidneys, so she began referring anyone under the age of 16 with urinary symptoms for specialist investigations. The advice was in print, and it was recent, so it must surely replace what had been standard practice – in this case, referring only the small minority of such children who display 'atypical' features.

This approach to clinical decision-making is still common, although the file of paper cuttings has usually been replaced by online articles that the clinician has bookmarked. How many clinicians do you know who justify their approach to a particular clinical problem by citing the results section of a single published study, even though they could not tell you anything at all about the methods used to obtain those results? Was the trial randomised and controlled (see section 'What are randomised controlled trials and why do they matter?' in Chapter 3)? How many patients, of what age, sex and disease severity, were involved (see section 'Who is the study about?' in Chapter 4)? How many withdrew from ('dropped out of') the study and why (see section 'Were preliminary statistical questions addressed?' in Chapter 4)? By what criteria were patients judged cured (see section 'Surrogate endpoints' in Chapter 6)? If the findings of the study appeared to contradict those of other researchers, what attempt was made to validate (confirm) and replicate (repeat) them (see section 'Ten questions to ask about a paper that claims to validate a diagnostic or screening test' in Chapter 8)? Were the statistical tests that allegedly proved the authors' point appropriately chosen and correctly performed (see Chapter 5)? Has the patient's perspective been systematically sought and incorporated via a shared decision-making tool (see Chapter 16)? Doctors (and nurses, midwifes, allied health professionals, medical managers, psychologists, medical students and consumer activists) who like to cite the results of medical research studies have a responsibility to ensure that they first go through a checklist of questions like these (more of which are listed in Appendix 1).

Decision-making by GOBSAT (good old boys sat around a table)

When Trisha wrote the first edition of this book in the mid-1990s, she was critical of the so-called 'GOBSAT (good old boys sat around a table) method for producing guidelines. Professor Cindy Mulrow [11], one of the founders of the science of systematic review (see Chapter 9) showed a few years ago that experts in a particular clinical field are *less* likely to provide an objective review of all the available evidence than a non-expert who approaches the literature with unbiased eyes, partly because non-evidence-based habits may get passed on unquestioningly from seniors to juniors in a specialty. Table 1.1 gives examples of practices that were at one time widely accepted as good clinical practice (and which would have made it into the GOBSAT guideline of the day) but which have subsequently been discredited by high-quality clinical trials. Indeed, one growth area in EBHC is using evidence to inform disinvestment in practices that were once believed to be evidence based [12].

While you should be wary of the 'GOBSAT' approach, there is increasing evidence that ignoring the views of subject experts entirely when constructing guidelines is not a sensible approach, for two reasons. Firstly, the embodied wisdom of people who have managed hundreds of patients with a condition can add great value to a thorough review of the published literature. And secondly, because evidence-based information is now much more readily available than it used to be, many subject experts these days have *both* clinical wisdom *and* up-to-date knowledge of the evidence base. Another growth area in EBHC is the science of how to use consensus processes in a systematic and objective manner rather than an opportunistic and partisan one. Chapter 19, new for this edition, explains a relatively new methodology for combining reviews of the evidence with tapping into experts' clinical wisdom.

Chapter 9 takes you through a checklist for assessing whether a 'systematic review of the evidence' produced to support recommendations for practice or policymaking really merits the description, and Chapter 10 discusses the harm that can be done by applying guidelines that are not evidence based.

Table 1.1 Examples of harmful practices once strongly supported by 'expert opinion'

Approximate time period	Clinical practice accepted by experts of the day	Practice shown to be harmful	Impact on clinical practice
From 500 BCE	Bloodletting (for just about any acute illness)	1820[a]	Bloodletting ceased around 1910
1957	Thalidomide for 'morning sickness' in early pregnancy led to the birth of over 8000 severely malformed babies worldwide	1960	The teratogenic effects of this drug were so dramatic that thalidomide was rapidly withdrawn when the first case report appeared
From at least 1900	Bed rest for acute low back pain	1986	Many doctors still advise people with back pain to 'rest up'
1960s	Benzodiazepines (e.g. diazepam) for mild anxiety and insomnia were initially marketed as 'non-addictive' but subsequently shown to cause severe dependence and withdrawal symptoms	1975	Benzodiazepine prescribing for these indications fell in the 1990s
1970s	Intravenous lignocaine in acute myocardial infarction, with a view to preventing arrhythmias, was subsequently shown to have no overall benefit and in some cases to *cause* fatal arrhythmias	1974	Lignocaine continued to be given routinely until the mid-1980s
Late 1990s	Rofecoxib (one of a new class of non-steroidal anti-inflammatory drug introduced for the treatment of arthritis) was later shown to increase the risk of heart attack and stroke	2004	Rofecoxib was quickly withdrawn following some high-profile legal cases in the USA, although new uses for cancer treatment (where risks may be outweighed by benefits) are now being explored

Table 1.1 (Continued)

Approximate time period	Clinical practice accepted by experts of the day	Practice shown to be harmful	Impact on clinical practice
2000s	Glitazones (a new class of drug for type 2 diabetes) were initially believed to produce better blood glucose control and improved cardiovascular risk compared with older classes of oral hypoglycaemic	2010	Rosiglitazone, for example, was withdrawn in Europe following post-marketing surveillance data showing increased risk of heart attack and death
2000s	Hydroxyethyl starch (HES) was standard practice for volume replacement in intensive care units	2013	Meta-analyses showed that not only does HES not improve survival but it is associated with adverse effects including bleeding, kidney damage, damage to organs (liver, lungs, spleen, bone marrow) and severe itching
2010s	Vaginal mesh implants for prolapse (a common complication after childbirth) were initially viewed as more effective and safer than traditional repair	2018	A review in UK in 2018 found that vaginal mesh implants were no more effective than standard repairs; adverse effects in some women required removal and, in some cases severe complications occurred, including (rare) deaths
2020s	Convalescent plasma was briefly hailed as potentially life-saving in the treatment of acute severe COVID-19 in early 2020 on the basis of non-randomised studies	2021	Randomised controlled trials showed that convalescent plasma had no benefit in most patients, except in rare cases where the plasma contained unusually high levels of neutralising antibodies. Some patients came to harm from transfusion reactions

[a] Interestingly, bloodletting was probably the first practice for which a randomised controlled trial was suggested. The physician van Helmont issued this challenge to his colleagues as early as 1662: 'Let us take 200 or 500 poor people that have fevers. Let us cast lots, that one half of them may fall to my share, and the others to yours. I will cure them without blood-letting, but you do as you know – and we shall see how many funerals both of us shall have' [13]. Thanks to Matthias Egger for this example.

Decision-making by cost minimisation

The popular press tends to be horrified when they learn that a treatment has been withheld from a patient for reasons of cost. Managers, politicians and, increasingly, doctors can count on being pilloried when a child with a rare cancer is not sent to a specialist unit in America or an elderly patient is denied a drug to stop her visual loss from macular degeneration. Yet, in the real world, all healthcare is provided from a limited budget and it is increasingly recognised that clinical decisions must take into account the economic costs of a given intervention. As Chapter 11 argues, clinical decision-making *purely* on the grounds of cost ('cost minimisation' – purchasing the cheapest option with no regard to how effective it is) is generally ethically unjustified and we are right to object vocally when this occurs.

Expensive interventions should not, however, be justified simply because they are new or because they ought to work in theory, or because the only alternative is to do nothing – but because they are very likely to save life or significantly improve its quality. How, though, can the benefits of a hip replacement in a 75-year-old be meaningfully compared with that of cholesterol-lowering drugs in a middle-aged man or infertility investigations for a couple in their twenties? Somewhat counterintuitively, there is no self-evident set of ethical principles or analytical tools that we can use to match limited resources to unlimited demand. As you can see in Chapter 11, the much-derided quality-adjusted life year or QALY and similar utility-based units are simply attempts to lend some objectivity to the illogical but unavoidable comparison of apples with oranges in the field of human suffering. In the UK, the National Institute for Health and Care Excellence (www.nice.org.uk) seeks to develop both evidence-based guidelines and fair allocation of NHS resources.

There is one more reason why some people find the term *evidence-based medicine* (or *healthcare*) unpalatable. This chapter has argued that EBHC is about coping with change, not about knowing all the answers before you start. In other words, it is not so much about what you have read in the past but about how you go about identifying and meeting your ongoing learning needs and applying your knowledge appropriately and consistently in new clinical situations. Doctors who were brought up in the old-school style of never admitting ignorance may find it hard to accept that a major element of scientific uncertainty exists in practically every clinical encounter, although, in most cases, the clinician fails to identify the uncertainty or to articulate it in terms of an answerable question (see next section). If you are interested in the research evidence on doctors' [lack of] questioning behaviour, see an excellent review by Swinglehurst [14].

The fact that none of us – not even the cleverest or most experienced – can answer all the questions that arise in the average clinical encounter means that the 'expert' is more fallible than they were traditionally cracked up to be. An evidence-based approach to ward rounds may turn the traditional medical hierarchy on its head when the staff nurse or junior doctor produces new evidence that challenges what the consultant taught everyone last week. For some senior clinicians, learning the skills of critical appraisal is the least of their problems in adjusting to an evidence-based teaching style!

Having defended EBHC against all the standard arguments put forward by clinicians, we should also acknowledge that a number of legitimate criticisms have been raised by philosophers and social scientists. Such arguments, summarised in Chapter 20, address the nature of knowledge and the question of how much medicine really rests on decisions at all. But please don't turn to that chapter (which is, philosophically speaking, a 'hard read') until you have fully grasped the basic arguments in the first few chapters of this book or you risk becoming confused!

Before you start: formulate the problem

When we ask medical students to write an essay about high blood pressure, they often produce long, scholarly and essentially correct statements on what high blood pressure is, what causes it and what the different treatment options are. On the day they hand their essays in, most of them know far more about high blood pressure than we do. They are certainly aware that high blood pressure is the single most common cause of stroke, and that detecting and treating everyone's high blood pressure would cut the incidence of stroke by almost half. Most of them are aware that stroke, although devastating when it happens, is a fairly rare event, and that blood pressure tablets have adverse effects such as tiredness, dizziness, impotence and getting 'caught short' when a long way from the lavatory.

But when we ask students a practical question such as 'Mrs Jones has developed light-headedness on these blood pressure tablets and she wants to stop all medication; what would you advise her to do?', they are often foxed. They sympathise with Mrs Jones' predicament, but they cannot distil from their pages of close-written text the one thing that Mrs Jones needs to know. As Smith (paraphrasing TS Eliot) asked a few years ago in a *BMJ* editorial: 'Where is the wisdom we have lost in knowledge, and the knowledge we have lost in information?'[15].

Experienced clinicians might think they can answer Mrs Jones' question from their own personal experience. But, as we showed in the previous section, few of them would be right. And even if they were right on this occasion, they would still need an overall system for converting the ragbag of information about a patient (an ill-defined set of symptoms, physical signs, test results and knowledge of what happened to this patient or a similar patient last time), the particular values and preferences (utilities) of the patient and other things that could be relevant (a hunch, a half-remembered article, the opinion of a more experienced colleague or a paragraph discovered by chance while flicking through a textbook) into a succinct summary of what the problem is and what specific additional items of information we need to solve that problem.

Sackett and colleagues, in a book subsequently revised by Straus et al. [16], have helped us by dissecting the parts of a good clinical question:

- First, define precisely *who* the question is about (i.e. ask 'How would I describe a group of patients similar to this one?').
- Next, define *which* manoeuvre you are considering in this patient or population (e.g. a drug treatment), and, if necessary, a comparison manoeuvre (e.g. placebo or current standard therapy).
- Finally, define the desired (or undesired) *outcome* (e.g. reduced mortality, better quality of life, and overall cost savings to the health service).

The second step may not concern a drug treatment, surgical operation or other intervention. The manoeuvre could, for example, be the exposure to a putative carcinogen (something that might cause cancer) or the detection of a particular surrogate endpoint in a blood test or other investigation. (A surrogate endpoint, as the section 'Surrogate endpoints' in Chapter 6 explains, is something that predicts, or is said to predict, the later development or progression of disease. In reality, there are very few tests that reliably act as crystal balls for patients' medical futures. The statement 'The doctor looked at the test results and told me I had six months to live' usually reflects either poor memory or irresponsible doctoring! In both these cases, the 'outcome' would be the development of cancer (or some other disease) several years later. In most clinical problems with individual patients, however, the 'manoeuvre' consists of a specific intervention initiated by a health professional.

Thus, in Mrs Jones's case, we might ask, 'In a 68-year-old white woman with essential (i.e. the most common form of) hypertension (high blood pressure), no coexisting illness, and no significant past medical history, whose blood pressure is currently X/Y, do the benefits of continuing therapy with ramipril (chiefly, reduced risk of stroke) outweigh the inconvenience?' Note that in framing the specific question, we have already established that Mrs Jones has never had a heart attack, stroke or early warning signs such as transient paralysis or loss of vision. If she had, her risk of subsequent stroke would be much higher and we would, rightly, load the risk–benefit equation to reflect this.

To answer the question we have posed, we must determine not just the risk of stroke in untreated hypertension but also the likely reduction in that risk which we can expect with drug treatment. This is, in fact, a rephrasing of a more general question (do the benefits of treatment in this case outweigh the risks?) which we should have asked before we prescribed bendroflumethiazide to Mrs Jones in the first place, and which all doctors should, of course, ask themselves every time they reach for their prescription pad.

Remember that Mrs Jones' alternative to staying on this particular drug is not necessarily to take no drugs at all; there may be other drugs with equivalent efficacy but less disabling adverse effects (as Chapter 6 argues, too many clinical trials of new drugs compare the product with placebo rather than with the best available alternative), or non-medical treatments such as exercise, salt restriction, homeopathy or yoga. Not all of these approaches would help Mrs Jones or be acceptable to her, but it would be quite appropriate to seek evidence as to *whether* they might help her – especially if she was asking to try one or more of these remedies.

We will probably find answers to some of these questions in the medical literature, and Chapter 2 describes how to search for relevant papers once you have formulated the problem. But before you start, give one last thought to your patient with high blood pressure. To determine her personal priorities (how does she value a 10% reduction in her risk of stroke in 5 years' time compared with the inability to go shopping unaccompanied today?), you will need to approach Mrs Jones, not a blood pressure specialist or the Medline database! Chapter 16 sets out some structured approaches for doing this.

Exercises based on this chapter

1. Go back to the fourth paragraph in this chapter, where examples of clinical questions are given. Decide whether each of these is a properly focused question in terms of:
   a. the patient or problem;
   b. the manoeuvre (intervention, prognostic marker, exposure);
   c. the comparison manoeuvre, if appropriate;
   d. the clinical outcome.
2. Now try the following:
   a. A 5-year-old child has been on high-dose topical steroids for severe eczema since the age of 20 months. The mother believes that the steroids are stunting the child's growth, and wishes to change to homeopathic treatment. What information does the dermatologist need to decide: (i) whether she is right about the topical steroids; and (ii) whether homeopathic treatment will be in this child's best interests?
   b. A woman who is 9 weeks pregnant calls out her general practitioner (GP) because of abdominal pain and bleeding. A previous ultrasound scan showed that the pregnancy was not ectopic. The GP decides that she might be having a miscarriage and tells her she must go into

hospital for a scan and, possibly, an operation to clear out the womb. The woman is reluctant. What information do they both need in order to establish whether hospital admission is medically necessary?

c. A 68-year-old man who is due for a COVID-19 booster vaccine, has got some information off the Internet which, he claims, proves that these vaccines are harmful and cause heart attacks. What information is needed to determine both the benefits and the potential harms of COVID-19 vaccination?

References

1. Sackett DL, Rosenberg WM, Gray J, et al. Evidence based medicine: what it is and what it isn't. *BMJ* 1996; **312**(7023): 71.
2. Sackett DL, Haynes RB. On the need for evidence-based medicine. *Evidence Based Medicine* 1995; **1**(1): 4–5.
3. Greenhalgh T. *How to Implement Evidence-based Healthcare.* Chichester: Wiley; 2019.
4. Sackett D, Ellis J, Mulligan I, et al. Inpatient general medicine is evidence based. *Lancet* 1995; **346**(8972): 407–10.
5. Runciman WB, Hunt TD, Hannaford NA, et al. CareTrack: assessing the appropriateness of health care delivery in Australia. *Medical Journal of Australia* 2012; **197**(10): 549.
6. Ebell MH, Sokol R, Lee A, Simons C, Early J. How good is the evidence to support primary care practice? *BMJ Evidence-Based Medicine* 2017; **22**: 88–92.
7. Treadwell JS, Wong G, Milburn-Curtis C, et al. GPs' understanding of the benefits and harms of treatments for long-term conditions: an online survey. *BJGP Open* 2020: **4**(1): bjgpopen20X101016.
8. Macnaughton J. Anecdote in clinical practice. In: Greenhalgh T, Hurwitz B, eds. *Narrative Based Medicine: Dialogue and discourse in clinical practice*, pp. 202–11. London: BMJ Publications, 1998.
9. Greenhalgh T. Narrative based medicine: narrative based medicine in an evidence-based world. *BMJ* 1999; **318**(7179): 323.
10. Greenhalgh T. Intuition and evidence – uneasy bedfellows? *British Journal of General Practice* 2002; **52**(478): 395.
11. Mulrow CD. Rationale for systematic reviews. *BMJ* 1994; **309**(6954): 597.
12. Harvey G, McInnes E. Disinvesting in ineffective and inappropriate practice: the neglected side of evidence-based health care? *Worldviews on Evidence-Based Nursing* 2015; **12**(6): 309–12.
13. van Helmont JA. *Oriatrike, or Physick Refined: The common errors therein refuted and the whole art reformed and rectified.* London: Lodowick-Loyd; 1662.
14. Swinglehurst DA. Information needs of United Kingdom primary care clinicians. *Health Information and Libraries Journal* 2005; **22**(3): 196–204.
15. Smith R. Where is the wisdom . . .? *BMJ* 1991; **303**(6806): 798.
16. Straus SE, Richardson WS, Glasziou P, et al. *Evidence-Based Medicine: How to practice and teach it (5th edn).* London: Elsevier; 2018.

Chapter 2 **Searching the literature**

The information jungle

Evidence is accumulating faster than ever before, and staying current is essential to ensure the best patient care.

Studies and reviews of studies of clinicians' information-seeking behaviour confirm that textbooks and personal contacts continue to be the most favoured sources for clinical information, followed by journal articles (see, e.g. Davies [1]). Use of the Internet as an information resource, especially the main database of medical articles PubMed/Medline, has increased dramatically in recent years, but the sophistication of searching and the efficiency in finding answers has not grown apace. Ask any medical librarian and you will hear tales of important clinical questions being addressed using unsystematic Google searches. While the need of healthcare professionals for information of the best quality has never been greater, barriers abound: lack of time, lack of facilities, lack of searching skills, lack of motivation and (perhaps worst of all) information overload [2].

The medical literature is far more of a jungle today than it was when the first edition of this book was published in 1996. The volume and complexity of published literature has grown: Medline alone has over 29 million references. While Medline is the flagship database for journal articles in the health sciences, it is a very conservative resource, and slow to pick up new journals or journals published outside the USA. Therefore, many thousands of high-quality papers that may be available via other databases are not on Medline. The proliferation of databases makes the information jungle that much more confusing, especially because each database covers its own range of journals and each has its own particular search protocols. How will you cope?

There is hope: in the past few years, the information 'jungle' has been tamed by means of information highways, high-speed transit systems, and platforms that employ artificial intelligence (AI) [3,4]. Knowing how to

How to Read a Paper: The Basics of Evidence-Based Healthcare, Seventh Edition.
Trisha Greenhalgh and Paul Dijkstra.

access these navigational wonders will save you time and improve your ability to find the best evidence. The purpose of this chapter is not to teach you to become an expert searcher but rather to help you recognise the kinds of resources that are available, choose intelligently among them and put them to work directly.

What are you looking for?

A searcher may approach medical (and, more broadly, health science) literature for three broad purposes:

1. Informally, almost recreationally, browsing to keep current and to satisfy our intrinsic curiosity.
2. Focused, looking for answers, perhaps related to questions that have occurred in clinic or that arise from individual patients and their questions.
3. Surveying the existing literature, perhaps before embarking on a research project, assignment or thesis.

Each approach involves searching in a very different way.

Browsing has an element of serendipity about it. In the old days, we would pick up our favourite journal and follow where our fancy took us. And if our fancy was informed with a few tools to help us discriminate the quality of papers we found, so much the better. These days, we can make use of new tools to help us with our browsing. We can browse electronic journals just as easily as paper journals; we can use alerting services to let us know when a new issue has been published and even tell us if articles matching our interest profile are in that issue. We can have rich site summary (RSS) feeds of articles from particular journals or on particular topics sent to our email addresses or our smartphones or personal blogs or podcasts, and we can participate in X (formerly Twitter) exchanges related to newly published papers. Almost every journal has links from its home page allowing at least one of these social networking services (e.g. *JOSPT Insights* for orthopaedic and sports physical therapists). These technologies are changing continuously. Those of us who have been faced with deluges of new offprints, photocopies and journal issues that we have been meaning to read will be happy to learn that we can create the same chaos electronically. That's what browsing serendipitously is all about, and it is a joy we should never lose, in whatever medium our literature may be published.

Looking for answers implies a much more focused approach, a search for an answer we can trust to apply directly to the care of a patient. When we find that trustworthy information, it is OK to stop looking – we don't need to beat the bush for absolutely every study that may have addressed this topic. This kind of query is increasingly well served by new synthesised information sources whose goal is to support evidence-based care and the transfer of research findings into practice. This is discussed further below.

Surveying the literature – preparing a detailed, broad-based and thoughtful literature review, for example, when writing an essay for an assignment, a thesis chapter or an article for publication – involves an entirely different process. The purpose here is less to influence patient care directly than to identify the existing body of research that has addressed a problem and clarify the gaps in knowledge that require further research. For this kind of searching, a strong knowledge of information resources and skill in searching them are fundamental. A simple PubMed search will not suffice. Multiple relevant databases need to be searched systematically, and citation chaining (see subsequent text) needs to be employed to assure that no stone has been left unturned. If this is your goal, you *must* consult with an information professional (health librarian, clinical informaticist, etc.).

Levels upon levels of evidence

The term *level of evidence* refers to what degree that information can be trusted, based on study design. Traditionally, and considering the most common type of question (relating to therapy), levels of evidence are represented as a pyramid with systematic reviews positioned grandly at the top, followed by well-designed randomised controlled trials (RCTs), then observational studies such as cohort studies or case–control studies, with case studies, bench (laboratory) studies and 'expert opinion' somewhere near the bottom (Figure 2.1). All this is described in more detail later in this book.

Our librarian colleagues, who are often keen on synthesised evidence and technical resources for decision support, remind us of a rival pyramid, with computerised decision support systems (abbreviated 'systems') at the top, above evidence-based practice guidelines, followed by systematic review synopses, with standard systematic reviews beneath these, and so on [5].

Others, proposing a 'circle of methods' [6], have challenged the evidence pyramid concept, and the superior position of RCTs [7] and systematic reviews [8]. See more about this in Chapter 3.

Whether we think in terms of the first (traditional) evidence pyramid or the second (more contemporary) one, or whether we feel challenged by evidence pyramids, RCTs and systematic reviews, the message is clear: all evidence, all information, is not necessarily equivalent. We need to keep a sharp eye out for the believability of whatever information we find, wherever we find it.

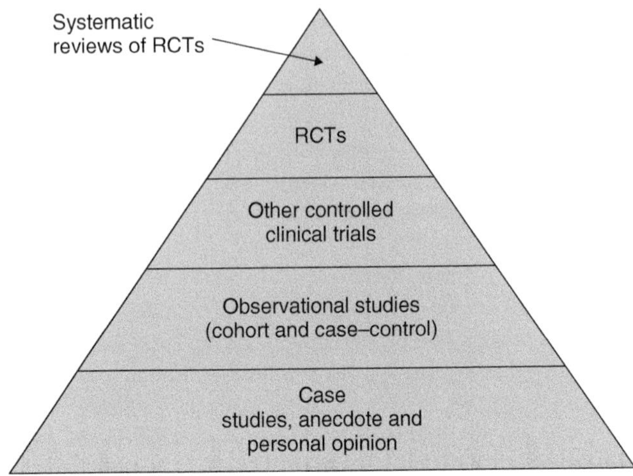

Figure 2.1 A simple hierarchy of evidence for assessing the quality of trial design in therapy studies.

Synthesised sources: systems, summaries and syntheses

Information resources synthesised from primary studies constitute a very high level of evidence indeed. These resources exist to help translate research into practice and inform clinician and patient decision-making. This kind of evidence is relatively new (at least, compared to traditional primary research studies, which have been with us for centuries), but their use is expected to grow considerably as they become better known.

Systematic reviews are perhaps the oldest and best known of the synthesised sources, having started in the 1980s under the inspiration of Archie Cochrane, who bemoaned the multiplicity of individual clinical trials whose information failed to provide clear messages for practice. The original efforts to search broadly for clinical trials on a topic and pool their results statistically grew into the Cochrane Library (www.cochranelibrary.com) in the mid-1990s; Cochrane reviews became the gold standard for systematic reviews and the Cochrane Collaboration the premier force for developing and improving review methodology [9].

There are many advantages to systematic reviews and a few cautions. On the plus side, systematic reviews are relatively easy to interpret. The systematic selection and appraisal of the primary studies according to an approved protocol means that bias is minimised. Smaller studies, which are all too common in some topic areas, may show a trend towards positive impact but lack statistical significance. But when data from several small studies are summed mathematically in a process called *meta-analysis*, the combined data may produce a statistically significant finding (see section 'Meta-analysis for the non-statistician'). Systematic reviews can help resolve contradictory findings among different studies on the same question. If the systematic review has been properly conducted, the results are likely to be robust and generalisable. On the negative side, systematic reviews can replicate and magnify flaws in the original studies (e.g. if all the primary studies considered a drug at subtherapeutic dose, the overall – misleading – conclusion may be that the drug has 'no effect'). Cochrane reviews can be a daunting read, but here's a tip. The bulk of a Cochrane review consists of methodological discussion: the gist of it can be gleaned by jumping to the 'plain language summary', always to be found directly following the abstract. Alternatively, you can gain a quick and accurate summary by looking at the pictures, especially something called a *forest plot*, which graphically displays the results of each of the primary studies along with the combined result. Chapter 9 explains systematic reviews in more detail.

Cochrane reviews are only published electronically, but other systematic reviews appear throughout the clinical literature. They are most easily accessed via the Cochrane Library, which publishes Cochrane reviews, the Database of Abstracts of Reviews of Effects (DARE), listed in Cochrane Library as 'other reviews'), and a database of health technology assessments (HTAs). DARE provides not only a bibliography of systematic reviews but also a critical appraisal of most of the reviews included, making this a 'pre-appraised source' for systematic reviews. HTAs are essentially systematic reviews but range further to consider economic and policy implications of drugs, technologies and health systems. All may be searched relatively simply and simultaneously via the Cochrane Library.

In the past, Cochrane reviews focused mainly on questions of therapy (see Chapter 6) or prevention but, since 2008, considerable effort has gone into producing other systematic reviews. These include systematic reviews of diagnostic tests (see Chapter 8), rapid reviews and qualitative systematic reviews (see Chapter 12).

Point-of-care resources are rather like electronic textbooks or detailed clinical handbooks, but are explicitly evidence-based, continuously updated and designed to be user-friendly – perhaps, the textbook of the future. Three popular ones are *Clinical Evidence*, *DynaMed* and *UpToDate*. All aspire to be firmly evidence-based, peer-reviewed, revised regularly and with links to the primary research incorporated into their recommendations.

- *BMJ Best Practice* (https://bestpractice.bmj.com/info), a British resource (for which a subscription is required), draws on systematic reviews to provide very quick information, especially on the comparative value of tests and interventions. Reviews are organised into sections, such as child health or skin disorders, or you can search the database by keyword (e.g. 'asthma') or by a full review list. In each clinical area, there are sections for doctors, nurses, pharmacists and patients.

- *DynaMed* (including *DynaMedex, DynaMed Decisions* and *Dynamic Health* (https://www.ebsco.com/health-care/clinical-decision-support), produced in the United States, is rather more like a handbook with chapters covering a wide variety of disorders, but with summaries of clinical research, levels of evidence and links to the primary articles. It covers causes and risks, complications and associated conditions (including differential diagnosis), what to look for in the history and physical examination, what diagnostic tests to do, prognosis, treatment, prevention and screening and links to patient information handouts. You can search very simply for the condition; the results include links to other chapters about similar conditions. This is a proprietary resource (i.e. you generally have to pay for it), although it may be provided free to those who offer to write a chapter themselves!
- *UpToDate* (https://www.wolterskluwer.com/en/solutions/uptodate), an evidence-based clinical decision support solution, has been around for more than 30 years. It is a subscription resource used by two million clinicians in more than 190 countries. Clinician authors, editors and peer reviewers collaborate to produce content on a wide range of topics, easy to access at the point of care and often integrated with electronic health systems.

All the above resources have applications ('apps') that allow use on smartphones, which improve their bedside usability for patient care.

New point-of-care resources are continually emerging, so it is very much a matter of individual preference which you use. The three listed were chosen because they are peer-reviewed, regularly updated and directly linked to the primary evidence.

Practice guidelines, covered in detail in Chapter 10, are 'systematically developed statements to assist practitioner and patient decisions about appropriate healthcare for specific clinical circumstances' [10]. In a good guideline, the scientific evidence is assembled systematically, the panel developing the guideline includes representatives from all relevant disciplines, including patients, and the recommendations are explicitly linked to the evidence from which they are derived [11]. Guidelines are a summarised form of evidence, very high on the hierarchy of pre-appraised resources, but the initial purpose of the guideline should always be kept in mind: guidelines for different settings and different purposes can be based on the same evidence but come out with different recommendations.

Guidelines are readily available from a variety of sources, including the following:

- *National Institute for Health and Care Excellence* (NICE; www.nice.org.uk) is a UK government-funded agency responsible for developing evidence-based guidelines and other evidence summaries to support national health policy. NICE Clinical Knowledge Summaries (http://cks.nice.org.uk), based closely on NICE guidelines, are designed especially for those working in primary healthcare.
- *World Health Organization* (https://www.who.int/publications/who-guidelines) develops global guidelines to ensure 'the appropriate use of evidence' on key topics like diphtheria [12], and lower back pain [13].
- *National Center for Complementary and Integrative Health Clinical Practice Guidelines* (https://www.nccih.nih.gov/health/providers/clinicalpractice) is a US Department of Health and Human Services resource with a list of guidelines (issued by third-party organisations) in several domain categories (e.g. allergy and immunology, cardiology, and family medicine).

A straightforward and popular way to search practice guidelines is via TRIP (Turning Research into Practice, www.tripdatabase.com), a federated search engine discussed below. For guidelines, look in the box panel to the left of the screen following a simple search on TRIP: a heading 'guidelines' appears, with subheadings for Australia and New Zealand, Canada, UK, United States, Europe, and Other, and a number indicting the number of guidelines found on that topic. NICE and National Guideline Clearinghouse are included among the guidelines searched.

Pre-appraised sources: synopses of systematic reviews and primary studies

If your topic is more circumscribed than those covered in the synthesised or summary sources listed above, or if you are simply browsing to keep current with the literature, consider one of the pre-appraised sources as a means of navigating through those millions of articles in our information jungle. The most common format is the digest of clinical research articles gleaned from core journals and deemed to provide important information for patient care: *BMJ Evidence-Based Medicine*, *ACP Journal Club*, *BMJ Mental Health*, *POEMS (Patient-Oriented Evidence that Matters)* and the Patient-Centered Outcomes Research Institute (PCORI) *Evidence Updates*. Some are free; some are available through institutions or memberships or private subscription. Most have a format that includes a structured abstract and a brief critical appraisal of the article's content. Studies included may be single studies or systematic reviews. Each is considered a pre-appraised source and, critical appraisal aside, simple inclusion has implications for the perceived quality and importance of the original article.

All these sources may be considered as small databases of select studies, which may be searched by keyword. Other services, such as PCORI's *Evidence Updates* (https://www.pcori.org/impact/evidence-updates), provide concise updates based on systematic reviews and other research studies to both patients and clinicians.

DARE was mentioned as a pre-appraised source for systematic reviews other than Cochrane reviews, in that it provides an augmented abstract and a brief critical appraisal for most systematic reviews in its database.

Another source that is considered pre-appraised, although it contains no appraisals, is the *Central Register of Controlled Trials* (CENTRAL), also part of the Cochrane Library. CENTRAL is a bibliography of studies included in Cochrane reviews, as well as in new studies on similar topics, maintained by the various Cochrane review groups. DARE, CENTRAL, the Cochrane Database of Systematic Reviews, Cochrane Clinical Answers, the HTA database and the NHS Economic Evaluation Database, which also includes critically appraised summaries of studies, may all be searched simultaneously in the Cochrane Library.

Specialised resources

Specialised information sources, organised (as the name implies) to assist the specialist clinician in a particular field, are often also useful for generalists and primary care clinicians. Most professional associations maintain excellent websites with practice guidelines, journal links and other useful information resources; most require membership of the association to access educational and practice materials. Some notable examples are:

- *GIDEON* (*Global Infectious Diseases and Epidemiology Network*, www.gideononline.com) is an evidence-based programme that assists with diagnosis and treatment of communicable diseases. In addition, GIDEON tracks incidence and prevalence of diseases worldwide and includes the spectrum covered by antibiotic agents.
- *Psychiatry Online* (https://psychiatryonline.org) is a compendium of core textbooks (including the *Diagnostic and Statistical Manual of Mental Disorders*, fifth edition), psychiatry journals and practice guidelines of the American Psychiatric Association, produced by the American Psychiatric Press.
- *LitCOVID* (https://www.ncbi.nlm.nih.gov/research/coronavirus), a literature hub run by the US National Library of Medicine, tracks up-to-date

scientific information about COVID-19. You could also check out collections on COVID-19 prepared by some of the leading medical journals, such as this one from the *Lancet* (https://www.thelancet.com/coronavirus/collection), to see how they compare in form and content.

These are only examples. Whatever your specialty (or specialist topic), there will usually be a similar resource maintained by a professional society. Ask a librarian or clinical informaticist to help you find the relevant one!

Primary studies: tackling the jungle

Whether through habit or through lack of familiarity with all the useful synthesised, summarised or pre-appraised sources described earlier, most healthcare practitioners still prefer a basic search of Medline/PubMed to answer their clinical information needs. Some simply prefer to assess the primary literature for themselves, without thumbnail critical appraisals or incorporation into larger disease management chapters. This, however, is easier said than done; paywalls prevent millions – clinicians and patients – from easy access to the primary literature.

Primary sources can be found in a variety of ways. You could look at the reference lists and hyperlinks from the secondary sources described. You could identify them from journals – for example, via RSS feeds, table-of-contents services or more focused topical information services. And you could search databases such as PubMed/Medline, EMBASE, PASCAL, Cochrane Library, CINAHL (Cumulated Index of Nursing and Allied Health Literature), SPORTDiscus, Biosis Previews, Web of Science, Scopus or Google or Google Scholar. Let's consider some of these databases.

PubMed

PubMed is the most frequently accessed Internet resource for most physicians and health professionals worldwide, probably because it is free and well known (just put 'PubMed' into Google and you will find it easily). Most people opt for the basic PubMed search, using two or three search text words at best – and characteristically turning up hundreds or thousands of references, of which they look at only the first couple of screens. This is certainly not the most efficient way to search, but it is the reality of how most people *do* search [14]. Interestingly, when just one or two more search terms are added, the efficiency of a basic PubMed search improves substantially [14].

Simple tools that are part of the Medline search engine can be used to help focus a search and produce better results for a basic search, but they are rarely used by medical students or doctors. One such tool is the '*limit*' function, allowing restrictions to such generic topics as gender, age group or study design, to language or to core clinical journals. The advanced search function on PubMed incorporates these limits into a single search page. Next time you are on the PubMed website with some time to spare, play with these tools and see how easily they can sharpen your search.

'*Clinical queries*', an option provided at the bottom of the basic PubMed screen, superimposes on the search a filter based on optimum study designs for best evidence, depending on the domain of the question and the degree to which one wishes to focus the question. For example, if you were searching for a therapy study for hypercholesterolaemia, the clinical query for therapy/narrow and specific would be rendered as '(hypercholesterolaemia) AND (randomised controlled trial [Publication Type] OR (randomised [Title/Abstract] AND controlled [Title/Abstract] AND trial [Title/Abstract]))'. This search resulted in 159 postings (in February 2024). Sometimes, the search might need further limits or perhaps the addition of a second term, such as a specific drug. In addition to clinical studies, PubMed has also added COVID-19 as a filter category.

Citation chaining (or, to use its alternative term, *citation tracking*) provides another means of following a topic. Let's say that, following your interest in hypercholesterolaemia, you wish to follow up a classic primary research study, the West of Scotland Coronary Prevention Study, originally published in the 1990s [15]. In your PubMed search, you found a study in the *New England Journal of Medicine* in 2007 that described a 10-year follow-up [16], but you now wonder if there has been anything further. The Web of Science (Clarivate) network, comprising Science Citation Index, Social Sciences Citation Index and the Arts and Humanities Citation Index online, provides a cited reference search feature. Entering the author's name (in this case I. Ford) and the year of publication (2007), we can trace the specific article and find that several hundred articles published since have cited it in their reference lists, including at least one 20-year follow-up study [17]. Citation searching can give a crude indication of the relative importance of a study, based on the number of times it has been cited (bearing in mind that one sometimes cites a paper when emphasising how bad it is!). A very simple (but somewhat less accurate) way of citation chaining is to use Google Scholar: simply put the article's title into this search engine and, when you have found it, select 'citations'.

SPORTDiscus

SPORTDiscus is a bibliographic database for sports and sports medicine research that includes records from several sports medicine journals, books, dissertations and more. It is one of more than 350 full-text databases hosted by EBSCO, a fee-based online research service (www.ebsco.com).

Google Scholar

Google Scholar, a very broad-based web browser, is increasingly popular and extremely handy, accessible as it is from the Google toolbar. For an obscure topic, Google Scholar can be an excellent resource on which to fall back, as it will identify papers that are listed on PubMed as well as those that aren't. Unfortunately, there are no quality filters (such as clinical queries), no limits (such as gender or age), so a search on a widely researched topic will tend to turn up a long list of hits that you have no alternative but to wade through.

One-stop shopping: federated search engines

Perhaps the simplest and most efficient answer for most clinicians searching for information for patient care is a federated search engine such as TRIP (www.tripdatabase.com), which searches multiple resources simultaneously and has the advantage of being free.

TRIP has a truly primitive search engine, but it searches synthesised sources (systematic reviews including Cochrane reviews), summarised sources (including practice guidelines from North America, Europe, Australia/New Zealand and elsewhere, as well as electronic textbooks) and pre-appraised sources (such as the journals *Evidence-Based Medicine* and *Evidence-Based Mental Health*), as well as searching all clinical query domains in PubMed simultaneously. Moreover, searches can be limited by discipline, such as paediatrics or surgery, helping both to focus a search and eliminate clearly irrelevant results and acknowledging the tendency of medical specialists to (rightly or wrongly) prefer the literature in their own journals. Given that most clinicians favour very simple searches, a TRIP search may well get you the maximum bang for your buck.

Using artificial intelligence to search the literature

Artificial intelligence technology to facilitate searching the health literature is promising. However, although resulting in a more focused literature search, there was no significant improvement in the number of results in this study [4]. Scite (https://scite.ai) is a subscription AI tool (with free resources like browser extension and Zotero plugin) that could speed up literature reviews [18]. Scite's advanced search feature allows you to search and filter metadata of publications and classifies citations by how they are 'talking' about a paper [18]. Scite's subscription features include an 'Assistant (an AI-powered 'research partner'), Search (to search citation statements directly for relevant facts and insights), Custom Dashboards to track trends and get insights from groups of papers, and Reference Check (screening manuscripts as you write to ensure that you are using high-quality references). Before you use an AI assistant to help you write an article or assignment, check the rules you're working under. Some journals and some educational providers either don't allow it at all or ask you to declare details. And remember, AI-supported searches have been known to hallucinate!

Asking for help and asking around

Healthcare professionals don't need to cope with the literature alone. Health librarians are readily available in universities, hospitals, government departments and agencies and professional societies. They know the databases available, they know the complexities of searching, they know the literature (even complex government documents and obscure data sets), and they usually know just enough about the topic to have an idea of what you are looking for and levels of evidence that are likely to be found. When one librarian can't find an answer, there are local and international colleagues with whom they could consult.

Asking people you know yourself or know about has its advantages. Experts in the field are often aware of unpublished research or reports commissioned by government or other agencies: notoriously hard to find 'grey' or 'fugitive' literature that is not indexed in any source. An international organised information-sharing organisation CHAIN (Contact, Help, Advice and Information Network, www.chain-network.org.uk) provides a useful online network for people working in health and social care who wish to share information. CHAIN can be joined for free and, once a member, you can pitch in a question and target it to a designated group of specialists.

In a field as overwhelming and complex as health information, asking colleagues and people you trust has always been a preferred source for information. In the early days of evidence-based medicine, asking around was seen as unsystematic and 'biased'. It remains true that asking around is insufficient for a search for evidence but, in the light of the ability of experts to locate obscure literature, can any search really be considered complete without it?

Online tutorials for effective searching

Many universities and other educational institutions now provide self-study tutorials, which you can access via computer, either on an intranet (for members of the university only) or the Internet (accessible to everyone). Here are some we found when revising this chapter for the seventh edition. Note that, as with all Internet-based sources, some sites will move or close down, so we apologise in advance if you find a dead link:

- *Finding the Evidence* from the University of Oxford's Centre for Evidence-Based Medicine. Some brief advice on searching key databases but relatively little in the way of teaching you how to do it. Perhaps best for those who have already been on a course and want to refresh their memory (https://www.cebm.net/2014/06/finding-the-evidence).
- *PubMed – Searching Medical Literature* from the Library at Georgia State University. As the title implies, this is limited to PubMed but offers some advanced tricks such as how to customise the PubMed interface to suit your personal needs (http://research.library.gsu.edu/pubmed).
- *PubMed Tutorial* from PubMed itself. Offers an overview of what PubMed does and doesn't do, as well as some exercises to get used to it (http://www.nlm.nih.gov/bsd/disted/pubmedtutorial).
- *How to undertake a literature search* from the Royal College of Nursing. They break the exercise of searching the literature down into ten steps, from identifying key concepts to choosing databases for your search and saving your results and search strategy. Each step is succinctly discussed with examples and suggestions of where to get help (https://www.rcn.org.uk/library/support/literature-searching-and-training/how-to-undertake-a-literature-search#steps).

There are many other similar tutorials accessible free on the Internet, but few of them cover much beyond searching for primary studies and systematic reviews in PubMed and the Cochrane Library.

Exercises based on this chapter

1. If you were a busy family physician and keen to stay updated on the latest developments in your specialty, which sources of evidence would you use? What would be the advantages and disadvantages of each of them?
2. Explore the TRIP database (www.tripdatabase.com or put 'Trip database' into Google) as an example of a powerful federated search engine. Put a term into the search box (for example 'gestational diabetes') and hit the search button. Now look down the left hand column and see what the site offers you in terms of systematic reviews, evidence-based synopses, guidelines and key primary research.
3. Explore the Cochrane Library and find a Cochrane review on a topic of your choice. The easiest way to get there is put 'Cochrane Library' into Google. On the home page, you can browse by broad category of topic, or you can use the search engine to look for more specific topics. Skim through an entire review (they are often very long) to get a feel for how these reviews are structured. Many of the recent ones have useful patient (lay) summaries which are short and relatively jargon free.

References

1. Davies K. The information-seeking behaviour of doctors: a review of the evidence. *Health Information and Libraries Journal* 2007; **24**: 78–94.
2. Del Fiol G, Workman TE, Gorman PN. Clinical questions raised by clinicians at the point of care: a systematic review. *JAMA Internal Medicine* 2014; **174**: 710–18.
3. Blaizot A, Veettil SK, Saidoung P, *et al.* Using artificial intelligence methods for systematic review in health sciences: a systematic review. *Research Synthesis Methods* 2022; **13**: 353–62.
4. Schoeb D, Suarez-Ibarrola R, Hein S, *et al.* Use of artificial intelligence for medical literature search: randomized controlled trial using the hackathon format. *Interactive Journal of Medical Research* 2020; **9**: e16606.
5. DiCenso A, Bayley L, Haynes RB. Accessing preappraised evidence: fine-tuning the 5S model into a 6S model. *Evidence Based Nursing* 2009; **12**(4): 99–101.
6. Tugwell P, Knottnerus JA. Is the 'evidence-pyramid' now dead? *Journal of Clinical Epidemiology* 2015; **68**: 1247–50.
7. Frieden TR. Evidence for health decision making: beyond randomized, controlled trials. *New England Journal of Medicine* 2017; **377**: 465–75.
8. Greenhalgh T, Thorne S, Malterud K. Time to challenge the spurious hierarchy of systematic over narrative reviews? *European Journal of Clinical Investigation* 2018; **48**(6): e12931.
9. Levin A. The Cochrane Collaboration. *Annals of Internal Medicine* 2001; **135**: 309–12.
10. US Institute of Medicine, Committee to Advise the Public Health Service on Clinical Practice Guidelines. *Clinical Practice Guidelines: Directions for a new program.* Washington, DC: National Academies Press; 1990. http://www.ncbi.nlm.nih.gov/books/NBK235751 (accessed 13 June 2023).
11. Grimshaw J, Freemantle N, Wallace S, *et al.* Developing and implementing clinical practice guidelines. *Quality and Safety in Health Care* 1995; **4**(1): 55–64.
12. World Health Organization. *Clinical Management of Diphtheria.* Geneva: WHO; 2024. https://www.who.int/publications/i/item/WHO-DIPH-Clinical-2024.1 (accessed 20 February 2024).
13. World Health Organization. *WHO Guideline for Non-Surgical Management of Chronic Primary Low Back Pain in Adults in Primary and Community Care Settings.* Geneva: WHO; 2023. https://www.who.int/publications/i/item/9789240081789 (accessed 20 February 2024).
14. Hoogendam A, Stalenhoef A, Robbé P de V, et al. Answers to questions posed during daily patient care are more likely to be answered by uptodate than PubMed. *Journal of Medical Internet Research* 2008; **10**: e1012.
15. Shepherd J, Cobbe SM, Ford I, et al. Prevention of coronary heart disease with pravastatin in men with hypercholesterolemia. *New England Journal of Medicine* 1995; **333**: 1301–8.
16. Ford I, Murray H, Packard CJ, et al. Long-term follow-up of the West of Scotland Coronary Prevention Study. *New England Journal of Medicine* 2007; **357**: 1477–86.

17. Ford I, Murray H, McCowan C, et al. Long-term safety and efficacy of lowering low-density lipoprotein cholesterol with statin therapy. *Circulation* 2016; **133**: 1073–80.
18. Scite. Using scite to speed up literature reviews and critical analysis [blog post]. https://scite.ai/blog/recite_using-scite-to-speed-up-literature-reviews-and-critical-analysis (accessed 20 February 2024).

Chapter 3 Getting your bearings: what is this paper about?

The science of 'trashing' papers

It usually comes as a surprise to students to learn that some (some purists have claimed up to 99% of) published articles belong in the bin, and should certainly not be used to inform practice. In 1979, the editor of the *British Medical Journal*, Dr Stephen Lock, wrote 'Few things are more dispiriting to a medical editor than having to reject a paper based on a good idea but with irremediable flaws in the methods used'. Fifteen years later, Altman was still claiming that only 1% of medical research was free of methodological flaws [1]; and in 2005 John Ioannidis published his classic, though controversial, paper, 'Why most published research findings are false' [2]. Box 3.1 shows the main flaws that lead to papers being rejected (and which are present to some degree in many that end up published).

Most papers appearing in medical journals these days are presented more or less in standard introduction, methods, research and discussion (IMRAD) format: Introduction (*why* the authors decided to do this particular piece of research), Methods (*how* they did it, and how they chose to analyse their results), Results (*what* they found) and Discussion (what they think the results *mean*). If you are deciding whether a paper is worth reading, you should do so on the design of the methods section, and not on the interest value of the hypothesis, the nature or potential impact of the results or the speculation in the discussion.

Conversely, bad science is bad science regardless of whether the study addressed an important clinical issue, whether the results are 'statistically significant', whether things changed in the direction you would have liked them to and whether the findings promise immeasurable benefits for patients or savings for the health service. Strictly speaking, *if you are going to trash a paper, you should do so before you even look at the results.*

How to Read a Paper: The Basics of Evidence-Based Healthcare, Seventh Edition.
Trisha Greenhalgh and Paul Dijkstra.

Box 3.1 Common reasons why papers are rejected for publication

1 The study did not address an important scientific issue (see section in this chapter 'Three preliminary questions to get your bearings').
2 The study was not original – that is, someone else has already performed the same or a similar study (see section 'Was the study original?').
3 The study did not actually test the authors' hypothesis (see section 'Three preliminary questions to get your bearings').
4 A different study design should have been used (see section 'What are randomised controlled trials and why do they matter?').
5 Practical difficulties (e.g. in recruiting participants) led the authors to compromise on the original study protocol (see section 'Was the design of the study sensible?').
6 The sample size was too small (see section 'Were preliminary statistical questions addressed?').
7 The study was uncontrolled or inadequately controlled (see section 'Was systematic bias avoided or minimised?').
8 The statistical analysis was incorrect or inappropriate (see Chapter 5).
9 The authors have drawn unjustified conclusions from their data.
10 There is a significant conflict of interest (e.g. one of the authors, or a sponsor, might benefit from the publication of the paper and insufficient safeguards were seen to be in place to guard against bias).
11 The paper is so badly written that it is incomprehensible.

It is much easier to pick holes in other people's work than to do a methodologically perfect piece of research oneself. But remember that scholarly *critique* is not the same as gratuitous *criticism*. There may be good practical reasons why the authors of the study have not performed a perfect study, and they know as well as you do that their work would have been more scientifically valid if this or that (anticipated or unanticipated) difficulty had not arisen during the course of the study.

Most good scientific journals send papers out to one or more referees for comments on their scientific validity, originality and importance before deciding whether to publish them. This process is known as *peer review*, and much has been written about it [3]. Common defects picked up by referees are listed in Box 3.1.

The assessment of methodological quality (critical appraisal) has been covered in detail in the widely cited series 'Users' Guides to the Medical Literature' originally published in *JAMA* (the journal of the American Medical Association). *JAMA*'s structured guides on how to read papers on therapy, diagnosis, screening, prognosis, causation, quality of care, economic analysis, systematic review, qualitative research and so on are regarded by many as the definitive checklists for critical appraisal. Appendix 1 lists some simpler checklists we have derived from the Users' Guides and the other sources cited at the end of this chapter, together with some ideas of our own. If you are an experienced journal reader, these checklists will be largely self-explanatory. But if you still have difficulty getting started when looking at a medical paper, try asking the preliminary questions in the next section.

Three preliminary questions to get your bearings

Question one: Why was the study needed and what was the research question? The introductory sentence of a research paper should state, in a nutshell, what the background to the research is. For example, 'One in ten children in UK has glue ear, and this condition is associated with significant delays in speaking and comprehension'. This statement should be followed by a brief review of the published literature; for example: 'The benefit–harm balance of grommet insertion is disputed, since grommets involve a surgical procedure under anaesthetic. The grommet may provide only temporary relief before becoming blocked, and in most children, glue ear resolves spontaneously. Bone conduction headphones, which provide partial restoration of hearing while the condition resolves, may provide a non-invasive alternative to grommet insertion.' It is irritatingly common for authors to forget to place their research in context, as the background to the problem is usually clear as daylight to them by the time they reach the writing-up stage.

The last sentence of the introduction (or occasionally somewhere early in the methods section) should state clearly the research question and/or the hypothesis that the authors have decided to test. For example: 'This study aimed to determine whether bone conduction headphones were more effective and safer than either immediate grommet insertion or watchful waiting'.

You may find that the research question has inadvertently been omitted or, more commonly, that the information is buried somewhere mid-paragraph. If the main research hypothesis is presented in the negative (which it usually is), such as 'The addition of pioglitazone to maximal dose metformin therapy will not improve the control of type 2 diabetes', it is known as a null hypothesis. The authors of a study rarely actually believe their null hypothesis when they embark on their research. Being human, they have usually set out to demonstrate a difference between the two arms of their study. But the way scientists do this is to say 'let's assume there's no difference; now let's try to disprove that theory'. If you adhere to the teachings of philosopher of science

Karl Popper, this hypotheticodeductive approach (setting up falsifiable hypotheses that you then proceed to test) is the very essence of the scientific method [4].

If you have not discovered what the authors' research question was by the time you are halfway through the methods section, you may find it in the first paragraph of the discussion. Remember, however, that not all research studies (even good ones) are set up to test a single definitive hypothesis. Qualitative research studies, which (as long as they are well-designed and well-conducted) are as valid and as necessary as the quantitative studies beloved by most evidence-based healthcare enthusiasts, aim to look at particular issues in a broad, open-ended way to illuminate issues, generate or modify hypotheses and prioritise areas to investigate. This type of research is discussed further in Chapter 12. Even quantitative research (which most of the rest of this book is about) is now seen as more than hypothesis testing. In general, it is preferable to talk about evaluating the strength of evidence around a particular issue than about proving or disproving hypotheses.

Question two: What was the research design?
First, decide whether the paper describes a primary or secondary study. Primary studies report research first hand, while secondary studies attempt to summarise and draw conclusions from previously published primary studies. Primary studies (sometimes known as *empirical studies*) are the stuff of most published research in medical journals. They include laboratory experiments, which can help elucidate the causal mechanism for an observed effect (Chapter 18), clinical trials (randomised or otherwise; Chapter 6), longitudinal cohort studies, including the increasingly popular 'big data' designs and others using artificial intelligence (Chapter 17), validation studies (e.g. of a new diagnostic test; Chapter 8), surveys (e.g. of people's attitudes; Chapter 13), qualitative research (e.g. to explore the patient's experience of illness; Chapter 12), genetic association studies (Chapter 15) and mixed-method case studies or organisational change (Chapter 14).

Secondary research includes various kinds of reviews, notably the *systematic* review (Chapter 9), which tries to cover all the literature on a particular topic in an objective and reproducible way. It also includes efforts to examine the costs of an intervention that has already been shown to be effective (Chapter 11), develop guidelines (Chapter 10) or reach consensus on a topic (Chapter 19).

Question three: Was the research design appropriate to the question?
Examples of the sort of questions that can reasonably be answered by different types of primary research study are given in the sections that follow. One question that frequently cries out to be asked is this: was a randomised controlled trial (RCT) the best method of addressing this particular research

Box 3.2 Broad fields of research

Most quantitative studies are concerned with one or more of the following:

- *Therapy*: testing the efficacy of drug treatments, surgical procedures, alternative methods of service delivery or other interventions. Preferred study design is RCT (see section 'What are randomised controlled trials and why do they matter?' and Chapters 6 and 7).
- *Diagnosis*: demonstrating whether a new diagnostic test is valid (can we trust it?) and reliable (would we get the same results every time?). Preferred study design is cross-sectional survey (see section 'What are cross-sectional surveys?' and Chapter 8).
- *Screening*: demonstrating the value of tests that can be applied to large populations and that pick up disease at a presymptomatic stage. Preferred study design is cross-sectional survey (see section 'What are cross-sectional surveys?' and Chapter 8).
- *Prognosis*: determining what is likely to happen to someone whose disease is picked up at an early stage. Preferred study design is longitudinal survey (see section 'What are cross-sectional surveys?').
- *Causation*: determining whether a putative harmful agent, such as environmental pollution, is related to the development of illness. Multiple study designs may be needed to gather sufficient evidence of causality, including cohort or case–control studies, depending on how rare the disease is (see sections 'What are cross-sectional surveys' and 'What are case reports?'), case reports (see section 'The traditional hierarchy of evidence') and mechanistic evidence of various kinds (see Chapter 18).
- *Attitudes and beliefs*: Usually studied using questionnaires (see Chapter 13).

Qualitative studies are discussed in Chapter 12.

question and, if the study was not an RCT, should it have been? Before you jump to any conclusions, decide what broad field of research the study covers (Box 3.2). Once you have done this, ask whether the study design was appropriate to this question.

What are randomised controlled trials and why do they matter?

In an RCT, participants in the trial are randomly allocated by a process equivalent to the flip of a coin to either one intervention (such as a drug treatment) or another (such as placebo treatment or, more commonly, best current therapy). Both groups (formally known as 'arms') are followed up for a prespecified time period and analysed in terms of specific outcomes defined at the outset of the study (e.g. death, heart attack, serum cholesterol level). Because, *on average*, the groups are identical apart from the intervention, any differences in outcome are, in theory, attributable to the intervention. In reality, however, not every RCT is a bowl of cherries.

Some papers that report trials comparing an intervention with a control group are not, in fact, randomised trials at all. The terminology for these is *other controlled clinical trials* – a term used to describe comparative studies in which participants were allocated to intervention or control groups in a non-random manner. This situation may arise, for example, when random allocation would be impossible, impractical or unethical; for example, when patients on ward A receive one diet while those on ward B receive a different diet. (Although this design is inferior to the RCT, it is much easier to execute, and was used successfully a century ago to demonstrate the benefit of brown rice over white rice in the treatment of beriberi [5].) The problems of non-random allocation are discussed further in section 'Was systematic bias avoided or minimised?' in relation to determining whether the two groups in a trial can reasonably be compared with one another on a statistical level.

Some trials count as a sort of halfway house between true randomised trials and non-randomised trials. In these types, randomisation is not performed truly at random (e.g. using sequentially numbered sealed envelopes each with a computer-generated random number inside) but by some method that allows the clinician to know which group the patient would be in *before they make a definitive decision to randomise the patient*. This allows subtle biases to creep in, as the clinician might be more (or less) likely to enter a particular patient into the trial if they believed that this individual would get active treatment. In particular, patients with more severe disease may be subconsciously withheld from the placebo arm of the trial. Examples of unacceptable methods include randomisation by last digit of date of birth (even numbers to group A, odds to group B), toss of a coin (heads to group A, tails to group B), sequential allocation (patient A to group 1; patient B to group 2, etc.) and date seen in clinic (all patients seen this week to group A; all those seen next week to group 2, etc.; Box 3.3).

Listed here are examples of clinical questions that would be best answered by an RCT, but note also the examples in the later sections of this chapter of situations where other types of studies could or must be used instead.

- Is this drug better than a placebo or a different drug for a particular disease?
- Is a new surgical procedure better than the currently favoured practice?
- Is a smartphone app offering cognitive behaviour therapy non-inferior to an in-person therapy from a psychologist in helping patients overcome phobia? (Note: many RCTs are designed not to demonstrate that a new, cheaper, treatment is superior to current practice, but merely that it is not inferior.)

Box 3.3 Advantages of the randomised controlled trial design

- Allows rigorous evaluation of a single variable (e.g. effect of drug treatment versus placebo) in a precisely defined patient group (e.g. postmenopausal women aged 50–60 years).
- Prospective design (i.e. data are collected on events which happen *after* you decide to do the study).
- Uses hypotheticodeductive reasoning (i.e. seeks to falsify, rather than confirm, its own hypothesis).
- Potentially eradicates bias by comparing two otherwise identical groups (but see subsequent text and section 'Was systematic bias avoided or minimised?' in Chapter 4).
- Allows for meta-analysis (combining the numerical results of several similar trials) at a later date.

RCTs are often said to be the gold standard in medical research. Up to a point, this is true (see section 'The traditional hierarchy of evidence') but only for certain types of clinical questions (see Box 3.2 and sections 'Cohort studies', 'Case–control studies', 'Cross-sectional surveys' and 'Case reports'). The questions that best lend themselves to the RCT design all relate to *interventions*, and are mainly concerned with therapy or prevention. It should be remembered, however, that even when we are looking at therapeutic interventions, and especially when we are not, there are a number of important disadvantages associated with randomised trials (Box 3.4).

Box 3.4 Disadvantages of the randomised controlled trial design

Expensive and time-consuming, hence, in practice:

- many RCTs are either never carried out, are performed on too few patients or are undertaken for too short a period
- most RCTs are funded by large research bodies (university or government-sponsored) or drug companies, so only questions important to them are addressed
- surrogate endpoints may not reflect outcomes that are important to patients (see section 'Surrogate endpoints' in Chapter 6).

May introduce 'hidden bias', especially through:

- imperfect randomisation (see examples in text)
- failure to randomise all eligible patients (clinicians only offer participation in the trial to patients they consider will respond well to the intervention)
- failure to blind assessors to randomisation status of patients (see section 'Was assessment 'blind'?' in Chapter 4).

Remember, too, that the results of an RCT may have limited applicability as a result of *selection bias* (selection of trial participants from a group that is unrepresentative of everyone with the condition), *uptake bias* (limited interest in the study, or ability to participate in it, from certain key groups), *performance bias* (differences in what is provided to the groups over and above the intervention being tested), *detection bias* (differences between the groups in how the outcomes are assessed), *attrition bias* (when one group has many more withdrawals or 'drop-outs' than the other) and *publication bias* (selective publication of positive results, often but not always because the organisation that funded the research stands to gain or lose depending on the findings) [6]. These biases are discussed further in Chapter 4.

Note also that analysis of only predefined 'objective' endpoints may exclude important qualitative aspects of the intervention (see Chapter 12) and may or may not include the outcomes that matter most to patients (see Chapter 16). Furthermore, RCTs can be well or badly managed [2] and, once published, their results are open to distortion by an over-enthusiastic scientific community or by a public eager for a new wonder drug. While all these problems might also occur with other trial designs, they may be particularly pertinent when an RCT is being sold to you as, methodologically speaking, whiter than white [7,8].

There are, in addition, many situations in which RCTs are unnecessary, impractical or inappropriate:

- RCTs are unnecessary:
  - when a clearly successful intervention for an otherwise fatal condition is discovered
  - when a previous RCT or meta-analysis has given a definitive result (either positive or negative). Arguably, it is actually unethical to ask patients to be randomised to a clinical trial without first conducting a systematic literature review to see whether the trial needs to be carried out at all.
- RCTs are impractical:
  - where the costs of a trial are unaffordable
  - where the number of participants needed to demonstrate a significant difference between the groups is prohibitively high.
- RCTs are inappropriate:
  - where the study is looking at the prognosis of a disease. For this analysis, the appropriate route to best evidence is a longitudinal survey of a properly assembled *inception cohort*
  - where the study is looking at the validity of a diagnostic or screening test. For this analysis, the appropriate route to best evidence is a *cross-sectional survey* of patients clinically suspected of harbouring the relevant disorder

- where the study is looking at a 'quality of care' issue in which the criteria for 'success' have not yet been established. For example, an RCT comparing medical versus surgical methods of abortion might assess 'success' in terms of number of patients achieving complete evacuation, amount of bleeding and pain level. The patients, however, might decide that other aspects of the procedure are important, such as knowing in advance how long the procedure will take, not seeing or feeling the abortus come out, and so on. For this analysis, the appropriate route to best evidence is *qualitative research methods* (see Chapter 12).

All these issues have been discussed in great depth by clinical epidemiologists and other scientists, who remind us that to turn our noses up at the non-randomised trial may indicate scientific naiveté and not, as many people routinely assume, intellectual rigour. You might also like to look up the emerging science of *pragmatic* RCTs – a methodology for taking account of practical, real-world challenges so that the findings of your trial will be more relevant to that real world when the trial is finished [9] (see also Chapter 6, where we introduce the Consolidated Standards of Reporting Trials statement, universally known as CONSORT, for presenting the findings of RCTs).

What are cohort studies?

In a cohort study, two (or more) groups of people are selected on the basis of differences in their exposure to a particular agent (such as a vaccine, a surgical procedure or an environmental toxin) and followed up to see how many in each group develop a particular disease, complication or other outcome. The follow-up period in cohort studies is generally measured in years (and sometimes in decades) because that is how long many diseases, especially cancer, take to develop. Note that RCTs are usually begun on people who already have a disease, whereas most cohort studies are begun on people who may or may not develop disease.

A special type of cohort study may also be used to determine the prognosis of a disease (i.e. what is likely to happen to someone who has it). A group of people who have all been diagnosed as having an early stage of the disease or a positive screening test (see Chapter 7) is assembled (the inception cohort) and followed up on repeated occasions to see the incidence (new cases per year) and time course of different outcomes. (Here is a definition that you should commit to memory if you can: *incidence* is the number of new cases of a disease per year, whereas *prevalence* is the overall proportion of the population who suffer from the disease.)

The world's most famous cohort study, whose authors all won knighthoods, was undertaken by Sir Austen Bradford Hill, Sir Richard Doll and, latterly,

Sir Richard Peto. They followed up 40 000 male British doctors divided into four cohorts (non-smokers, and light, moderate and heavy smokers) using both all-cause (any death) and cause-specific (death from a particular disease) mortality as outcome measures. Publication of their 10-year interim results in 1964 [10], which showed a substantial excess in both lung cancer mortality and all-cause mortality in smokers, with a 'dose–response' relationship (i.e. the more you smoke, the worse your chances of getting lung cancer), went a long way to demonstrating that the link between smoking and ill health was causal rather than coincidental. The 20-year [11], 40-year [12] and 50-year [13] results of this momentous study (which achieved an impressive 94% follow-up of those recruited in 1951 and not known to have died) illustrate both the perils of smoking and the strength of evidence that can be obtained from a properly conducted cohort study.

Given here are clinical questions that should be addressed by a cohort study:

- Does smoking cause lung cancer?
- Does the contraceptive pill 'cause' breast cancer? Note, once again, that the word 'cause' is a loaded and potentially misleading term. As John Guillebaud argued in his excellent book, *The Pill. . .*[14], if a thousand women went on the oral contraceptive pill tomorrow, some of them would get breast cancer. But some of those would have got it anyway. The question that epidemiologists try to answer through cohort studies is, 'what is the additional risk of developing breast cancer which this woman would run by taking the pill, over and above the baseline risk attributable to her own hormonal balance, family history, diet, alcohol intake, and so on?'.
- Does high blood pressure get better over time?
- What happens to infants who have been born very prematurely, in terms of subsequent physical development and educational achievement?

Since the first edition of this book appeared, cohort studies have undergone a quiet revolution, due partly to the exponential increase in computer power that has occurred in the past generation (and particularly the facility to link with electronic patient records; see Chapter 17 on 'artificial intelligence' (including big data studies) and partly to the emergence of population genetics (see Chapter 15). Whereas 20 years ago, respectability in research circles seemed to be based almost exclusively on whether one was currently conducting a randomised controlled trial and while such trials are still very important, these days, the well-dressed quantitative researcher is also expected to talk about their 'cohort', which is usually known by a catchy acronym and includes several thousand patients being followed up over time. Professor Richard Hobbs, for example, is a quantitative researcher based at the University of Oxford. His collection of cohorts includes OXVASC (around 10 000 people who have had an acute stroke), OXVALVE (6000 older people with screen-detected heart valve problems) and OXREN (3250 older people with chronic kidney disease). Google them to find out more!

What are case–control studies?

In a case–control study, patients with a particular disease or condition are identified and 'matched' with controls (e.g. someone the same age and gender with some other disease, or no disease, randomly picked from a general practitioner's list). Data are then collected (e.g. by searching back through these people's medical records or by asking them to recall their own history) on past exposure to a possible causal agent for the disease. Like cohort studies, case–control studies are generally concerned with the aetiology of a disease (i.e. what causes it) rather than its treatment. They lie lower down the conventional hierarchy of evidence (in other words, they are a weaker form of evidence than RCTs or cohort studies), but this design is usually the only option when studying rare conditions – and it also offers options in genetic association studies (see Chapter 15). An important source of difficulty (and potential bias) in a case–control study is the precise definition of who counts as a 'case', because one misallocated individual may substantially influence the results (see section 'Was systematic bias avoided or minimised?'). In addition, a case–control study cannot demonstrate causality; in other words, the *association* of A with B in a study of this design does not prove that A has *caused* B.

Clinical questions that could be addressed by a case–control study include:

- Does the prone sleeping position increase the risk of cot death (sudden infant death syndrome) in babies?
- Does whooping cough vaccine cause brain damage?
- Did eating at a particular pizza restaurant in a particular time period cause hepatitis A?

What are cross-sectional surveys?

We have probably all been asked to take part in a survey, even if it was only a person in the street asking us which brand of toothpaste we prefer. Surveys conducted by epidemiologists are run along essentially the same lines but more rigorously: a representative sample of participants is recruited and then interviewed, examined or otherwise studied to gain answers to a specific clinical (or other) question. In cross-sectional surveys, data are collected at a single time point but may refer retrospectively to health experiences in the past; for example, a survey of patients' medical records to see how often their blood pressure has been recorded in the past 5 years.

A cross-sectional survey should address the following clinical questions:

- What is the 'normal' height of a 3-year-old child? This, like other questions about the range of normality, can be answered simply by measuring the height of enough healthy 3-year-olds. But such an exercise does not answer the related clinical question 'when should an unusually short child be investigated for disease?' because, as in almost all biological measurements, the physiological (normal) overlaps with the pathological (abnormal). This problem is discussed further in the section 'Likelihood ratios'.
- What do psychiatric nurses believe about the value of antidepressant drugs and talking therapies in the treatment of severe depression?
- Is it true that 'half of all cases of diabetes are undiagnosed'? This an example of the more general question, 'What is the prevalence (proportion of people with the condition) of this disease in this community?' The only way of finding the answer is to do the definitive diagnostic test on a representative sample of the population.

What are case reports?

A case report describes the medical history of a single patient in the form of a story ('Mrs B is a 54-year-old secretary who developed chest pain in June 2010. . .'). Case reports are often run together to form a *case series*, in which the medical histories of more than one patient with a particular condition are described to illustrate an aspect of the condition, the treatment or, most commonly these days, adverse reaction to treatment.

Although this type of research is traditionally considered to be weak scientific evidence, a great deal of information that would be lost in a clinical trial or survey can be conveyed in a case report. In addition, case reports are immediately understandable by non-academic clinicians and by the lay public. They can, if necessary, be written up and published within days, which gives them a definite edge over clinical trials (whose gestation period can run into years) or meta-analyses (even longer). And the clinical case is the unit of learning (doctors learn medicine, and nurses nursing, by accumulating and reflecting on individual cases). There are certainly good theoretical grounds for the reinstatement of the humble case report as a useful and valid contribution to medical science, not least because the story is one of the best vehicles for *making sense* of a complex clinical situation.

The following are clinical situations in which a case report or case series is an appropriate type of study.

- A doctor notices that two babies born in their hospital have absent limbs (phocomelia). Both mothers had taken a new drug (thalidomide) in early pregnancy. The doctor wishes to alert his colleagues worldwide to the possibility of drug-related damage as quickly as possible [15]. (Anyone who thinks 'quick and dirty' case reports are never scientifically justified should remember this example.)
- A patient who went undiagnosed with chronic pain and fatigue for years was subsequently found to be suffering from an unusual presentation of a rare disease. The team caring for her decide to write this story up as a lesson for other clinicians [16].

The traditional hierarchy of evidence

As mentioned briefly in Chapter 2, standard notation for the relative weight carried by the different types of primary study when making decisions about clinical interventions (the 'hierarchy of evidence') puts them in the following order:

1. Systematic reviews and meta-analyses;
2. RCTs with definitive results (i.e. confidence intervals that do not overlap the threshold clinically significant effect; see section 'Probability and confidence')
3. RCTs with non-definitive results (i.e. a point estimate that suggests a clinically significant effect but with confidence intervals overlapping the threshold for this effect; see section 'Probability and confidence')
4. Cohort studies, including 'big data' studies, in which large numbers of people are followed using entries on their medical records;
5. Case–control studies
6. Cross-sectional surveys
7. Case reports.

The pinnacle of the hierarchy is, quite properly, reserved for secondary research papers, in which all the primary studies on a particular subject have been hunted out and critically appraised according to rigorous criteria (see Chapter 9). Note, however, that not even the most hard-line protagonist of EBM would place a sloppy meta-analysis or an RCT that was seriously methodologically flawed above a large, well-designed cohort study. And as Chapter 12 shows, many important and valid studies in the field of qualitative research do not feature in this particular hierarchy of evidence at all.

In other words, evaluating the potential contribution of a particular study to medical science requires considerably more effort than is needed to check off its basic design against the above-mentioned 7-point scale. A more complex representation of the hierarchy of evidence geared to the domain of the question (therapy/prevention, diagnosis, harm, prognosis) was drawn up by a group of us in 2011 [17] and is available for download on the Centre for Evidence-Based Medicine website (https://www.cebm.ox.ac.uk/resources/levels-of-evidence/ocebm-levels-of-evidence). But before you look up these more advanced tools, make sure you are clear on the traditional (basic) hierarchy described in this section.

The take-home message is, don't apply the hierarchy of evidence mechanically; it's only a rule of thumb. In the next chapter, we go into more detail about how to assess the methodological quality of published papers.

Exercises based on this chapter

1. In the opening section of this chapter, we suggested that if you are going to trash a paper, you should do so without even looking at the results section. When you have read through the rest of the chapter, list the arguments for assessing a paper's merits on the basis of the research question, study design and methods (but not the results).
2. Which study design is most appropriate for answering the following kinds of question:
   a. Assessing the benefits of a treatment?
   b. Evaluating a diagnostic or screening test?
   c. Determining the course and prognosis of a disease?
   d. Determining whether a particular agent is likely to have a damaging effect?
   e. Measuring people's attitudes to a topic?
3. List five different kinds of bias that can occur in randomised controlled trials. How would you try to reduce each of these?

References

1. Altman DG. The scandal of poor medical research. *BMJ* 1994; **308**: 283.
2. Ioannidis, John PA. Why most published research findings are false. *PLoS Medicine* 2005; **2**.8: e124.
3. Stahel PF, Moore. EE Peer review for biomedical publications: we can improve the system. *BMC Medicine* 2014; **12**: 179.
4. Popper KR. *The Logic of Scientific Discovery*. Abingdon: Psychology Press; 2002.
5. Fletcher W. Rice and beriberi: preliminary report of an experiment conducted at the Kuala Lumpur Lunatic Asylum. *Lancet* 1907; **1**: 1776.
6. Cochrane Collaboration. *The Cochrane Handbook for Systematic Reviews of Interventions*. Oxford: Cochrane Collaboration; 2022. https://training.cochrane.org/handbook (accessed 7 July 2023).
7. Kaptchuk TJ. The double-blind, randomized, placebo-controlled trial: gold standard or golden calf? *Journal of Clinical Epidemiology* 2001; **54**: 541–9.

8. Greenhalgh T, Howick J, Maskrey N. Evidence-based medicine: a movement in crisis? *BMJ* 2014; **348**: g3725.
9. Eldridge S. Pragmatic trials in primary health care: what, when and how? *Family Practice* 2010; **27**: 591–2.
10. Doll R, Hill AB. Mortality in relation to smoking: ten years' observations of British doctors. *BMJ* 1964; **1**: 1399.
11. Doll R, Peto R. Mortality in relation to smoking: 20 years' observations on male British doctors. *BMJ* 1976; **2**: 1525.
12. Doll R, Peto R, Wheatley K, et al. Mortality in relation to smoking: 40 years' observations on male British doctors. *BMJ* 1994; **309**: 901–11.
13. Doll R, Peto R, Boreham J, et al. Mortality in relation to smoking: 50 years' observations on male British doctors. *BMJ* 2004; **328**: 1519.
14. Guillebaud J, MacGregor A. *The Pill and other Forms of Hormonal Contraception*. USA: Oxford University Press, 2009.
15. McBride WG. Thalidomide and congenital abnormalities. *Lancet* 1961; **2**: 1358.
16. Cohen, S., & Markham, F. Ehlers–Danlos hypermobility type in an adult with chronic pain and fatigue: a case study. *Clinical Case Reports* 2017; **5**: 1248–51.
17. Howick J, Chalmers I, Glasziou P, et al. *The 2011 Oxford CEBM Levels of Evidence (Introductory Document)*. Oxford: Oxford Centre for Evidence-Based Medicine; 2011.

Chapter 4 **Assessing methodological quality**

As we argued in the previous chapter, a paper will sink or swim on the strength of its methods section. This chapter considers five essential questions which should form the basis of your decision to 'bin' it outright (because of fatal methodological flaws), interpret its findings cautiously (because the methods were less than robust) or trust it completely (because you can't fault the methods at all). Five important questions are considered in turn:

- Was the study original?
- Who is it about?
- Was it well designed?
- Was systematic bias avoided (e.g. was the study adequately 'controlled')?
- Was it large enough and continued for long enough to make the results credible?

Was the study original?

There is, in theory, no point in testing a scientific hypothesis that someone else has already proved one way or the other. But, in real life, science is seldom so cut and dried. Only a tiny proportion of medical research breaks entirely new ground, and an equally tiny proportion repeats exactly the steps of previous workers. The majority of research studies will tell us (if they are methodologically sound) that a particular hypothesis is slightly more or less likely to be correct than it was before we added our piece to the wider jigsaw. Hence, it may be perfectly valid to do a study that is, on the face of it, 'unoriginal'. Indeed, the whole science of meta-analysis depends on there being more than one study in the literature that have addressed the same question in pretty much the same way.

How to Read a Paper: The Basics of Evidence-Based Healthcare, Seventh Edition.
Trisha Greenhalgh and Paul Dijkstra.

The practical question to ask, then, about a new piece of research, is not 'has anyone ever conducted a similar study before?' but 'does this new research add to the literature in any way?' A list of such examples is given here:

1. Is this study bigger, continued for longer or otherwise more substantial than the previous one(s)?
2. Are the methods of this study any more rigorous (in particular, does it address any specific methodological criticisms of previous studies)?
3. Will the numerical results of this study add significantly to a meta-analysis of previous studies?
4. Is the population studied different in any way (e.g. has the study looked at different ethnic groups, ages or genders than have previous studies)?
5. Is the clinical issue addressed of sufficient importance, and does there exist sufficient doubt in the minds of the public or key decision-makers to make new evidence 'politically' desirable even when it is not strictly scientifically necessary?

Who is the study about?

In a previous edition of this book, Trisha mentioned that one of the first papers that ever caught her eye was entitled 'But will it help *my* patients with myocardial infarction?' [1]. This article opened her eyes to the fact that research on someone else's patients may not have a take-home message for one's own practice. This is not mere xenophobia. The main reasons why the participants in a clinical trial or survey might differ from patients in 'real life' are listed here:

- They were more, or less, ill than the patients you see.
- They were from a different age or ethnic group, or lived a different lifestyle, from your own patients.
- They received more (or different) attention during the study than you could ever hope to give your patients.
- Unlike most real-life patients, they had nothing wrong with them apart from the condition being studied.
- None of them smoked, drank alcohol or were taking the contraceptive pill.

Hence, before swallowing the results of any paper whole, here are some questions that you should ask yourself.

1. *How were the participants recruited?* If you wanted to do a questionnaire survey of the views of users of the hospital casualty department, you could recruit respondents by putting an advert in the local newspaper or your hospital's social media. However, this method would be a good example of *recruitment bias* because the sample you obtained would be skewed in favour of users who were highly motivated to answer your

questions, liked to read newspapers or followed the hospital social media accounts. You would do better to issue a questionnaire to every user (or to a one in ten sample of users) who turned up on a particular day.

2. *Who was included in the study?* In the past, clinical trials routinely excluded people with coexisting illness, those who did not speak English, those taking certain other medication and people who could not read the consent form. This approach may be experimentally clean but because clinical trial results will be used to guide practice in relation to wider patient groups, it is actually scientifically flawed. The results of pharmacokinetic studies of new drugs in 23-year-old healthy male volunteers will clearly not be applicable to women over 80 (most of whom have at least one other coexisting illness). A number of papers (see, for example, this one from oncology by Hamaker et al. [2]) have revealed the biases against older people and those with comorbidities in the design of clinical trials. As a result, in most conditions we still don't have a reliable evidence base for how to treat the over-80s. In healthcare research, sex and gender bias is rife! Steuernagel et al. [3], an analysis paper in the *BMJ*, argues that sex and gender bias are interdependent, resulting in under-representation; the authors propose solutions to counter these imbalances.
3. *Who was excluded from the study?* For example, a randomised controlled trial (RCT) may be restricted to patients with moderate or severe forms of a disease such as heart failure – a policy that could lead to false conclusions about the treatment of *mild* heart failure. This has important practical implications when clinical trials performed with hospital outpatients are used to dictate 'best practice' in primary care, where the spectrum of disease is generally milder.
4. *Were the participants studied in 'real-life' circumstances?* For example, were they admitted to hospital purely for observation? Did they receive lengthy and detailed explanations of the potential benefits of the intervention? Were they given the telephone number of a key research worker? Did the company who funded the research provide new equipment that would not be available to the ordinary clinician? These factors would not invalidate the study, but they may cast doubts on the applicability of its findings to your own practice.

Was the design of the study sensible?

Although the terminology of research trial design can be forbidding, much of what is grandly termed *critical appraisal* is plain common sense. Personally, we assess the basic design of a clinical trial via two questions:

1. *What specific intervention or other manoeuvre was being considered, and what was it being compared with?* This is one of the most fundamental questions in appraising any paper. It is tempting to take published

statements at face value, but remember that authors may misrepresent (usually subconsciously rather than deliberately) what they actually did, and overestimate its originality and potential importance. In the examples in Table 4.1, we have used hypothetical statements so as not to cause offence, but they are all based on similar mistakes seen in print.

2. *What outcome was measured, and how?* If you had an incurable disease, for which a pharmaceutical company claimed to have produced a new wonder drug, you would measure the efficacy of the drug in terms of whether it made you live longer (and, perhaps, whether life was *worth* living, given your condition and any adverse effects of the medication). You would not be too interested in the levels of some obscure enzyme in your blood that the

Table 4.1 Examples of problematic descriptions in the methods section of a paper

What the authors said	What they should have said (or done)	An example of
'We measured how often GPs ask patients whether they smoke'	'We looked in patients' medical records and counted how many had had their smoking status recorded'	Assumption that medical records are 100% accurate
'We measured how doctors treat low back pain'	'We measured what doctors *say* they do when faced with a patient with low back pain'	Assumption that what doctors say they do reflects what they actually do
'We compared a nicotine-replacement patch with placebo'	'Participants in the intervention group were asked to apply a patch containing 15 mg nicotine twice daily; those in the control group received identical-looking patches'	Failure to state dose of drug or nature of placebo
'We asked 100 teenagers to participate in our survey of sexual attitudes'	'We approached 147 white American teenagers aged 12–18 (85 males) at a summer camp; 100 of them (31 males) agreed to participate'	Failure to give sufficient information about participants (note that, in this example, the figures indicate a recruitment bias towards women)
'We randomised patients to either "individual care plan" or "usual care"'	'The intervention group were offered an individual care plan consisting of . . .; control patients were offered . . .'	Failure to give sufficient information about intervention (enough information should be given to allow the study to be replicated by other researchers)

Table 4.1 (Continued)

What the authors said	What they should have said (or done)	An example of
'To assess the value of an educational leaflet, we gave the intervention group a leaflet and a telephone helpline number. Controls received neither'	If the study is purely to assess the value of the leaflet, both groups should have had the helpline number	Failure to treat groups equally apart from the specific intervention
'We measured the use of vitamin C in the prevention of the common cold'	A systematic literature search would have found numerous previous studies on this subject	Unoriginal study

manufacturer assured you were a reliable indicator of your chances of survival. The use of such *surrogate endpoints* is discussed further in Chapter 6.

The measurement of symptomatic (e.g. pain), functional (e.g. mobility), psychological (e.g. anxiety) or social (e.g. inconvenience) effects of an intervention is fraught with even more problems. The methodology of developing, administering and interpreting such 'soft' outcome measures is beyond the scope of this book. But, in general, you should always look for evidence in the paper that the outcome measure has been objectively validated. In other words, someone has demonstrated that the 'outcome measure' used in the study does actually measure what it purports to measure, and that changes in this outcome measure adequately reflect changes in the status of the patient. Remember that what is important in the eyes of the doctor may not be valued so highly by the patient, and vice versa. One of the most exciting developments in evidence-based medicine (EBM) in recent years is the emerging science of patient-reported outcomes measures (see section 'Patient-reported outcome measures' in Chapter 16').

Was bias avoided or minimised?

Bias is defined by epidemiologists as anything that systematically influences the conclusions about groups and distorts comparisons [4]. Whether the design of a study is an RCT, a non-randomised comparative trial, a cohort study or a case–control study, the aim should be for the groups being compared to be as like one another as possible except for the particular difference being examined. They should, as far as possible, receive the same explanations, have the same contacts with health professionals, and be assessed the same number of times by the same assessors, using the same outcome measures [5–7]. Different study designs call for different steps to reduce systematic bias.

Sources of bias in randomised controlled trials

In an RCT, systematic bias is (in theory) avoided by selecting a sample of participants from a particular population and allocating them randomly to the different groups. The section 'What are randomised controlled trials and why do they matter?' in Chapter 3 describes some ways in which bias can creep into even this gold standard of clinical trial design, and Figure 4.1 summarises particular sources to check for.

Sources of bias in non-randomised controlled clinical trials

Trisha once chaired a seminar in which a multidisciplinary group of students from the medical, nursing, pharmacy and allied professions were presenting the results of several in-house research studies. All but one of the studies presented were of comparative, but non-randomised, design – that is, one group of patients (say, hospital outpatients with asthma) had received one intervention (say, an educational leaflet), while another group (say, patients attending general practitioner surgeries with asthma) had received another

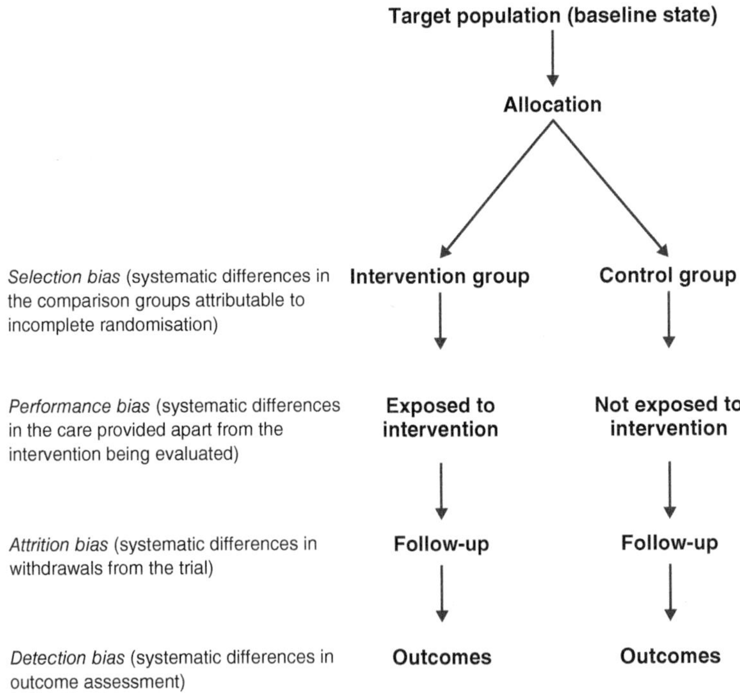

Figure 4.1 Sources of bias to check for in a randomised controlled trial.

intervention (say, group educational sessions). It was surprising how many of the presenters believed that their study was, or was equivalent to, an RCT. In other words, these commendably enthusiastic and committed young researchers were blind to the most obvious bias of all: they were comparing two groups that had inherent, self-selected differences even before the intervention was applied (as well as having all the additional potential sources of bias listed in Figure 4.1 for RCTs).

As a general rule, if the paper you are looking at is a non-randomised controlled clinical trial, you must decide if the baseline differences between the intervention and control groups are likely to have been so great as to invalidate any differences ascribed to the effects of the intervention. This is, in fact, almost always the case. Sometimes, the authors of such a paper will list the important features of each group (such as mean age, sex ratio and markers of disease severity) in a table to allow you to compare these differences yourself. For a formal checklist on assessing the quality of non-randomised comparative studies, see Deeks et al. [8].

Sources of bias in cohort studies

In the previous chapter, we mentioned the 'quiet revolution' in cohort studies that has occurred in recent times. It remains the case that the RCT is *ideally* the best way to assess whether treatment A is better than treatment B. But for various reasons (cost being one, computer power being another), observational studies in which nobody is randomised have become more popular. In the expanding field of comparative effectiveness studies (assessing which of two or more treatments is best in a particular condition) for example, observational studies comparing one naturally occurring cohort to another are now commonplace. For a discussion on the benefits and trade-offs of such studies, see Nallamothu et al.[9] and Berger et al. [10].

The selection of a comparable control group is one of the most difficult decisions facing the authors of an observational (cohort or case–control) study. Ideally, the single difference between groups should be their exposure to the agent being studied. Few cohort studies, however, succeed in identifying two groups of subjects who are equal in age, gender mix, socioeconomic status, presence of coexisting illness and so on. In practice, much of the 'controlling' in cohort studies occurs at the analysis stage, where complex statistical adjustment is made for baseline differences in key variables. Unless this is performed adequately, statistical tests of probability and confidence intervals (see Chapter 5) will be dangerously misleading.

This problem is illustrated by the various cohort studies on the risks and benefits of alcohol, which have consistently demonstrated a J-shaped relationship between alcohol intake and mortality. The best outcome (in terms of premature death) lies with the cohort group who are moderate drinkers [11].

Self-confessed teetotallers, it seems, are significantly more likely to die young than the average person who drinks three or four drinks a day.

But can we assume that teetotallers are, *on average*, identical to moderate drinkers except for the amount they drink? We certainly can't. As we all know, the teetotal population includes those who have been ordered to give up alcohol on health grounds ('sick quitters'), those who, for health or other reasons, have cut out a host of additional items from their diet and lifestyle, those from certain religious or ethnic groups which would be under-represented in the other cohorts (notably Muslims and Seventh Day Adventists) and those who drink like fish but choose to lie about it.

The details of how these different features of teetotalism were controlled for by the epidemiologists are discussed elsewhere [10,11]. Interestingly, when Trisha was writing the third edition of this book in 2005, the conclusion at that time was that even when due allowance was made in the analysis for potential confounding variables in people who described themselves as non-drinkers, these individuals' increased risk of premature mortality remained (i.e. the 'J curve' was a genuine phenomenon) [11].

By the time that Trisha wrote the fourth edition in 2010, though, a more sophisticated analysis of the various cohort studies (i.e. which controlled more carefully for 'sick quitters') had been published [12]. It showed that, all other things being equal, teetotallers are no more likely to contract heart disease than moderate drinkers (hence, the famous 'J curve' may have been an artefact all along). Subsequently, a new meta-analysis purported to show that the J curve was a genuine phenomenon and alcohol was indeed protective in small quantities [13], but a year later a new analysis of the same primary studies came to the opposite conclusion, having placed more weight on so-called methodological flaws [14]. And a further meta-analysis a few years later by the same authors suggests that this conclusion still holds [15]. But for this (seventh) edition of *How to Read a Paper* the evidence has changed again! An updated systematic review and meta-analysis published in March 2023 by the same authors suggests that daily low or moderate alcohol intake is not significantly associated with all-cause mortality risk [16]. Interestingly, increased risk was evident at higher consumption levels and started at lower levels for women compared with men. The protective effect of moderate alcohol intake is one of the best examples of the challenges of correcting for bias in non-randomised studies; you might like to discuss it with your EBM colleagues over a beer.

Guides for authors of protocols for observational epidemiological studies vary highly in format and content [17]. If you're looking for a definitive checklist for reporting observational studies (both cohort and case-control), we recommend the STROBE (Strengthening the Reporting of Observational Studies in Epidemiology) statement [18], and several STROBE extensions that might be relevant to you. For example, the International Olympic Committee consensus statement: methods for recording and reporting of epidemiological data on injury and illness in sport 2020 (including STROBE Extension for Sport Injury and Illness Surveillance, STROBE-SIIS) [19].

Large prospective cohort studies are extremely useful for prediction algorithms. To estimate the 10-year risk of cardiovascular disease in women and men using QRISK®3 (www.qrisk.org), 981 general practices in England (7.89 million patients aged 25–84 years) were used to develop scores and a separate set of 328 practices (2.67 million patients) were used to validate the scores [20].

Sources of bias in case–control studies

In case–control studies (in which the experiences of individuals with and without a particular disease are analysed retrospectively to identify exposure to possible causes of that disease), the process most open to bias is not the assessment of outcome, but the diagnosis of 'caseness' and the decision as to *when* the individual became a case.

A good example of this occurred a few years ago when legal action was brought against the manufacturers of the whooping cough (pertussis) vaccine, which was alleged to have caused neurological damage in a number of infants [21]. To answer the question, 'Did the vaccine cause brain damage?' a case–control study had been undertaken in which a 'case' was defined as an infant who, previously well, had exhibited fits or other signs suggestive of brain damage within 1 week of receiving the vaccine. A control was an infant of the same age and sex taken from the same immunisation register, who had received immunisation and who may or may not have developed symptoms at some stage.

New onset of features of brain damage in apparently normal babies is extremely rare, but it does happen, and the link with recent immunisation could conceivably be coincidental. Furthermore, heightened public anxiety about the issue could have biased the recall of parents and health professionals so that infants whose neurological symptoms predated, or occurred some time after, the administration of pertussis vaccine, might be wrongly classified as cases. The judge in the court case ruled that misclassification of three such infants as 'cases' rather than controls led to the overestimation of the harm attributable to whooping cough vaccine by a factor of three. Although this ruling has subsequently been challenged, the principle stands: that assignment of 'caseness' in a case–control study must be performed rigorously and objectively if systematic bias is to be avoided.

Was assessment 'blind'?

Even the most rigorous attempt to achieve a comparable control group will be wasted effort if the people who assess outcome (e.g. those who judge whether someone is still clinically in heart failure, or who say whether an x-ray is 'improved' from last time) know to which group the patient they are assessing was allocated. If you believe that the evaluation of clinical signs and the interpretation of diagnostic tests such as ECGs and x-rays is 100% objective, you haven't been in the game very long [22].

The chapter 'The clinical examination' in Sackett and colleagues' book *Clinical Epidemiology: A basic science for clinical medicine* [23] provides substantial evidence that, when examining patients, doctors find what they expect and hope to find. It is rare for two competent clinicians to reach complete agreement for any given aspect of the physical examination or interpretation of any diagnostic test. The level of agreement beyond chance between two observers can be expressed mathematically as the kappa score, with a score of 1.0 indicating perfect agreement. Kappa scores for specialists in the field assessing the height of a patient's jugular venous pressure, classifying diabetic retinopathy from retinal photographs and interpreting a mammogram x-ray were, respectively, 0.42, 0.55 and 0.67 [23].

This digression into clinical disagreement should have persuaded you that efforts to keep assessors 'blind' (or to avoid offence to the visually impaired, *masked*), to the group allocation of their patients are far from superfluous. If, for example, you knew that a patient had been randomised to an active drug to lower blood pressure rather than to a placebo, you might be more likely to recheck a reading that was surprisingly high. This is an example of *performance bias*, which, along with other pitfalls for the unblinded assessor, are listed in Figure 4.1.

An excellent example of controlling for bias by adequate 'blinding' was published in the *Lancet* in 1996 [24]. Majeed and colleagues performed an RCT that demonstrated, in contrast with the findings of several previous studies, that the recovery time (days in hospital, days off work and time to resume full activity) after laparoscopic removal of the gallbladder (the 'keyhole surgery' approach) was no quicker than that associated with the traditional open operation. The discrepancy between this trial and its predecessors may have been because of the authors' meticulous attempt to reduce bias (Figure 4.1). The patients were not randomised until after induction of general anaesthesia. Neither the patients nor their carers were aware of which operation had been performed, as all patients left the operating theatre with identical dressings (complete with blood stains!). These findings challenge previous authors to ask themselves whether it was expectation bias, rather than swifter recovery, which spurred doctors to discharge the laparoscopic surgery group earlier. The ethical issues surrounding sham operations are complex; see Savulescu et al. [25] for more detail on that topic.

Were preliminary statistical questions addressed?

As non-statisticians, we tend only to look for three numbers in the methods section of a paper. While, strictly speaking, many other things are also important, these three will get you started:

- the size of the sample
- the duration of follow-up; and
- the completeness of follow-up.

Sample size

One crucial prerequisite before embarking on a clinical trial is to perform a sample size ('power') calculation. A trial should be big enough to have a high chance of detecting, as statistically significant, a worthwhile effect if it exists, and thus to be reasonably sure that no benefit exists if it is not found in the trial.

To calculate sample size, the researcher must ascertain two things.

1. The level of difference between the two groups that would constitute a *clinically significant* effect. Note that this may not be the same as a statistically significant effect. To cite an example from a famous clinical trial of hypertension therapy, you could administer a new drug that lowered blood pressure by around 10 mmHg and the effect would be a statistically significant lowering of the chances of developing stroke (i.e. the odds are less than 1 in 20 that the reduced incidence occurred by chance) [26]. However, if the people being asked to take this drug had only mildly raised blood pressure and no other major risk factors for stroke (i.e. they were relatively young, not diabetic, had normal cholesterol levels, etc.), this level of difference would only prevent around one stroke in every 850 patients treated – a clinical difference in risk that many patients would classify as not worth the hassle of taking the tablets. This was shown over 20 years ago and has been confirmed by numerous studies since (see the Cochrane review by Wright et al. [27]). Yet far too many doctors still treat their patients according to the *statistical* significance of the findings of mega trials rather than the clinical significance for their patient.
2. The mean and the standard deviation (abbreviated SD) of the principal outcome variable.

If the outcome in question is an event (such as hysterectomy) rather than a quantity (such as blood pressure), the items of data required are the proportion of people experiencing the event in the population and an estimate of what might constitute a clinically significant change in that proportion.

Once these items of data have been ascertained, the minimum sample size can be easily computed using standard formulae, nomograms or tables, which may be obtained from published papers [28], textbooks [29], free access websites (try http://www.macorr.com/ss_calculator.htm) or commercial statistical software packages (see, e.g. www.ncss.com/pass). Hence, the researchers can, *before the trial begins*, work out how large a sample they will need to have a moderate, high or very high chance of detecting a true difference between the groups. The likelihood of detecting a true difference is known as the *power* of the study. It is common for studies to stipulate a power of between 80% and 90%. Hence, when reading a paper about an RCT, you should look for a sentence that reads something like this (which is taken from Majeed and colleagues' cholecystectomy paper described earlier) [24]:

> *For a 90% chance of detecting a difference of one night's stay in hospital using the Mann–Whitney U-test [see Chapter 5, Table 5.1], 100 patients were needed in each group (assuming a SD of two nights). This gives a power greater than 90% for detecting a difference in operating times of 15 minutes, assuming a SD of 20 minutes.*

If the paper you are reading does not give a sample size calculation *and* it appears to show that there is no difference between the intervention and control arms of the trial, you should extract from the paper (or directly from the authors) the information in 1 and 2 above and do the calculation yourself. Underpowered studies are ubiquitous in the medical literature, usually because the authors found it harder than they anticipated to recruit their participants. Such studies typically lead to a type II or β error – that is, the erroneous conclusion that an intervention has no effect. (In contrast, the rarer type I or α error is the conclusion that a difference is significant when, in fact, it is because of sampling error.)

Duration of follow-up

Even if the sample size itself was adequate, a study must be continued for long enough for the effect of the intervention to be reflected in the primary outcome variable. If the authors were looking at the effect of a new painkiller on the degree of postoperative pain, their study may only have needed a follow-up period of 48 hours. On the other hand, if they were looking at the effect of nutritional supplementation in the preschool years on final adult height, follow-up should have been measured in decades.

Even if the intervention has demonstrated a significant difference between the groups after, say, 6 months, that difference may not be sustained. As many dieters know from bitter experience, strategies to reduce obesity often show dramatic results after 2 or 3 weeks, but if follow-up is continued for a year or more, the unfortunate participants have (more often than not) put most of the weight back on.

Completeness of follow-up

It has been shown repeatedly that participants who withdraw from research studies are less likely to have taken their tablets as directed, more likely to have missed their interim check-ups and more likely to have experienced adverse effects on any medication than those who do not withdraw (incidentally, don't use the term *drop out* as this is pejorative). People who fail to complete questionnaires may feel differently about the issue (and probably less strongly) than those who email them back. People on a weight-reducing programme are more likely to continue coming back if they are actually losing weight. If you want to read more, this paper by Skea and colleagues [30] explored participant-reported factors influencing non-retention within a clinical trial context.

The following are among the reasons patients withdraw (or are withdrawn by the researchers) from clinical trials.

1. Incorrect entry of patient into trial (i.e. researcher discovers during the trial that the patient should not have been randomised in the first place because they did not fulfil the entry criteria).
2. Suspected adverse reaction to the trial drug. Note that you should never look at the 'adverse reaction' rate in the intervention group without comparing it with that on placebo. Inert tablets bring people out in a rash surprisingly frequently.
3. Loss of participant motivation ('I don't want to take these tablets any more' – but more often 'I don't want to keep coming back to clinic and filling out long questionnaires').
4. Clinical reasons (e.g. concurrent illness, pregnancy).
5. Loss to follow-up (e.g. participant moves away).
6. Death. Clearly, people who die will not attend for their outpatient appointments, so unless specifically accounted for they might be misclassified as withdrawals. This is one reason why studies with a low follow-up rate (say, below 70%) are generally considered untrustworthy.

Ignoring everyone who has failed to complete a clinical trial will bias the results, usually in favour of the intervention. It is, therefore, standard practice to analyse the results of comparative studies on an *intention-to-treat* basis. This means that all data on participants originally allocated to the intervention arm of the study, including those who withdrew before the trial finished, those who did not take their tablets and even those who subsequently received the control intervention for whatever reason, should be analysed, along with data on the patients who followed the protocol throughout. Conversely, withdrawals from the placebo arm of the study should be analysed with those who faithfully took their placebo. If you look hard enough in a paper, you will usually find the sentence, 'results were analysed on an intention-to-treat basis', but you should not be reassured until you have checked and confirmed the figures yourself.

There are, in fact, a few situations when intention-to-treat analysis is, rightly, not used. The most common is the *efficacy* (*or per-protocol*) *analysis*, which is to explain the effects of the intervention itself and is therefore of the treatment actually received. But even if the participants in an efficacy analysis are part of an RCT, for the purposes of the analysis they effectively constitute a cohort study (see section 'What are cohort studies?' in Chapter 3).

A note on ethical considerations

In earlier editions of this book, Trisha wrote about her experience as a junior doctor of possible research misconduct by colleagues:

> *I got a job in a world-renowned teaching hospital. One of my humble tasks was seeing the geriatric (elderly) patients in casualty. I was soon invited out to lunch by two charming mid-career doctors, who (I later realised) were seeking my help with their research. In return for getting my name on the paper, I was to take a rectal biopsy (i.e. cut out a small piece of tissue from the rectum) on any patient over the age of 90 who had constipation. I asked for a copy of the consent form that patients would be asked to sign. When they assured me that the average 90-year-old would hardly notice the procedure, I smelt a rat and refused to cooperate with their project. At the time, I was naïvely unaware of the seriousness of the offence being planned by these doctors.*

Doing *any* research, particularly that which involves invasive procedures, on vulnerable and sick patients without full consideration of ethical issues is both a criminal offence and potential grounds for a doctor to be 'struck off' the medical register. Getting formal ethical approval for one's research study (for UK readers, the Health Research Authority, www.hra.nhs.uk) and ensuring that the research is properly run and adequately monitored (a set of tasks and responsibilities known as *research governance*) can be an enormous bureaucratic hurdle. Ethical issues were, sadly, sometimes ignored in the past in research in babies, the elderly, those with learning difficulties and those unable to protest (e.g. prisoners and the military), leading to some infamous research scandals.

These days, most editors routinely refuse to publish research that has not been approved by a research ethics committee. Note, however, that heavy-handed approaches to research governance by official bodies may be ethically questionable. Neurologist and researcher Professor Charles Warlow argued some years ago that the overemphasis on 'informed consent' by well-intentioned research ethics committees has been the kiss of death to research into head injuries, strokes and other acute brain problems (in which, clearly, the person is in no position to consider the personal pros and cons of taking part in a research study) [31]. In 2012, exasperated researchers published a salutary tale entitled 'Bureaucracy stifles medical research in Britain' [32]. Ten years later, and bureaucracy seems to be even worse [33]. The bottom-line message for this book is: make sure that the study you are reading about has had ethical approval, while also sympathising with researchers who have had to 'jump through hoops' to get it.

Summing up

Having worked through the methods section of a paper, you should be able to tell yourself in a short paragraph what sort of study was performed, on how many participants, where the participants came from, what treatment or other intervention was offered, how long the follow-up period was (or, if a survey, what the response rate was) and what outcome measure(s) were used. You should also, at this stage, identify what statistical tests, if any, were used to analyse the data (see Chapter 5 for more on statistics). If you are clear about these things before reading the rest of the paper, you will find the results easier to understand, interpret and, if appropriate, reject. You should be able to come up with descriptions such as those given here:

> *This paper describes an unblinded randomised trial, concerned with therapy, in 267 hospital outpatients aged between 58 and 93 years, in which four-layer compression bandaging was compared with standard single-layer dressings in the management of uncomplicated venous leg ulcers. Follow-up was six months. Percentage healing of the ulcer was measured from baseline in terms of the surface area of a tracing of the wound taken by the district nurse and calculated by a computer scanning device. Results were analysed using the Wilcoxon matched-pairs test.*
>
> *This is a questionnaire survey of 963 general practitioners randomly selected from throughout the UK, in which they were asked their year of graduation from medical school and the level at which they would begin treatment for essential hypertension. Response options on the structured questionnaire were 'below 89 mm Hg', '90–99 mm Hg' and '100 mm Hg or greater'.*

Results were analysed using a Chi-squared test on a 3 × 2 table to see whether the threshold for treating hypertension was related to whether the doctor graduated from medical school before or after 2005. This is a case report of a single patient with a suspected fatal adverse drug reaction to the newly released hypnotic drug Sleepol.

When you have had a little practice in looking at the methods section of research papers along the lines suggested in this chapter, you will find that it is only a short step to start using the checklists in Appendix 1, or the more comprehensive guides you will find in more advanced texts. We will return to many of the issues discussed here in Chapter 6, in relation to evaluating papers on trials of drug therapy and other simple interventions.

Exercises based on this chapter

1. Find a recent paper describing an RCT. Make careful notes on the paper, extracting data on the following:
   a. What was the research question and what hypothesis were the authors attempting to test?
   b. Who was included in the trial and who was excluded?
   c. What was the primary outcome measure?
   d. In your opinion, was the trial large enough, complete enough and continued for long enough to make you confident in the result?
   e. Do you think the trial needs to be repeated? If so, why?
2. Look back at the story in this chapter about the J-curve linking alcohol intake with mortality. Do you believe that the J-curve relationships has now been disproved? To answer this, you will need to get hold of the full text of the referenced papers and read the detailed arguments. If you don't believe the authors of the latest meta-analysis, can you craft a counter-argument?
3. Find the paper on development and validation of QRISK3 risk prediction algorithms to estimate future risk of cardiovascular disease. Why is it important to use two different populations to develop and validate a prediction model? You might be interested in three recent papers published on clinical prediction models [34–36].

References

1. Mitchell JR. 'But will it help my patients with myocardial infarction?' The implications of recent trials for everyday country folk. *BMJ* 1982; **285**: 1140–8.
2. Hamaker ME, Stauder R, van Munster BC. Exclusion of older patients from ongoing clinical trials for hematological malignancies: an evaluation of the National Institutes of Health Clinical Trial Registry. *Oncologist* 2014; **19**: 1069–75.

3. Steuernagel CR, Lam CSP, Greenhalgh T. Countering sex and gender bias in cardiovascular research requires more than equal recruitment and sex disaggregated analyses. *BMJ* 2023; **382**: e075031.
4. Coggon D, Rose G, Barker D. *Epidemiology for the Uninitiated*. Chichester: Wiley; 2009.
5. Cuff A. Sources of bias in clinical trials [blog post]. *Applying Criticality* 19 June 2013. https://applyingcriticality.wordpress.com/2013/06/19/sources-of-bias-in-clinical-trials (accessed 3 September 2023).
6. Delgado-Rodriguez M, Llorca J. Bias. *Journal of Epidemiology and Community Health* 2004; **58**: 635–41.
7. University of Oxford Centre for Evidence-Based Medicine. *Catalog of Bias*. https://catalogofbias.org (accessed 2 September 2023).
8. Deeks JJ, Dinnes J, D'Amico R, et al. Evaluating non-randomised intervention studies. *Health Technoogyl Assessment* 2003; **7**: iii–x, 1–173.
9. Nallamothu BK, Hayward RA, Bates ER. Beyond the randomized clinical trial. *Circulation* 2008; **118**: 1294–303.
10. Berger ML, Dreyer N, Anderson F, et al. Prospective observational studies to assess comparative effectiveness: The ISPOR good research practices task force report. *Value in Health* 2012; **15**: 217–30.
11. Rimm EB, Williams P, Fosher K, et al. Moderate alcohol intake and lower risk of coronary heart disease: meta-analysis of effects on lipids and haemostatic factors. *BMJ* 1999; **319**: 1523–8.
12. Fillmore KM, Stockwell T, Chikritzhs T, et al. Moderate alcohol use and reduced mortality risk: systematic error in prospective studies and new hypotheses. *Annals of Epidemiology* 2007; **17**: S16–23.
13. Ronksley PE, Brien SE, Turner BJ, et al. Association of alcohol consumption with selected cardiovascular disease outcomes: a systematic review and meta-analysis. *BMJ* 2011; **342**: d671.
14. Stockwell T, Greer A, Fillmore K, et al. How good is the science? *BMJ* 2012; **344**: e2276.
15. Stockwell T, Zhao J, Panwar S, et al. Do 'moderate' drinkers have reduced mortality risk? A systematic review and meta-analysis of alcohol consumption and all-cause mortality. *Journal of Studies on Alcohol and Drugs* 2016; **77**: 185–98.
16. Zhao J, Stockwell T, Naimi T, et al. Association between daily alcohol intake and risk of all-cause mortality: a systematic review and meta-analyses. *JAMA Network Open* 2023; **6**: e236185.
17. Malmsiø D, Frost A, Hróbjartsson A. A scoping review finds that guides to authors of protocols for observational epidemiological studies varied highly in format and content. *Journal of Clinical Epidemiology* 2023; **154**: 156–66.
18. von Elm E, Altman DG, Egger M, et al. The Strengthening the Reporting of Observational Studies in Epidemiology (STROBE) Statement: Guidelines for Reporting Observational Studies. *PLoS Med.* 2007;4. doi: 10.1371/journal.pmed.0040296
19. Bahr R, Clarsen B, Derman W, et al. International Olympic Committee consensus statement: methods for recording and reporting of epidemiological data on injury

and illness in sport 2020 (including STROBE Extension for Sport Injury and Illness Surveillance (STROBE-SIIS)). *British Journal of Sports Medicine* 2020; **54**: 372–89.

20. Hippisley-Cox J, Coupland C, Brindle P. Development and validation of QRISK3 risk prediction algorithms to estimate future risk of cardiovascular disease: prospective cohort study. *BMJ* 2017; **357**: j2099.
21. Bowie C. Lessons from the pertussis vaccine court trial. *Lancet* 1990; **335**: 397–9.
22. Gawande A. *Complications: A surgeon's notes on an imperfect science.* London: Profile Books; 2010.
23. Sackett DL, Haynes RB, Tugwell P. *Clinical Epidemiology: A basic science for clinical medicine.* Boston, MA: Little, Brown; 1985.
24. Majeed AW, Troy G, Smythe A, et al. Randomised, prospective, single-blind comparison of laparoscopic versus small-incision cholecystectomy. *Lancet* 1996; **347**: 989–94.
25. Savulescu J, Wartolowska K, Carr A. Randomised placebo-controlled trials of surgery: ethical analysis and guidelines. *Journal of Medical Ethics* 2016; **42**: 776–83.
26. Medical Research Council Working Party. Medical Research Council trial of treatment of hypertension in older adults: principal results. *BMJ* 1992; **304**: 405–12.
27. Wright JM, Musini VM, Gill R. First-line drugs for hypertension. *Cochrane Database of Systematic Reviews* 2018;**4**(4):CD001841.
28. Charles P, Giraudeau B, Dechartres A, et al. Reporting of sample size calculation in randomised controlled trials: review. *BMJ* 2009; **338**: b1732.
29. Machin D, ed. *Sample Size Tables for Clinical Studies.* 3rd edn. Oxford: Wiley-Blackwell; 2008.
30. Skea ZC, Newlands R, Gillies K. Exploring non-retention in clinical trials: a meta-ethnographic synthesis of studies reporting participant reasons for drop out. *BMJ Open* 2019; **9**: e021959.
31. Warlow C. Over-regulation of clinical research: a threat to public health. *Clinical Medicine (London)* 2005; **5**: 33–8.
32. Snooks H, Hutchings H, Seagrove A, et al. Bureaucracy stifles medical research in Britain: a tale of three trials. *BMC Medical Research Methodology* 2012; **12**: 122.
33. Snooks H, Khanom A, Ballo R, et al. Is bureaucracy being busted in research ethics and governance for health services research in the UK? Experiences and perspectives reported by stakeholders through an online survey. *BMC Public Health* 2023; **23**: 1119.
34. Collins GS, Dhiman P, Ma J, et al. Evaluation of clinical prediction models (part 1): from development to external validation. *BMJ* 2024; **384**: e074819.
35. Riley RD, Archer L, Snell KIE, et al. Evaluation of clinical prediction models (part 2): how to undertake an external validation study. *BMJ* 2024; **384**: e074820.
36. Riley RD, Snell KIE, Archer L, et al. Evaluation of clinical prediction models (part 3): calculating the sample size required for an external validation study. *BMJ* 2024; **384**: e074821.

Chapter 5 **Statistics for the non-statistician**

How can non-statisticians evaluate statistical tests?

In this age where healthcare leans increasingly on mathematics, no clinician can afford to leave the statistical aspects of a paper entirely to the 'experts'. If, like us, you believe yourself to be somewhat innumerate, remember that you do not need to be able to build a car to drive one. What you do need to know (at a basic level, to get you started) is which is the best test to use for common types of statistical questions. You need to be able to describe in words what the test does and in what circumstances it becomes invalid or inappropriate. And you need to know enough vocabulary to be able to converse with a statistician. Box 5.1 shows some frequently used 'tricks of the trade', of which all of us need to be aware (in our own as well as other people's practice).

The summary checklist in Appendix 1, explained in detail in the subsequent sections, constitutes our own method for assessing the adequacy of a statistical analysis, which some readers might find too simplistic. If you do, please skip this section and turn either to a more comprehensive presentation for the non-statistician: the 'Basic Statistics for Clinicians' series in the *Canadian Medical Association Journal* [1–4] or to a more mainstream statistical textbook. Popular statistics textbooks (including those preferred when Trisha asked her X (formerly Twitter) followers for a previous edition of this book) include Altman [5], Bland [6] and Kirkwood et al. [7]. If you find statistics impossibly difficult, take the sections below one at a time and return to read the next section only when you feel comfortable with the previous ones. None of the sections presupposes a detailed knowledge of the actual calculations involved.

The first question to ask, by the way, is, 'Have the authors used any statistical tests at all?' If they are presenting numbers and claiming that these numbers mean something, without using statistical methods to prove it, they are almost certainly skating on thin ice.

How to Read a Paper: The Basics of Evidence-Based Healthcare, Seventh Edition.
Trisha Greenhalgh and Paul Dijkstra.

Box 5.1 Ten ways you could cheat on statistical tests when writing up results

1 Throw all your data into a computer (statistical software) and report as significant any relationship where '$p < 0.05$' (see section 'Have *p*-values been calculated and interpreted appropriately?').

2 If baseline differences between the groups favour the intervention group, remember not to adjust for them (see section 'Have they determined whether their groups are comparable, and, if necessary, adjusted for baseline differences?').

3 Do not test your data to see if they are normally distributed. If you do, you might be stuck with non-parametric tests, which aren't as much fun (see section 'What sort of data have they got, and have they used appropriate statistical tests?').

4 Ignore all withdrawals ('drop-outs') and non-responders, so the analysis only concerns subjects who fully complied with treatment (see section 'Were preliminary statistical questions addressed?').

5 Always assume that you can plot one set of data against another and calculate an *r*-value (Pearson correlation coefficient; see section 'Has correlation been distinguished from regression, and has the correlation coefficient (*r*-value) been calculated and interpreted correctly?') and that a 'significant' *r*-value proves causation (see section 'Have assumptions been made about the nature and direction of causality?').

6 If outliers (points that lie a long way from the others on your graph) are messing up your calculations, just rub them out. But if outliers are helping your case, even if they appear to be spurious results, leave them in (see section 'Were "outliers" analysed with both common sense and appropriate statistical adjustments?').

7 If the confidence intervals of the difference between the groups in your results overlap zero, leave them out of your report. Better still, mention them briefly in the text but don't draw them in on the graph and ignore them when drawing your conclusions (see section 'Have confidence intervals been calculated, and do the authors' conclusions reflect them?').

8 If the difference between two groups becomes significant 4.5 months into a 6-month trial, stop the trial and start writing up. Alternatively, if at 6 months the results are 'nearly significant', extend the trial for another 3 weeks (see section 'Have the data been analysed according to the original study protocol?').

9 If your results prove uninteresting, ask the computer to go back and see if any particular subgroups behaved differently. You might find that your intervention worked after all in Chinese women aged 52–61 (see section 'Have the data been analysed according to the original study protocol?').

10 If analysing your data the way you planned to does not give the result you wanted, rerun the analysis through a selection of other tests (see section 'If the statistical tests in the paper are obscure, why have the authors chosen to use them and have they included a reference?').

Have the authors set the scene correctly?

Have they determined whether their groups are comparable and, if necessary, adjusted for baseline differences?

Most comparative clinical trials include either a table or a paragraph in the text showing the baseline characteristics of the groups being studied (i.e. their characteristics *after* random allocation, for trials, to a specific group but *before* the trial or observational study was begun). Such a table should demonstrate that both the intervention and control groups are similar in terms of age and sex distribution and key prognostic variables (such as the average size of a cancerous lump). If there are important differences in these baseline characteristics, even though they may be due to chance, it can pose a challenge to your data analysis and interpretation of results. In this situation, you can carry out certain statistical adjustments to allow for these differences and hence strengthen your argument. To find out how to make such adjustments, see the relevant section in any of the mainstream biostatistics textbooks – but don't try to memorise the formulae!

What sort of data do they have and have they used appropriate statistical tests?

Numbers are often used to label the properties of things. We can assign a number to represent our height, weight and so on. For properties like these, the measurements can be treated as actual numbers. We can, for example, calculate the average weight and height of a group of people by averaging the measurements. But consider a different example, in which we use numbers to label the property 'city of origin', where 1 means London, 2 means Manchester, 3 means Birmingham and so on. We could still calculate the average of these numbers for a particular sample of cases but the result would be meaningless. The same would apply if we labelled the property 'liking for *x*', with 1, not at all, 2, a bit and 3, a lot. Again, we could calculate the 'average liking' but the numerical result would be uninterpretable unless we knew that the difference between 'not at all' and 'a bit' was exactly the same as the difference between 'a bit' and 'a lot'.

The statistical tests used in medical papers are generally classified as either parametric (i.e. they assume that the data were sampled from a particular form of distribution, such as a normal distribution) or non-parametric (i.e. they do not assume that the data were sampled from a particular type of distribution).

The non-parametric tests focus on the *rank order* of the values and ignore the absolute differences between them (if we arrange the data in ascending order and then rank them as a 1, 2, 3 . . ., non-parametric tests will use ranks to analyse data instead of the actual data). As you might imagine, statistical significance is more difficult to demonstrate with rank order tests (indeed, some statisticians are cynical about the value of the latter) and this tempts researchers to use statistics such as the *r*-value (explained below) inappropriately. Not only is the *r*-value (parametric) easier to calculate than an equivalent rank order statistic such as Spearman's ρ (pronounced 'rho') but it is also much more likely to give (apparently) significant results. Unfortunately, it will also give an entirely spurious and misleading estimate of the significance of the result, unless the data are appropriate to the test being used. More examples of parametric tests and their rank order equivalents (if present) are given in Table 5.1.

Another consideration is the shape of the distribution from which the data were sampled. When Trisha was at school, her class plotted the amount of pocket money received against the number of children receiving that amount. The results formed a histogram approximately the same shape as in Figure 5.1 – a 'normal' distribution. (The term *normal* refers to the shape of the graph and is used because many biological phenomena show this pattern of distribution.) Some biological variables, such as body weight show, skew distribution, as shown in Figure 5.2. (Figure 5.2, in fact, shows a negative skew, whereas body weight would be positively skewed. The average adult male body weight is around 80 kg and people exist who are 160 kg but nobody weighs less than nothing, so the graph cannot possibly be symmetrical.)

Non-normal (skewed) data can sometimes be *transformed* to give a normal-shape graph by plotting the logarithm of the skewed variable or performing some other mathematical transformation (such as square root or reciprocal). Some data, however, cannot be transformed into a smooth pattern, and the significance of this is discussed below. Deciding whether data are normally distributed is important, because it will determine what type of statistical tests to use. For example, linear regression (see below) will give misleading results unless the points on the scatter graph form a particular distribution about the regression line; that is, the residuals (the perpendicular distance from each point to the line) should themselves be normally distributed. Transforming data to achieve a normal distribution (if this is indeed achievable) is not 'cheating'. It simply ensures that data values are given appropriate emphasis in assessing the overall effect. Using tests based on the normal distribution to analyse non-normally distributed data is very

Table 5.1 Some commonly used statistical tests

Parametric test	DV and IV types	Example of equivalent non-parametric (rank order) test	Purpose of test	Example
Two sample (unpaired) *t*-test	DV: scale/continuous IV: categorical (only 2 groups)	Mann–Whitney *U*-test	Compares 2 independent samples drawn from the same population	To compare girls' heights with boys' heights
One-sample (paired) *t*-test	DV: scale/continuous IV: condition (only 2 levels, e.g. pre and post)	Wilcoxon matched-pairs test	Compares 2 sets of observations on a single sample (tests the hypothesis that the mean difference between 2 measurements is 0)	To compare weight of obese adults before and after an intervention
One way ANOVA	DV: scale/continuous IV: categorical (3 or more groups)	Analysis of variance by ranks (e.g. Kruskall–Wallis test)	Compares the means of 3 or more groups to determine if there are significant differences among them	To compare the average blood pressure in three ethnic groups (Asian, African, white)
Repeated measures one-way ANOVA	DV: scale/continuous IV: condition (3 or more levels)	Friedman test	Designed to handle situations where data is collected across multiple time points or conditions on the same subjects	To determine how plasma glucose level changes 1, 2 or 3 hours after a meal
Two-way ANOVA	DV: scale/continuous IV1: categorical (2 or more groups) IV1: categorical (2 or more groups)	No direct equivalent	Useful when you need to simultaneously analyse the influence of 2 factors on a single outcome, examining their main effects and potential interaction	To determine if diet type (low carb vs standard diet) and exercise level (moderate vs. high) have a significant impact on blood glucose levels in patients with type 2 diabetes
Repeated measure two-way ANOVA	DV: scale/continuous IV1: condition (2 or more levels) IV1: condition (2 or more levels)	No direct equivalent	Suitable when you want to assess the combined effects of interventions and time on outcomes investigating both main effects and potential interaction	Does the new drug compared with standard have a significant effect on patients' blood pressure over 3 measurement points (1, 2 and 3 months)?

(*Continued*)

Table 5.1 (Continued)

Parametric test	DV and IV types	Example of equivalent non-parametric (rank order) test	Purpose of test	Example
No direct equivalent	DV: categorical IV: categorical	χ^2 test	Tests the null hypothesis that the proportions of variables estimated from two (or more) independent samples are the same	To assess whether acceptance into medical school is more likely if the applicant was born in the UK
No direct equivalent	DV: categorical IV: categorical	McNemar's test	Tests the null hypothesis that the proportions estimated from a paired sample are the same	To determine whether a new drug significantly reduced symptoms compared with a standard treatment in same group of patients
Product moment correlation coefficient (Pearson's r)	DV: scale/continuous IV: scale/continuous	Spearman's rank correlation coefficient (ρ)	Assesses the *strength* of association between two continuous variables	To assess whether and to what extent plasma HbA1c level is correlated to plasma triglyceride level in patients with diabetes
Linear Regression	DV: scale/continuous IV: scale/continuous	No direct equivalent	Describes the numerical relation between two quantitative variables, allowing one value to be predicted from the other	To see how peak expiratory flow rate varies with height
Multiple regression	DV: scale/continuous IV1: scale/continuous IV2 or more: scale/ continuous/binary	No direct equivalent	Describes the numerical relation between a dependent variable after adjusting for one or more predictor variables (covariates)	To determine whether and to what extent a person's age, determines their blood pressure after adjusting for body fat and sodium intake

ANOVA, analysis of variance; DV, dependent variable; HbA1c, glycated haemoglobin; IV, independent variable.

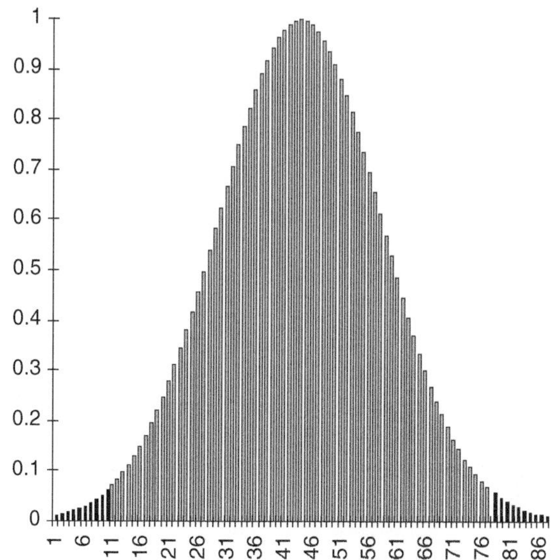

Figure 5.1 Example of a normal curve.

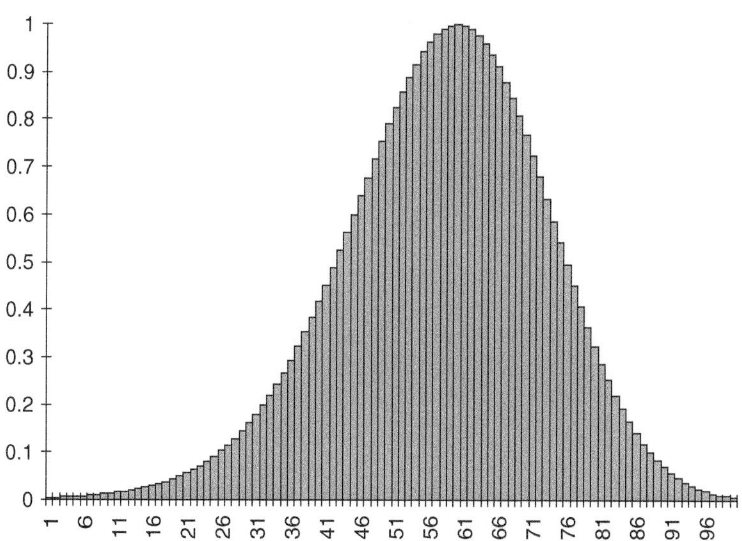

Figure 5.2 Example of a skew curve.

definitely cheating. Cheating is, of course, a strong word. Sometimes 'cheating' is not deliberate but is done out of ignorance or a lack of (statistical) knowledge. Biostatisticians are therefore key members of the research team, as this paper argues [8].

If the statistical tests in the paper are obscure, why have the authors chosen to use them, and have they included a reference?

There sometimes seems to be an infinite number of possible statistical tests. In fact, most basic clinical studies can be analysed using a formulary of about a dozen. The rest are small print and should be reserved for special indications. If the paper you are reading appears to describe a standard set of data that have been collected in a standard way but the test used is unpronounceable and not listed in a basic statistics textbook, you should smell a rat. The authors should, in such circumstances, state why they have used this test, and give a reference (with page numbers) for a definitive description of it.

Have the data been analysed according to the original study protocol?

Even if you are not interested in the statistical justification, common sense should tell you why points 8 and 9 in Box 5.1 amount to serious cheating. If you trawl for long enough, you will inevitably find some category of participants who appear to have done particularly well or badly. However, each time you look to see if a particular subgroup is different from the rest, you greatly increase the likelihood that you will eventually find one that appears to be so, even though the difference is entirely due to chance.

Similarly, if you play coin toss with someone, no matter how far you fall behind, there will come a time when you are one ahead. Most people would agree that to stop the game then would not be a fair way to play. So it is with research. If you make it inevitable that you will (eventually) obtain an apparently positive result, you will also make it inevitable that you will be misleading yourself about the justice of your case. Terminating an intervention trial prematurely for ethical reasons when participants in one arm are faring particularly badly is different, and is discussed elsewhere [9].

Going back and raking over your data to look for 'interesting' or 'unplanned' results (retrospective subgroup analysis or, more colloquially, data dredging) is known as data-dredging bias and can lead to false conclusions [10,11]. In an early study on the use of aspirin in the prevention of stroke in predisposed patients, the results showed a significant effect in both sexes combined, and a retrospective subgroup analysis appeared to show that the effect was confined to men [12]. This conclusion led to aspirin being withheld from women for many years until the results of other studies (including a large meta-analysis [13]) showed this subgroup effect to be spurious.

This and other examples are given in a paper by Oxman and Guyatt [14], 'A consumer's guide to subgroup analysis', which reproduces a useful checklist for deciding whether apparent differences in subgroup response are real.

Paired data, tails and outliers

Were paired tests performed on paired data?

Students often find it difficult to decide whether to use a paired or unpaired statistical test to analyse their data. There is, in fact, no great mystery about this. If you measure something twice on each participant (e.g. lying and standing blood pressure), you will probably be interested not just in the average difference in lying versus standing blood pressure in the entire sample but also in how much each individual's blood pressure changes with position. In this situation, you have what are called *paired* data, because each measurement in one position is paired with a measurement on the same person in a different position.

In this example, it is having the same person on both occasions that makes the pairings, but there are other possibilities (e.g. any two measurements made of bed occupancy of the same hospital ward). In these situations, it is likely that the two sets of values will be significantly correlated (e.g. my blood pressure next week is likely to be closer to my blood pressure last week than to the blood pressure of a randomly selected adult last week). In other words, we would expect two randomly selected 'paired' values to be closer to each other than two randomly selected 'unpaired' values. Unless we allow for this, by carrying out the appropriate 'paired' sample tests, we can end up with a biased estimate of the significance of our results.

Was a two-tailed test performed whenever the effect of an intervention could conceivably be a negative one?

Reflecting a possible general aversion to statistics, the concept of a test with tails might cause some researchers to think of devils or snakes. In fact, the term *tail* refers to the extremes of the distribution – the dark areas in Figure 5.1. Let's say that a graph represents the diastolic blood pressures of a group of individuals of which a random sample are about to be put on a low-sodium diet. If you assume that a low-sodium diet has a significant lowering effect on blood pressure, subsequent blood pressure measurements on these participants would be more likely to lie within the left-hand 'tail' of the graph. Hence, we would analyse the data with one-tailed statistical tests because we assumed a fall in diastolic blood pressure.

But on what grounds might we assume that a low-sodium diet could only conceivably put blood pressure down but could never put it *up*? Even if there are valid physiological reasons why that might be the case in this particular example, it is certainly not good science always to assume that you know the *direction* of the effect that your intervention will have. A new drug intended to relieve nausea, for example, might actually exacerbate it; and an educational leaflet intended to reduce anxiety might increase it. Hence, your statistical analysis should, in general, test the hypothesis that either high *or* low values in your outcome variable dataset have arisen by chance. In the language of the statisticians, this means you need a two-tailed statistical test unless you have very convincing evidence that the difference can only be in one direction.

Were 'outliers' analysed with both common sense and appropriate statistical adjustments?

Unexpected results may reflect idiosyncrasies in the participant (e.g. unusual metabolism), errors in measurement (e.g. faulty equipment), errors in interpretation (e.g. misreading a meter reading) or errors in calculation (e.g. misplaced decimal points). Only the first of these is a 'real' result that deserves to be included in the analysis. A result that is many orders of magnitude away from the others is less likely to be genuine, but it may be. A few years ago, while doing a research project, Trisha measured a number of different hormone levels in about 30 participants. One participant's growth hormone levels came back about 100 times higher than everyone else's. Trisha assumed that this result was a transcription error, so she moved the decimal point two places to the left. Some weeks later, she met the technician who had analysed the specimens and he asked 'Whatever happened to that chap with acromegaly?'.

A right course of action should have been to contact the lab technician and to verify the accuracy of the data from the original source. Outliers are easily detected using graphs such as histograms and box plots. This often leads to skewed distribution of data and you are inclined to use non-parametric statistical tests. However, some transformations (such a log transformation or reciprocal as mentioned before) can convert the same data to appear normally distributed. We can then use parametric statistical tests.

Statistically correcting for outliers (e.g. to modify their effect on the overall result) is quite a sophisticated statistical manoeuvre. If you are interested, try the relevant section in your favourite statistics textbook.

Correlation, regression and causation

Has correlation been distinguished from regression, and has the correlation coefficient (*r*-value) been calculated and interpreted correctly?

For many non-statisticians, the terms *correlation* and *regression* are synonymous and refer vaguely to a mental image of a scatter plot with dots sprinkled messily along a diagonal line sprouting from the intercept of the axes. You would be right in assuming that, if two things are not correlated, it will be meaningless to attempt a regression. But regression and correlation are both precise statistical terms that serve different functions [4].

The *r*-value (or to give it its official name, 'Pearson's product–moment correlation coefficient') is among the most overused statistical instruments in the book. Strictly speaking, the *r*-value is not valid unless certain criteria are fulfilled:

1. The data (or, more accurately, the population from which the data are drawn) should be normally distributed. If they are not, non-parametric tests of correlation should be used instead (see Table 5.1).
2. The two variables should be structurally independent (i.e. one should not be forced to vary with the other). If they are not, a paired t or other paired test should be used instead.
3. Only a single pair of measurements should be made on each participant, as the measurements made on successive participants need to be statistically independent of each other if we are to end up with unbiased estimates of the population parameters of interest.
4. Every *r*-value should be accompanied by a *p*-value, which expresses how likely an association of this strength would be to have arisen by chance, or (better) a confidence interval, which expresses the range within which the 'true' *R*-value is likely to lie. (Note that lower case '*r*' represents the correlation coefficient of the sample, whereas upper case '*R*' represents the correlation coefficient of the entire population; *p*-values and confidence intervals are discussed in more detail below).

Remember, too, that even if the *r*-value is an appropriate value to calculate from a set of data, it does not tell you whether the relationship, however strong, is causal.

The term *regression* refers to a mathematical *equation* that allows one variable (the *target* variable) to be predicted from another (the *independent* variable). Regression, then, implies a direction of influence, although, as the next section will argue, it does not prove causality. In the case of multiple regression, a far more complex mathematical equation (which, thankfully, usually remains the secret of the computer that calculated it) allows the target variable to be predicted from two or more independent variables (often known as *covariables*).

The simplest regression equation, which you may remember from your school days, is $y = a + bx$, where y is the dependent variable (plotted on the vertical axis), x is the independent variable (plotted on the horizontal axis), a is the y-intercept and b is a constant. Not many biological variables can be predicted with such a simple equation. The weight of a group of people, for example, varies with their height, but not in a linear way. In the first edition of this book, Trisha gave the example, 'I am twice as tall as my son and three times his weight, but although I am four times as tall as my newborn nephew I am much more than six times his weight'. Both son and nephew now tower over Trisha, but the example will hold. Weight probably varies more closely with the square of someone's height than with height itself, so a quadratic rather than a linear regression would be more appropriate.

Even when you have fed sufficient height–weight data into a computer for it to calculate the regression equation that best predicts a person's weight from their height, your predictions would still be pretty poor, as weight and height are not all that closely *correlated*. There are other things that influence weight in addition to height, and we could, to illustrate the principle of multiple regression, enter data on age, sex, daily calorie intake and physical activity level into the computer and ask it how much each of these covariables contributes to the overall equation (or model).

The elementary principles described here, particularly the numbered points earlier, should help you spot whether correlation and regression are being used correctly in the paper you are reading. A more detailed discussion on the subject can be found in statistical textbooks listed at the end of this chapter [5–7] and in the fourth article in the Basic Statistics for Clinicians series [4].

Have assumptions been made about the nature and direction of causality?

Remember the ecological fallacy: just because a town has a large number of unemployed people and a very high crime rate, it does not necessarily follow that the unemployed are committing the crimes! In other words, the presence of an *association* between A and B tells you nothing at all about either the presence or the direction of causality. To demonstrate that A has caused B (rather than B causing A, or A and B both being caused by C), you need more than a correlation coefficient. Box 5.2 gives some criteria, originally developed by Sir Austin Bradford Hill [15], which should be met before assuming causality. We explore these criteria further in Chapter 18.

Probability and confidence

Have *p*-values been calculated and interpreted appropriately?

One of the first values a student of statistics learns to calculate is the *p*-value; that is, the probability that any particular outcome would have arisen by chance. Standard scientific practice, which is essentially arbitrary, usually deems a *p*-value of less than 1 in 20 (expressed as $p < 0.05$ and equivalent to a betting odds of 20 to 1) as 'statistically significant' and a *p*-value of less than 1 in 100 ($p < 0.01$) as 'statistically highly significant'.

By definition, then, 1 chance association in 20 (this must be around one major published result per journal issue) will appear to be significant when it

Box 5.2 Tests for causation

1 Is there evidence from true experiments in humans?
2 Is the association strong?
3 Is the association consistent from study to study?
4 Is the temporal relationship appropriate (i.e. did the postulated cause precede the postulated effect)?
5 Is there a dose–response gradient (i.e. does more of the postulated effect follow more of the postulated cause)?
6 Does the association make epidemiological sense?
7 Does the association make biological sense?
8 Is the association specific?
9 Is the association analogous to a previously proven causal association?

Source: Adapted from Hill [15].

isn't, and 1 in 100 will appear highly significant when it is really what Trisha's children call a 'fluke'. Hence, if the researchers have made multiple comparisons, they ought to make a correction to try to allow for them. The most widely known procedure for doing this is probably the Bonferroni test (described in most standard statistical textbooks), although a reviewer of earlier editions of this book described this as 'far too severe' and offered several others. Rather than speculate on tests that we don't personally understand, we recommend asking a statistician's advice if the paper you are reading makes multiple comparisons.

A result in the statistically significant range ($p < 0.05$ or $p < 0.01$, depending on what you have chosen as the cutoff) suggests that the authors should reject the null hypothesis (i.e. the hypothesis that there is no real difference between two groups). But as we have argued earlier (see section 'Were preliminary statistical questions addressed?'), a p-value in the non-significant range tells you that *either* there is no difference between the groups *or* there were too few participants to demonstrate such a difference if it existed. It does not tell you which.

The p-value has a further limitation. Guyatt and colleagues [1] conclude thus, in the first article of their 'Basic Statistics for Clinicians' series on hypothesis testing using p-values:

> *Why use a single cut-off point [for statistical significance] when the choice of such a point is arbitrary? Why make the question of whether a treatment is effective a dichotomy (a yes–no decision) when it would be more appropriate to view it as a continuum?*

For this, we need confidence intervals, which are considered next.

Have confidence intervals been calculated and do the authors' conclusions reflect them?

A confidence interval, which a good statistician can calculate on the result of just about any effect size of interest (proportion, the *r*-value, the odds ration [OR], the absolute risk reduction [ARR], the number needed to treat and the sensitivity, specificity and other key features of a diagnostic test), allows you to estimate for both 'positive' trials (those that show a statistically significant difference between two arms of the trial) and 'negative' ones (those that appear to show no difference), whether the strength of the evidence is strong or weak, and whether the study is *definitive* (i.e. obviates the need for further similar studies). The calculation of confidence intervals has been covered with great clarity in the classic book *Statistics with Confidence* [16] and their interpretation has been covered by Guyatt et al. [2] and Sedgwick [17].

If you repeated the same clinical trial hundreds of times, you would not obtain exactly the same result each time. But, *on average*, you would establish a particular level of difference (or lack of difference) between the two arms of the trial. In 90% of the trials, the difference between two arms would lie within certain broad limits, and in 95% of the trials, it would lie between certain, even broader, limits.

Now, if, as is usually the case, you only conducted one trial, how do you know how close the result is to the 'real' difference between the groups? The answer is that you don't. But by calculating, say, the 95% confidence interval around your result, you will be able to say that there is a 95% chance that the 'real' difference lies between these two limits. The sentence to look for in a paper should read something like this one:

> *In a trial of the treatment of heart failure, 33% of the patients randomised to ACE inhibitors died, whereas 38% of those randomised to hydralazine and nitrates died. The point estimate of the difference between the groups [the best single estimate of the benefit in lives saved from the use of an ACE inhibitor] is 5%. The 95% confidence interval around this difference is −1.2% to +12%.*

More likely, the results would be expressed in the following shorthand: 'The ACE inhibitor group had a 5% (95% CI −1.2 to +12) higher survival'.

In this particular example, the 95% confidence interval overlaps zero difference and, if we were expressing the result as a dichotomy (i.e. is the hypothesis 'proven' or 'disproven'?), we would classify it as a negative trial. Yet, as Guyatt and colleagues argue [2], there probably is a real difference, and it *probably* lies closer to 5% than either −1.2% or +12%. A more useful conclusion from these results is that 'all else being equal, an angiotensin-converting enzyme (ACE) inhibitor is probably the appropriate choice for patients with heart failure, but the strength of that inference is weak' [2].

As section 'Ten questions to ask about a paper that claims to validate a diagnostic or screening test' in Chapter 8 argues, the larger the trial (or the larger the pooled results of several trials), the narrower the confidence interval, and, therefore, the more likely the result is to be definitive.

In interpreting 'negative' trials, one important thing you need to know is 'would a much larger trial be likely to show a significant benefit?'. To answer this question, look at the *upper* 95% confidence interval of the result. There is only one chance in 40 (i.e. a 2.5% chance, as the other 2.5% of extreme results will lie below the *lower* 95% confidence interval) that the real result will be this much or more. Now ask yourself: 'Would this level of difference be *clinically* significant?' and if it wouldn't, you can classify the trial as not only negative but also definitive. If, on the other hand, the upper 95% confidence interval represented a clinically significant level of difference between the groups, the trial may be negative but it is also non-definitive.

Until fairly recently, the use of confidence intervals was relatively uncommon in medical papers. Fortunately, most trials in journals that follow Consolidated Standards of Reporting Trials or CONSORT guidelines (see Chapter 6) now include these routinely, but even so, many authors do not interpret their confidence intervals correctly. You should check carefully in the discussion section to see whether the authors have correctly concluded: (i) whether and to what extent their trial supported their hypothesis, and (ii) whether any further studies need to be done.

The bottom line (quantifying the chance of benefit and harm)

Have the authors expressed the effects of an intervention in terms of the likely benefit or harm that an individual patient can expect?

It is all very well to say that a particular intervention produces a 'statistically significant difference' in outcome but if you were being asked to take a new medicine, you would want to know how much better your chances would be (in terms of any particular outcome) compared with your chances if you didn't take the new medicine. Three simple calculations (and we promise you they are simple: if you can add, subtract, multiply and divide you will be able to follow this section) will enable you to answer this question objectively and in a way that means something to the non-statistician. The calculations are the relative risk reduction, the ARR and the number needed to treat.

To illustrate these concepts, and to persuade you that you need to know about them, let us tell you about a survey that Fahey and his colleagues [18] conducted a few years ago. They wrote to 182 board members of district health authorities in England (all of whom would be in some way responsible for making important health service decisions) and put the following data to them about four different rehabilitation programmes for heart attack victims. They asked which one they would prefer to fund:

- Programme A – which reduced the rate of deaths by 20%.
- Programme B – which produced an absolute reduction in deaths of 3%.
- Programme C – which increased patients' survival rate from 84% to 87%.
- Programme D – which meant that 31 people needed to enter the programme to avoid one death.

Of the 140 board members who responded, only 3 spotted that all 4 'programmes' in fact related to the same set of results. The other 137 participants all selected one of the programmes in preference to one of the others, thus revealing (as well as their own ignorance) the need for better basic training in epidemiology for healthcare policymakers. In fact, 'Programme A' is the relative risk reduction; 'Programme B' is the ARR; 'Programme C' is another way of expressing the ARR and 'Programme D' is the number needed to treat.

Let's continue with this example, which Fahey and colleagues reproduced from a study by Yusuf and colleagues [19]. We have expressed the figures as a two by two table giving details of which treatment the patients received in their randomised trial and whether they were dead or alive 10 years later (Table 5.2).

Simple maths tells you that patients on medical therapy have a 404/1325 = 0.305 or 30.5% chance of being dead at 10 years. This is the *absolute* risk of death for the control (medical therapy) group: let's call it x. Patients randomised to coronary artery bypass grafting (CABG) have a 350/1324 = 0.264 or 26.4% chance of being dead at 10 years. This is the absolute risk of death for the intervention (CABG) group: let's call it y.

The *relative risk* of death in patients treated with CABG compared with medical intervention controls – is y/x or 0.264/0.305 = 0.87 (87%).

Table 5.2 Data from a trial of medical therapy versus coronary artery bypass grafting (CABG) after heart attack [18,19]

	Outcome at 10 years		Total number of patients randomised in each group
Treatment	Dead	Alive	
Medical therapy	404	921	1325
CABG	350	974	1324

The *relative risk* reduction (i.e. the amount by which the risk of death is reduced in the CABG group compared with the control group) is 100 – 87% $(1 - y/x) = 13\%$.

The *ARR* (or risk difference) – that is, the absolute amount by which CABG reduces the risk of death at 10 years – is 30.5 – 26.4% = 4.1% (0.041).

The *number needed to treat* (i.e. how many patients need a CABG to prevent, on average, one death by 10 years) is the reciprocal of the ARR, 1/ARR = 1/0.041 = 24. In other words, while CABG was more effective than medical therapy, 24 people would need to have one to prevent one additional death.

The general formulae for calculating these 'bottom line' effects of an intervention are reproduced in Appendix 2. For a discussion on which of these values is most useful in which circumstances, see Jaeschke and colleagues' article in the 'Basic Statistics for Clinicians' series [3].

Summary

It is possible to be seriously misled by taking the statistical competence (and/or the intellectual honesty) of authors for granted. Statistics can be an intimidating science, and understanding its finer points often calls for expert help. But we hope that this chapter has shown you that the statistics used in most medical research papers can be evaluated – at least up to a point – by the non-expert using a simple checklist such as that in Appendix 1. In addition, you might like to check the paper you are reading (or writing) against the common errors given in Box 5.1. If you are hungry for more on statistics and their issues and misinterpretation, and guidelines for statistical reporting, try these three papers: (1) the classic paper 'Statistical tests, P values, confidence intervals, and power: a guide to misinterpretations' by Sander Greenland and colleagues [20]; (2) Riley and colleagues' paper on the 12 most common issues encountered during statistical peer review in the *BMJ* – 'On the 12th day of Christmas, a statistician sent to me. . .' [21]; and (3) Assel and colleagues' 'Guidelines for reporting of statistics for clinical research in urology' [22]. It is very likely that these guidelines could be transferable to research in other healthcare fields.

Exercises based on this chapter

1. Take a current clinical journal and select four or five (perhaps all the research papers in one issue) that describe an intervention trial. Now, taking each paper in turn, list all the statistical tests used in the study. Can you justify why each test was used? What value did each test add?
2. Using the same set of papers, find the estimate of benefit and the estimate of harm from each treatment. Express these as number needed to treat. If this figure is not given in the paper, try to calculate it from the raw data.

3. Go back to the section on non-parametric (rank order) statistics. Now, find a paper which uses one of the non-parametric tests in Table 5.1. Why did the authors choose a non-parametric test instead of a more powerful parametric test?

References

1. Guyatt G, Jaeschke R, Heddle N, et al. Basic statistics for clinicians: 1. Hypothesis testing. *CMAJ* 1995; **152**: 27–32.
2. Guyatt G, Jaeschke R, Heddle N, et al. Basic statistics for clinicians: 2. Interpreting study results: confidence intervals. *CMAJ* 1995; **152**: 169–73.
3. Jaeschke R, Guyatt G, Shannon H, et al. Basic statistics for clinicians: 3. Assessing the effects of treatment: measures of association. *CMAJ* 1995; **152**: 351–7.
4. Guyatt G, Walter S, Shannon H, et al. Basic statistics for clinicians: 4. Correlation and regression. *CMAJ* 1995; **152**: 497–504.
5. Altman DG. *Practical Statistics for Medical Research*. 2nd edn. London: Chapman & Hall; 2020.
6. Bland M. *An Introduction to Medical Statistics*. 4th edn. Oxford: Oxford University Press; 2015.
7. Kirkwood BR, Sterne JAC, Kirkwood BR. *Essential Medical Statistics*. 2nd edn. New Malden, MA: Blackwell Science; 2003.
8. Casals M, Finch CF. Sports biostatistician: a critical member of all sports science and medicine teams for injury prevention. *British Journal of Sports Medicine* 2018; **52**: 1457–61.
9. Pocock SJ. When (not) to stop a clinical trial for benefit. *JAMA* 2005; **294**: 2228–30.
10. Erasmus A, Holman B, Ioannidis JPA. Data-dredging bias. *BMJ Evidence-Based Medicine* 2022; **27**: 209–11.
11. Delgado-Rodriguez M, Llorca J. Bias. *Journal of Epidemiology and Community Health* 2004; **58**: 635–41.
12. Canadian Cooperative Study Group. A randomized trial of aspirin and sulfinpyrazone in threatened stroke. *New England Journal of Medicine* 1978; **299**: 53–9.
13. Antiplatelet Trialists' Collaboration. Secondary prevention of vascular disease by prolonged antiplatelet treatment. *British Medical Journal* 1988; **296**: 320–31.
14. Oxman AD, Guyatt GH. A consumer's guide to subgroup analyses. *Annals of Internal Medicine* 1992; **116**: 78–84.
15. Hill AB. The environment and disease: association or causation? *Proceedings of the Royal Society of Medicine* 1965; **58**: 295–300.
16. Altman DG, Machin D, Bryant TN, et al., eds. *Statistics With Confidence: Confidence intervals and statistical guidelines*. 2nd edn. London: BMJ Books; 2011.
17. Sedgwick P. Understanding confidence intervals. *BMJ* 2014; **349**: g6051.
18. Fahey T, Griffiths S, Peters TJ. Evidence based purchasing: understanding results of clinical trials and systematic reviews. *BMJ* 1995; **311**: 1056–9.
19. Yusuf S, Zucker D, Passamani E, et al. Effect of coronary artery bypass graft surgery on survival: overview of 10-year results from randomised trials by the

Chapter 5

Coronary Artery Bypass Graft Surgery Trialists Collaboration. *Lancet* 1994; **344**: 563–70.

20. Greenland S, Senn SJ, Rothman KJ, et al. Statistical tests, *P* values, confidence intervals, and power: a guide to misinterpretations. *European Journal of Epidemiology* 2016; **31**: 337–50.
21. Riley RD, Cole TJ, Deeks J, et al. On the 12th day of Christmas, a statistician sent to me. . . *BMJ* 2022; **379**: e072883.
22. Assel M, Sjoberg D, Elders A, et al. Guidelines for reporting of statistics for clinical research in urology. *BJU International* 2019; **123**: 401–10.

Chapter 6 Papers that report clinical trials of simple interventions

What is a clinical trial?

This chapter is about papers that report clinical trials, specifically trials of *simple interventions* – interventions that are well demarcated (see Chapter 7 to find out about *complex interventions*, which aren't). A clinical trial is usually (but not always) a randomised controlled trial (RCT), a key study design that we introduced in Chapter 3 (see section 'What are randomised controlled trials and why do they matter?') and explained more about in Chapter 4 (see subsection 'Sources of bias in randomised controlled trials'). Here, we build on those introductory sections and discuss the most common kind of simple intervention trial, the RCT of drug therapy. We also consider how to make a decision about therapy and the curse of surrogate endpoints. Finally, we introduce the Consolidated Standards of Reporting Trials (CONSORT) statement, which lists what information you should expect to find in a paper reporting an RCT of simple intervention.

As mentioned in the introductory sections on RCTs in Chapters 3 and 4, clinical trials compare the effects of one treatment with another. They may involve patients, healthy people, or both [1]. Many clinicians and researchers consider clinical trials to be the gold standard method for evaluation of healthcare interventions, with inherent advantages over non-randomised observational studies [2]. Clinical trials aim to generate high-quality evidence about the most effective treatment or preventative strategy for patients with a specific condition (such as established coronary heart disease) or people with risk factors (such as high serum cholesterol levels) who are at risk of developing a condition in the future. Clinical trials are generally expensive, lengthy and complicated. Unnecessary clinical trials (e.g. ones that repeat definitive studies already in the literature) are therefore wasteful of scarce human and monetary resources (not to mention a waste of everyone's time, including the patients who volunteer for the study). The first – and probably

How to Read a Paper: The Basics of Evidence-Based Healthcare, Seventh Edition.
Trisha Greenhalgh and Paul Dijkstra.

most important – question you should ask is whether the trial reported in the paper you are reading was really necessary. Did the state of knowledge and uncertainty about the condition actually merit a new trial at the time of this study was commenced?

Drug trials: 'evidence' and marketing

If you are a clinical doctor, nurse practitioner or pharmacist (i.e. if you prescribe or dispense drugs), the pharmaceutical and medical devices industries are interested in you, and spend a proportion of their multimillion pound annual advertising budget trying to influence you (Box 6.1); however, as a past editor of the *BMJ*, Fiona Godlee states in this editorial:

> *it takes two to tango. It's time for the profession to take a lead. This means saying no to gifts and hospitality, ensuring that research and clinical collaborations are transparent and unbiased in their design and reporting, refusing to be a guest or ghost author, declining the role of paid opinion leader, paying our way for information and education, and refusing industry support unless it is entirely transparent and in patients' or the public's best interests [3].*

Even if you are a mere patient, the industry might, in some countries where it is legal, target you directly through direct-to-consumer advertising (DTCA) [4]. Robert Shmerling has described how DTCA could 'hook us'; he gives examples of advertising words that should sound alarm bells [5]. When Trisha wrote the first edition of this book in 1995, the standard management of vaginal thrush (*Candida* infection) was for a doctor to prescribe clotrimazole pessaries. By the time the second edition was published in 2001, these pessaries were available over the counter in pharmacies. For the past 15 years, clotrimazole has been advertised on prime-time TV – thankfully after the nine o'clock watershed – and more recently the manufacturers of this and other powerful drugs are advertising directly to consumers via the Internet and social media [6]. In case you were wondering, such advertising is often biased; for example, it tends to place more emphasis on benefits than risks and it tends to imply that the condition isn't going to get better on its own [7].

One of the most effective ways of changing the prescribing habits of a clinician is still via a pharmaceutical sales representative (known to most of us in the UK as the 'drug rep' and to our North American colleagues as the 'detailer'), who travels round with a briefcase full of 'evidence' in support of their wares [8]. Indeed, as we discuss in more detail in Chapters 14 and 15, the evidence-based medicine movement has learnt a lot from the drug industry in recent years about changing the behaviour of physicians, and now uses

Box 6.1 Ten tips for the pharmaceutical industry: how to present your product in the best light

1. Think up a plausible physiological mechanism for why the drug works and become slick at presenting it. Preferably, find a surrogate endpoint that is heavily influenced by the drug (see section 'Making decisions about therapy').
2. When designing clinical trials, select a patient population, clinical features and trial length that reflect the maximum possible response to the drug.
3. If possible, compare your product only with placebos. If you must compare it with a competitor, make sure the latter is given at a sub-therapeutic dose.
4. Include the results of pilot studies in the figures for definitive studies, so it looks as if more patients have been randomised than is actually the case.
5. Omit mention of any trial that had a fatality or serious adverse drug reaction in the treatment group. If possible, don't publish such studies.
6. Have your graphics department maximise the visual impact of your message. It helps not to label the axes of graphs or say whether scales are linear or logarithmic. Make sure you do not show individual patient data or confidence intervals.
7. Become master of the hanging comparative ('better' – but better than what?).
8. Invert the standard hierarchy of evidence so that anecdote takes precedence over randomised trials and meta-analyses.
9. Name at least three local opinion leaders who use the drug and offer 'starter packs' for the doctor to try.
10. Present a 'cost-effectiveness' analysis which shows that your product, even though more expensive than its competitor, 'actually works out cheaper' (see section 'The great guidelines debate').

the same sophisticated techniques of persuasion in what is known as *academic detailing* of individual health professionals [9]. Interestingly, DTCA often works by harnessing the persuasive power of the patient, who effectively becomes an unpaid 'rep' for the pharmaceutical industry. If you think you'd be able to resist a patient more easily than a real rep, you're probably wrong – as Becker and Midoun's systematic review of DTCA in psychiatric conditions showed [10]. Pharmaceutical companies also know the significant DTCA potential of big sport events like the Super Bowl, as Gray and colleagues' study illustrates [11].

Before you agree to meet a pharmaceutical rep (or when a patient attends with a newspaper article, Internet download or a ChatGPT summary recommending the drug or device), remind yourself of some basic rules of research design. As Chapter 3 argued, questions about the benefits of therapy should ideally be addressed with RCTs. But preliminary questions about pharmacokinetics (i.e. how the drug behaves while it is getting to its site of action), particularly those relating to bioavailability, require a straight dosing experiment in healthy (and, if ethical and practicable, sick) volunteers. Similarly, a medical device needs to go through a careful design phase to optimise its functionality and usability before being tested in a clinical trial. This is also the case for artificial intelligence (AI) systems as we discuss in the chapter on AI.

In relation to drugs, common (and hopefully mild) adverse reactions may be picked up, and their incidence quantified, in the RCTs undertaken to demonstrate efficacy. But rare (and usually more serious) adverse drug reactions require both pharmacovigilance surveys (collection of data prospectively on patients receiving a newly licensed drug) and case–control studies (see section 'What are cohort studies?' in Chapter 3) to establish association. Ideally, individual rechallenge experiments (where the patient who has had a reaction considered to be caused by the drug is given the drug again in carefully supervised circumstances) should be performed to establish causation [12].

Pharmaceutical reps do not tell nearly as many lies as they used to (drug marketing has become an altogether more sophisticated science), but as Goldacre [13] has shown in his book *Bad Pharma*, they probably still provide information that is at best selective and at worst overtly biased. It often helps their case, for example, to present the results of uncontrolled trials and express them in terms of before-and-after differences in a particular outcome measure. Reference to the section 'What are cross-sectional surveys?' in Chapter 3 and the literature on placebo effects [14,15] should remind you why uncontrolled before-and-after studies are the stuff of teenage magazines, not hard science. In fact, they are discouraged [16].

The late Dr Andrew Herxheimer, who edited the *Drug and Therapeutics Bulletin* for many years, undertook a survey of 'references' cited in advertisements for pharmaceutical products in the leading UK medical journals. He once told Trisha that a high proportion of such references cite 'data on file' and many more refer to publications written, edited and published entirely by the industry. Evidence from these sources has sometimes (although by no means invariably) been shown to be of lower scientific quality than that which appears in independent, peer-reviewed journals. And let's face it, if you worked for a drug company that had made a major scientific breakthrough, you would probably submit your findings to a publication such as the *Lancet* or the *New England Journal of Medicine* before publishing them in-house. In other words, you don't need to 'trash' papers about drug trials because of where they have been published, but you do need to look closely at the methods and statistical analysis of such trials.

Making decisions about therapy

Sackett and colleagues [12], in their classic textbook *Clinical Epidemiology: A basic science for clinical medicine*, argued that before starting a patient on a drug, the doctor should:

1. Identify *for this patient* the ultimate objective of treatment (cure, prevention of recurrence, limitation of functional disability, prevention of later complications, reassurance, palliation, symptomatic relief, etc.).
2. Select the *most appropriate* treatment using all available evidence (this includes addressing the question of whether the patient needs to take any drug at all).
3. Specify the *treatment target* (how will you know when to stop treatment, change its intensity or switch to some other treatment?).

For example, in the treatment of high blood pressure, the doctor might decide that:

1. the *ultimate objective of treatment* is to prevent (further) target organ damage to brain, eye, heart, kidney and so on (and thereby prevent serious complications such as stroke and, ultimately, death)
2. the *choice of specific treatment* is between the various classes of antihypertensive drugs selected on the basis of randomised, placebo-controlled and comparative trials – as well as between non-drug treatments such as salt restriction; and
3. the *treatment target* might be a phase V diastolic blood pressure (right arm, sitting) of less than 90 mmHg, or as close to that as tolerable in the face of drug adverse effects.

Note that in some situations (e.g. terminal care), the ultimate objective of treatment may not be to prolong life but, whatever it is, it should be stated and the drug regimen organised to achieve it. If Sackett et al.'s three steps are not followed, therapeutic chaos can result. For example, in old (> 74 years) adults, unless your patient has type 2 diabetes, statin treatment will likely not reduce atherosclerotic cardiovascular disease or all-cause mortality [17]. In a veiled slight on surrogate endpoints (see below), Sackett and his team remind us that the choice of specific therapy should be determined by evidence of what *does* work, and not on what *seems* to work or *ought* to work. 'Today's therapy', they warn, 'when derived from biologic facts or uncontrolled clinical experience, may become tomorrow's bad joke' [12].

Surrogate endpoints

If you are a practising (and non-academic) clinician, your main contact with research papers might not be through peer reviewed journals but through what gets fed to you by industry: 'industry reps', DTCA or indeed industry-sponsored trials with surrogate endpoints. Industry is a slick player at the surrogate endpoint game, and we make no apology for labouring the point that such outcome measures must be evaluated very carefully.

We will define a surrogate endpoint as:

> *a variable which is relatively easily measured and which predicts a rare or distant outcome of either a toxic stimulus (e.g. pollutant) or a therapeutic intervention (e.g. drug, surgical procedure, piece of advice), but which is not itself a direct measure of either harm or clinical benefit.*

The growing interest in surrogate endpoints in medical research reflects two important features of their use:

- They can considerably reduce the *sample size*, *duration* and, therefore, *cost*, of clinical trials.
- They can allow treatments to be assessed in situations where the use of primary outcomes would be excessively *invasive* or *unethical.*

In the evaluation of pharmaceutical products, commonly used surrogate endpoints include:

- pharmacokinetic measurements (e.g. concentration–time curves of a drug or its active metabolite in the bloodstream)
- *in vitro* (i.e. laboratory) measures such as the mean inhibitory concentration of an antimicrobial against a bacterial culture on agar
- macroscopic appearance of tissues (e.g. gastric erosion seen at endoscopy)
- change in levels of (alleged) 'biological markers of disease' (e.g. microalbuminuria in the measurement of diabetic kidney disease)
- radiological appearance (e.g. shadowing on a chest x-ray or, in a more contemporary setting, functional magnetic resonance imaging).

Surrogate endpoints have a number of drawbacks. First and foremost, the surrogate endpoint may not closely reflect the treatment target – in other words, it may not be valid or reliable. Second, a change in the surrogate endpoint does not itself answer the essential preliminary questions: 'What is the objective of treatment in this patient?' and 'What, according to valid and reliable research studies, is the best available treatment for this condition?' Third, the use of a surrogate endpoint has the same limitations as the use of any other single measure of the success or failure of therapy – it ignores all the other measures! Over-reliance on a single surrogate endpoint as a measure of therapeutic success usually reflects a narrow or naïve clinical perspective.

Finally, surrogate endpoints are often developed in animal models of disease because changes in a specific variable can be measured under controlled conditions in a well-defined population. However, extrapolation of these findings to human disease is liable to be invalid [18], for these reasons:

- In animal studies, the population being studied has fairly uniform biological characteristics and may be genetically inbred.
- Both the tissue and the disease being studied may vary in important characteristics (e.g. susceptibility to the pathogen, rate of cell replication) from the parallel condition in human subjects.
- The animals are kept in a controlled environment, which minimises the influence of lifestyle variables (e.g. diet, exercise, stress) and concomitant medication.
- Giving high doses of chemicals to experimental animals may distort the usual metabolic pathways and thereby give misleading results. Animal species best suited to serve as a surrogate for humans vary for different chemicals.

The ideal features of a surrogate endpoint are shown in Box 6.2. If the 'rep' who is trying to persuade you about the value of the drug or modality cannot justify the endpoints used, you should challenge them to produce additional evidence [19].

If you are interested in pursuing some real examples of surrogate endpoints that led to misleading practices and recommendations, try these:

- The controversial granting of accelerated approval by the US Food and Drug Administration (FDA) in June 2021 to aducanumab for treating Alzheimer's disease, based on a surrogate end point: the drug's amyloid-reducing effects [20]. This was despite evidence that shrinkage of β-amyloid protein plaques does not predictably delay cognitive impairment in patients [21]. As a result of this approval, three advisors to the FDA resigned [22]. In December 2021, the European Medicines Agency (EMA) rejected aducanumab for medical use in the European Union [23]. Biogen has since withdrawn its application for a marketing authorization of aducanumab for the treatment of Alzheimer's disease [24].

Box 6.2 Ideal features of a surrogate endpoint

1 The surrogate endpoint should be reliable, reproducible, clinically available, easily quantifiable, affordable and exhibit a 'dose–response' effect (i.e. the higher the level of the surrogate endpoint, the greater the probability of disease).

2 It should be a true predictor of disease (or risk of disease) and not merely express exposure to a covariable. The relationship between the surrogate endpoint and the disease should have a biologically plausible explanation.

3 It should be sensitive – that is, a 'positive' result in the surrogate endpoint should pick up all or most patients at increased risk of adverse outcome.

4 It should be specific – that is, a 'negative' result should exclude all or most of those without increased risk of adverse outcome.

5 There should be a precise cut-off point between normal and abnormal values.

6 It should have an acceptable positive predictive value – that is, a 'positive' result should always or usually mean that the patient thus identified is at increased risk of adverse outcome (see section 'Ten questions to ask about a paper describing a complex intervention').

7 It should have an acceptable negative predictive value – that is, a 'negative' result should always or usually mean that the patient thus identified is not at increased risk of adverse outcome (see section 'Ten questions to ask about a paper describing a complex intervention').

8 It should be amenable to quality control monitoring.

9 Changes in the surrogate endpoint should rapidly and accurately reflect the response to therapy – in particular, levels should normalise in states of remission or cure.

- A study of a new 'cure' for vaginal dryness, whose efficacy was measured in terms of proportion of parabasal cells in the 'vaginal maturation index', along with vaginal pH [25]. The parabasal cell index perked up and vaginal pH improved in the intended direction, allowing the researchers to claim that the drug was effective, but in reality the women in the study didn't feel significantly less dry (we were not surprised to find that the study was funded by the drug's manufacturer). In another industry-sponsored study using the same surrogate endpoints and patient outcome for vaginal dryness, women did feel significantly less dry [26]. Interestingly, the authors argued that the 'most bothersome symptom' (MBS; an FDA-recommended patient-reported endpoint for clinical trials) 'may not adequately evaluate or address the multiple symptoms associated with vulvovaginal atrophy (VVA) in postmenopausal women.' They continued 'MBS is a subjective, patient-reported endpoint that may be influenced by a greater placebo effect than more objective endpoints.' Their 'objective endpoints' are actually surrogate endpoints!

- The use of ECG findings instead of clinical outcomes (syncope, death) in deciding the efficacy and safety of anti-arrhythmia drugs [27].
- The use of albuminuria instead of the overall clinical benefit–harm balance to evaluate the usefulness of dual renin–angiotensin blockade in hypertension [28,29]. In this example, the intervention was based on a hypothetical argument that blocking the renin–angiotensin pathway at two separate stages would be doubly effective, and the surrogate marker confirmed that this seemed to be the case, but the combination was also doubly effective at producing the potentially fatal adverse effect of hypokalaemia!

It would be unsporting to suggest that the pharmaceutical industry always develops surrogate endpoints with the deliberate intention of misleading the licensing authorities and health professionals. In early research into HIV and AIDS, for example, a surrogate endpoint (the CD4 count) was used instead of mortality to accelerate the introduction of highly effective anti-HIV drugs into clinical practice, thereby saving thousands of lives [30]. But this rush to 'save lives' in potentially fatal diseases can lead to an overuse of surrogate endpoints and premature licensing of dubious drugs, as a balanced review of the use of surrogate endpoints in cancer research showed [31]. Walia and colleagues' 2022 review warned that oncological drugs approved on the basis of surrogate outcomes that are not associated with clinically meaningful outcomes can cause significant harm to patients [32]. In short, the industry has a vested interest in overstating its case on the strength of these endpoints [13], so use caution when you read a paper whose findings are not based on hard, patient-relevant outcomes.

There is currently no guideline for the reporting of RCTs using surrogate endpoints; the SPIRIT/CONSORT-SURROGATE project group aims to change this. They are developing SPIRIT (Standard Protocol Items: Recommendations for Interventional Trials) and CONSORT extensions to improve the reporting of these trials [33]. You can follow their work on the project website [34]. Surrogate endpoints are only one of many ways in which industry-sponsored trials may give a misleading impression of the efficacy of a drug. Other subtle (and not so subtle) influences on research design, such as framing the question in a particular way or selective reporting of findings, have been described in a 2017 Cochrane review of how industry-sponsored trials tend to favour industry products [35].

What information to expect in a paper describing a randomised controlled trial: the CONSORT statement

Drug trials are an example of a 'simple intervention'; that is, an intervention that is well demarcated (i.e. it's easy to say what the intervention comprises) and lends itself to an 'intervention on' versus 'intervention off' research design. In Chapters 3 and 4, we gave some preliminary advice on assessing the methodological quality of research studies. Here's some more detail. In 1996, an international working group produced a standard checklist, known as CONSORT, for reporting RCTs in medical journals, which has now been updated several times, the latest in 2010 [36].There is now also a CONSORT statement for non-drug treatments [37], for interventions involving AI (CONSORT-AI) [38] and the reporting of harms in randomised trials [39]. Without doubt, the use of such checklists has increased the quality and consistency of reporting of trials in the medical literature [40]. A checklist based on the CONSORT statement is reproduced in Table 6.1. Please do not try to learn this table off by heart (we certainly couldn't reproduce it ourselves from memory) but do refer to it if you are asked to critically appraise a paper to which it applies or if you are planning on writing up a randomised trial yourself.

Incidentally, one important way to reduce bias in drug marketing is to ensure that every trial that is begun is also written up and published [41]. Otherwise, the drug industry (or anyone else with a vested interest) could withhold publication of any trial that did not support their own belief in the efficacy and/or cost-effectiveness of a particular product. Goldacre [13] covers the topic of compulsory trial registration at inception (and the reluctance of some drug companies to comply with it) in his book.

Getting worthwhile evidence from pharmaceutical representatives

Any doctor who has ever given an audience to a 'rep' who is selling a non-steroidal anti-inflammatory drug will recognise the gastric erosion example. The question to ask them is not 'what is the incidence of gastric erosion on your drug?', but 'what is the incidence of potentially life-threatening gastric bleeding?'. Other questions to ask 'drug reps', based on an early article in the *Drug and Therapeutics Bulletin* [42], are listed here:

1. See representatives only by appointment. Choose to see only those whose product interests you and confine the interview to that product.
2. Take charge of the interview. Do not hear out a rehearsed sales routine but ask directly for the information.

Table 6.1 Checklist for a randomised controlled trial based on the CONSORT statement

Title/abstract	Do the title and abstract say how participants were allocated to interventions (e.g. 'random allocation', 'randomised' or 'randomly assigned')?
Introduction	Is the scientific background and rationale for the study adequately explained?
Methods	
Objectives	Were the specific objectives and/or hypothesis to be tested stated explicitly?
Participants and setting	Does the paper state the eligibility criteria for participants and the settings and locations where the data were collected?
Interventions	Does the paper give precise details of the intervention(s) and the control intervention(s) and how and when they were administered?
Outcomes	Have the primary and secondary outcome measures been clearly defined? When applicable, have the methods used to enhance the quality of measurements (e.g. multiple observations, training of assessors) been set out?
Sample size	How was sample size determined? When applicable, were any interim analyses and/or rules for stopping the study early explained and justified?
Blinding (masking)	Does the paper state whether or not participants, those administering the interventions and those assessing the outcomes were blinded to group assignment? How was the success of blinding assessed?
Statistical methods	Were the statistical methods used to compare groups for primary and secondary outcome(s) and any subgroup analyses, appropriate?
Details of randomisation	
Sequence generation	Was the method used to generate the random allocation sequence, including details of any restrictions (e.g. blocking, stratification), clearly described?
Allocation concealment	Was the method used to implement the random allocation sequence (e.g. numbered containers or central telephone) stated, and was it made clear whether the sequence was concealed until interventions were assigned?
Implementation	Does the paper say who generated the allocation sequence, who enrolled participants and who assigned participants to their groups?
Results	
Flow diagram	Is a clear diagram included showing the flow of participants through the trial? This should report, for each group, the numbers of participants randomly assigned, receiving intended treatment, completing the study protocol and analysed for the primary outcome.
Protocol deviations	Are all deviations from the original study protocol explained and justified?
Recruitment dates	Have the authors given the date range during which participants were recruited to the study?

Table 6.1 (Continued)

Title/abstract	Do the title and abstract say how participants were allocated to interventions (e.g. 'random allocation', 'randomised' or 'randomly assigned')?
Baseline data	Are the baseline demographic and clinical characteristics of each group described?
Numbers analysed	Is the number of participants (denominator) in each group included in each analysis, and is the analysis by 'intention to treat'?
Outcomes and estimation	For each primary and secondary outcome, is there a summary of results for each group, and the estimated effect size and its precision (e.g. 95% confidence interval)?
Ancillary analyses	Are all additional analyses described and justified, including subgroup analyses, both prespecified and exploratory?
Adverse events	Have the authors reported and discussed all important adverse events?
Discussion	
Interpretation	Is the interpretation of the results justified, taking into account study hypotheses, sources of potential bias or imprecision and the dangers of multiple comparisons?
Generalisability	Have the authors made defensible estimate of the generalisability (external validity) of the trial findings?

Source: Reproduced from Schulz et al. [36] with permission of BMJ Publishing Group Ltd.

Chapter 6

3. Request independent published evidence from reputable peer-reviewed journals.
4. Do not look at promotional brochures, which often contain unpublished material, misleading graphs and selective quotations.
5. Ignore anecdotal 'evidence' such as the fact that a medical celebrity is prescribing the product.
6. Using the 'STEP' acronym, ask for evidence in four specific areas:
   - Safety – that is, likelihood of long-term or serious adverse effects caused by the drug (remember that rare but serious adverse reactions to new drugs may be poorly documented).
   - Tolerability, which is best measured by comparing the pooled withdrawal rates between the drug and its most significant competitor.
   - eEficacy, of which the most relevant dimension is how the product compares with your current favourite.
   - Price, which should take into account indirect as well as direct costs (see section 'Ten questions to ask about an economic analysis').
7. Evaluate the evidence stringently, paying particular attention to the power (sample size) and methodological quality of clinical trials and the use of surrogate endpoints. Apply the CONSORT checklist (Table 6.1). Do not accept theoretical arguments in the drug's favour (e.g. 'longer half life') without direct evidence that this translates into clinical benefit.

8. Do not accept the newness of a product as an argument for changing to it. Indeed, there are good scientific arguments for doing the opposite.
9. Decline to try the product via starter packs or by participating in small-scale, uncontrolled 'research' studies.
10. Record in writing the content of the interview and return to these notes if the rep requests another audience.

For more sophisticated advice on how to debunk sponsored clinical trial reports that attempt to blind you with statistics, see Montori and colleagues' helpful users' guide [43] and (more tangentially but worth noting) Goldacre's blockbuster on the corporate tricks of 'big pharma' [13].

A note on vaccine trials

Vaccine trials, a form of RCT designed to test the efficacy of a vaccine in preventing disease, have been around for decades, but fast-track vaccine trials (in which a new vaccine is rapidly developed in a race against time during an epidemic or pandemic) came into the spotlight in 2020 with the rapid development of several coronavirus disease 2019 (COVID-19) vaccines which saved millions of lives worldwide. (You can read the story of the Oxford vaccine on the COVID-19 Oxford Vaccine Trial website: https://www.research.ox.ac.uk/area/coronavirus-research/vaccine). In April 2020, the UK Government rapidly set up a Vaccine Taskforce and tasked NHS Digital develop a service for the public to register their interest in participating in COVID-19 vaccine RCTs. This was done through NHS DigiTrials (https://digital.nhs.uk/services/nhs-digitrials), a digital platform which provides a service to support and accelerate clinical trials, and reduce the effort and cost of developing new drugs and vaccines.

Vaccine trials also paved the way for new treatments. The success of mRNA vaccines against COVID-19, for example, has sparked renewed interest in mRNA as a means of delivering therapeutic proteins [44]. But fast-track vaccines against COVID-19 were not a panacea, and they generated a number of controversies. A detailed discussion of all these controversies is beyond the scope of this book, but we share one here because it illustrates an important basic point about RCTs: that while an experimental trial is a very good way of testing the *efficacy* of a drug or vaccine, it's not a rock-solid way of detecting rare harms. This is because RCTs are powered to detect a clinically important difference in efficacy (that is, answering the question 'How well does the drug or vaccine work?'). They are therefore almost always underpowered to detect a serious adverse effect that happens only once in several thousand patients (in other words, an RCT is less good for answering the question 'is the drug or vaccine 100% safe?').

While the benefits of the different vaccines against COVID-19 outweighed the risks of harm in most people, some troubling findings began to appear in 2021: the Oxford/AstraZeneca vaccine became linked to very rare but occasionally serious and even fatal blood clots in young women. This finding was unexpected and puzzling, and had not been suspected, despite several large and well-conducted clinical trials. The mystery was solved by Professor Marie Scully, a consultant haematologist at University College London hospitals, who identified the *mechanism* for this rare adverse effect – a combination of increased tendency for the blood to clot and low platelets – and a test for it (the PF4 test). Based on an understanding of the underlying mechanism, doctors now know how to diagnose and treat this rare adverse effect. Young people (especially women under the age of 30) in whom the risks of this particular vaccine may outweigh the benefits may now choose to have an alternative vaccine. You can read more about this remarkable story in Bosley [45], Scully et al. [46] and Perry et al. [47]. We discuss the importance of mechanistic evidence further in Chapter 18.

Exercises based on this chapter

1. Get hold of some advertisements for drugs, from medical journals and in publicly oriented sources (DTCA). What claims are being made for these products? Are the outcomes 'hard' or surrogate? Are the claims made to consumers different from those made to doctors? What questions would you ask a drug rep if they were trying to persuade you to prescribe the drug?
2. Using search methods described in Chapter 2, search the literature for evidence on the management of female sexual dysfunction. Look for review articles (especially systematic reviews). What pharmaceutical products are recommended for this condition? What outcomes are measured in studies? To what extent is the efficacy of drugs for female sexual dysfunction attributable to: (a) a placebo effect, and (b) the use of surrogate outcomes?
3. Review the publications on the controversial granting of accelerated approval (by the US FDA in June 2021) to aducanumab for treating Alzheimer's disease. Can you describe why the surrogate end point, the drug's amyloid-reducing effects, was problematic? Base your answer on the ideal features of a surrogate end point listed in Box 6.2.

References

1. NHS England. Clinical trials. 2022. https://www.nhs.uk/conditions/clinical-trials (accessed 4 September 2023).
2. National In statute for Health and Care Research. Clinical Trials Guide, version 2. 2019. https://www.nihr.ac.uk/documents/clinical-trials-guide/20595 (accessed 4 September 2023).

3. Godlee F. Doctors, patients, and the drug industry. *BMJ* 2009; **338**: b463.
4. Liang BA, Mackey T. Direct-to-consumer advertising with interactive internet media: global regulation and public health issues. *JAMA* 2011; **305**: 824–5.
5. Shmerling RH. Harvard Health Ad Watch: How direct-to-consumer ads hook us. Harvard Health [blog post]. 3 March 2022. https://www.health.harvard.edu/blog/harvard-health-ad-watch-what-you-should-know-about-direct-to-consumer-ads-2019092017848 (accessed 4 September 2023).
6. Mackey TK, Cuomo RE, Liang BA. The rise of digital direct-to-consumer advertising? Comparison of direct-to-consumer advertising expenditure trends from publicly available data sources and global policy implications. *BMC Health Services Research* 2015; **15**: 236.
7. Kaphigst KA, Dejong W, Rudd RE, et al. A content analysis of direct-to-consumer television prescription drug advertisements. *Journal of Health Communication* 2004; **9**: 515–28.
8. Spurling GK, Mansfield PR, Montgomery BD, et al. Information from pharmaceutical companies and the quality, quantity, and cost of physicians' prescribing: a systematic review. *PLoS Medicine* 2010; **7**: e1000352.
9. O'Brien MA, Rogers S, Jamtvedt G, et al. Educational outreach visits: effects on professional practice and health care outcomes. *Cochrane Database of Systematic Reviews* 2007(**4**): CD000409.
10. Becker SJ, Midoun MM. Effects of direct-to-consumer advertising on patient prescription requests and physician prescribing: a systematic review of psychiatry-relevant studies. *Journal of Clinical Psychiatry* 2016; **77**: e1293–300.
11. Gray MP, San-Juan-Rodriguez A, Chen N, et al. Impact of direct-to-consumer drug advertising during the Super Bowl on drug utilization. *Research in Social Administrative Pharmacy* 2020; **16**: 1136–9.
12. Sackett DL, Haynes RB, Tugwell P. *Clinical Epidemiology: A basic science for clinical medicine*. Boston, MA: Little Brown; 1985.
13. Goldacre B. *Bad Pharma: How medicine is broken, and how we can fix it*. London: Fourth Estate; 2013.
14. Tavel ME. The placebo effect: the good, the bad, and the ugly. *American Journal of Medicine* 2014; **127**: 484–8.
15. Howick J, Friedemann C, Tsakok M, et al. are treatments more effective than placebos? a systematic review and meta-analysis. *PLoS One* 2013; **8**: e62599.
16. Goodacre S. Uncontrolled before-after studies: discouraged by Cochrane and the EMJ. *Emergency Medicine Journal* 2015; **32**: 507–8.
17. Ramos R, Comas-Cufí M, Martí-Lluch R, et al. Statins for primary prevention of cardiovascular events and mortality in old and very old adults with and without type 2 diabetes: retrospective cohort study. *BMJ* 2018; **362**: k3359.
18. Gøtzsche PC, Liberati A, Torri V, et al. Beware of surrogate outcome measures. *International Journal of Technology Assessment in Health Care* 1996; **12**: 238–46.
19. Habibi R, Lexchin J, Mintzes B, et al. Unwarranted claims of drug efficacy in pharmaceutical sales visits: are drugs approved on the basis of surrogate outcomes promoted appropriately? *British Journal of Clinical Pharmacology* 2017; **83**: 2549–56.
20. Dawoud D, Naci H, Ciani O, et al. Raising the bar for using surrogate endpoints in drug regulation and health technology assessment. *BMJ* 2021; **374**: n2191.

21. Ackley SF, Zimmerman SC, Brenowitz WD, et al. Effect of reductions in amyloid levels on cognitive change in randomized trials: instrumental variable meta-analysis. *BMJ* 2021; **372**: n156.
22. Mahase E. Three FDA advisory panel members resign over approval of Alzheimer's drug. *BMJ* 2021; **373**: n1503.
23. Roxby P. Alzheimer's drug aducanumab not approved for use in EU. *BBC News* 17 December 2021. https://www.bbc.com/news/health-59699907 (accessed 11 September 2023).
24. European Medicines Agency. Aduhelm (application withdrawn). 2022. https://www.ema.europa.eu/en/medicines/human/withdrawn-applications/aduhelm (accessed 11 September 2023).
25. Portman D, Palacios S, Nappi RE, et al. Ospemifene, a non-oestrogen selective oestrogen receptor modulator for the treatment of vaginal dryness associated with postmenopausal vulvar and vaginal atrophy: a randomised, placebo-controlled, phase III trial. *Maturitas* 2014; **78**: 91–8.
26. Archer DF, Goldstein SR, Simon JA, et al. Efficacy and safety of ospemifene in postmenopausal women with moderate-to-severe vaginal dryness: a phase 3, randomized, double-blind, placebo-controlled, multicenter trial. *Menopause* 2019; **26**: 611–21.
27. Connolly SJ. Use and misuse of surrogate outcomes in arrhythmia trials. *Circulation* 2006; **113**: 764–6.
28. Messerli FH, Staessen JA, Zannad F. Of fads, fashion, surrogate endpoints and dual RAS blockade. *European Heart Journal* 2010; **31**: 2205–8.
29. Harel Z, Gilbert C, Wald R, et al. The effect of combination treatment with aliskiren and blockers of the renin-angiotensin system on hyperkalaemia and acute kidney injury: systematic review and meta-analysis. *BMJ* 2012; **344**: e42.
30. Maguire S. Discourse and adoption of innovations: a study of HIV/AIDS treatments. *Health Care Management Review* 2002; **27**: 74.
31. Kemp R, Prasad V. Surrogate endpoints in oncology: when are they acceptable for regulatory and clinical decisions, and are they currently overused? *BMC Medicine* 2017; **15**: 134.
32. Walia A, Haslam A, Prasad V. FDA validation of surrogate endpoints in oncology: 2005–2022. *Journal of Cancer Policy* 2022; **34**: 100364.
33. Ciani O, Manyara AM, Chan A-W, et al. Surrogate endpoints in trials: a call for better reporting. *Trials* 2022; **23**: 991.
34. SPIRIT/CONSORT-SURROGATE reporting group. *SPIRIT/CONSORT-SURROGATE Reporting Guidelines for Surrogate Endpoints*. Glasgow: Medical Research Council/Chief Scientist Office Social and Public Health Sciences Unit, University of Glasgow. https://www.gla.ac.uk/schools/healthwellbeing/research/mrccsosocialandpublichealthsciencesunit/programmes/complexity/methods-development/spirit-consort-surrogate (accessed 11 September 2023).
35. Lundh A, Lexchin J, Mintzes B, et al. Industry sponsorship and research outcome. *Cochrane Database of Systematic Reviews*. 2017; **(2)**: MR000033.
36. Schulz KF, Altman DG, Moher D, et al. CONSORT 2010 statement: updated guidelines for reporting parallel group randomised trials. *BMJ* 2010; **340**: c332.

37. Boutron I, Altman DG, Moher D, et al. CONSORT Statement for Randomized Trials of Nonpharmacologic Treatments: A 2017 update and a CONSORT extension for nonpharmacologic trial abstracts. *Annals of Internal Medicine* 2017; **167**: 40–7.
38. Liu X, Rivera SC, Moher D, et al. Reporting guidelines for clinical trial reports for interventions involving artificial intelligence: the CONSORT-AI Extension. *BMJ* 2020; **370**: m3164.
39. Junqueira DR, Zorzela L, Golder S, et al. CONSORT Harms 2022 statement, explanation, and elaboration: updated guideline for the reporting of harms in randomised trials. *BMJ* 2023; **381**: e073725.
40. Turner L, Shamseer L, Altman DG, et al. Does use of the CONSORT Statement impact the completeness of reporting of randomised controlled trials published in medical journals? A Cochrane review. *Systematic Reviews* 2012; **1**: 60.
41. Chalmers I, Glasziou P, Godlee F. All trials must be registered and the results published. *BMJ* 2013; **346**: f105.
42. Herxheimer A. Getting good value from drug reps. *Drug and Therapeutics Bulletin* 1983; **21**: 13–15.
43. Montori VM, Jaeschke R, Schünemann HJ, et al. Users' guide to detecting misleading claims in clinical research reports. *BMJ* 2004; **329**: 1093–6.
44. Rohner E, Yang R, Foo KS, et al. Unlocking the promise of mRNA therapeutics. *Nature Biotechnology* 2022; **40**: 1586–600.
45. Boseley S. How UK doctor linked rare blood-clotting to AstraZeneca Covid jab. *The Guardian* 13 April 2021. https://www.theguardian.com/society/2021/apr/13/how-uk-doctor-marie-scully-blood-clotting-link-astrazeneca-covid-jab-university-college-london-hospital (accessed 21 February 2024).
46. Scully M, Singh D, Lown R, et al. Pathologic antibodies to platelet factor 4 after ChAdOx1 nCoV-19 vaccination. *New England Journal of Medicine* 2021; **384**: 2202–11.
47. Perry RJ, Tamborska A, Singh B, et al. Cerebral venous thrombosis after vaccination against COVID-19 in the UK: a multicentre cohort study. *Lancet* 2021; **398**: 1147–56.

Chapter 7 **Papers that report trials of complex interventions**

Complex interventions

In Chapter 6, we defined a simple intervention (such as a drug) as one that is well demarcated (i.e. it is easy to say what the intervention comprises) and lends itself to an 'intervention on' versus 'intervention off' research design. A complex intervention is one that is not well demarcated (i.e. it is hard to say precisely what the intervention is) and which poses implementation challenges for researchers. Complex interventions generally involve multiple interacting components and may operate at more than one level (e.g. both individual and organisational) [1]. They include:

- advice or education for patients
- education or training for health care staff
- interventions that seek active and ongoing input from the participant (e.g. physical activity, dietary interventions, lay support groups or psychological therapy delivered either face to face or online)
- a medical device or smartphone application that requires the patient to use it in a particular way and perhaps enter data to be sent remotely to the clinician
- organisational interventions intended to increase the uptake of evidence-based practice (e.g. audit and feedback), which are discussed in more detail in a separate book, *How to Implement Evidence-Based Healthcare* [2].

Professor Penny Hawe and her colleagues [3] have argued that a complex intervention can be thought of as a 'theoretical core' (the components that make it what it is, which researchers must therefore implement faithfully) and additional non-core features that may (indeed, should) be adapted flexibly to local needs or circumstances. For example, if the intervention is providing feedback to doctors on how closely their practice aligns with an

How to Read a Paper: The Basics of Evidence-Based Healthcare, Seventh Edition.
Trisha Greenhalgh and Paul Dijkstra.

evidence-based hypertension guideline, the *core* of the intervention might be information on what proportion of patients in a given time period achieved the guideline's recommended blood pressure level. The *non-core* elements might include how the information is given (orally, by letter and by email), whether the feedback is given as numbers or as a diagram, whether it is given confidentially or in a group-learning situation and so on.

Complex interventions need to go through a development phase so that the different components can be optimised before being tested in a full-scale randomised controlled trial (RCT) [4]. Typically, there is an initial *development* phase of qualitative interviews or observations, and perhaps a small survey to find out what people would find acceptable, which feed into the design the intervention. This is followed by a small-scale *pilot trial* (effectively a 'dress rehearsal' for a full-scale trial, in which a small number of participants are randomised to see what practical and operational issues come up), and finally the full, definitive trial [1].

Here's an example. One of Trisha's research students, a doctor, wanted to study the impact of yoga classes on the control of diabetes. She initially spent some time interviewing people with diabetes and yoga teachers who worked with clients who had diabetes. She designed a small questionnaire to ask people with diabetes if they were interested in yoga, and found that some, but not all, were. All this was part of her *development phase*. The previous research literature on the therapeutic use of yoga gave her some guidance on core elements of the intervention; for example, there appeared to be good theoretical reasons why the focus should be on relaxation-type exercises rather than the more physically demanding strength or flexibility postures.

The student's initial interviews and questionnaires gave her a great deal of useful information, which she used to design the non-core elements of the yoga intervention. She knew, for example, that her potential participants were reluctant to travel very far from home, that they did not want to attend more than twice a week, that the subgroup most keen to try yoga were the recently retired (age 60–69 years) and that many potential participants described themselves as 'not very bendy' and were anxious not to overstretch themselves. All this information helped her design the detail of the intervention, such as who would do what, where, how often, with whom, for how long and using what materials or instruments.

Disappointingly, when the carefully designed complex intervention was tested in an RCT, it had no impact on diabetes control compared with waiting list controls [5]. In the discussion section of the paper reporting the findings of the yoga trial, we offered two alternative interpretations. The first interpretation was that, contrary to previous non-randomised study findings, yoga has no effect on diabetes control. The second interpretation was that yoga may have an impact but despite our efforts in the development phase,

Box 7.1 Examples of complex intervention studies

- A complex intervention to help women with depression in contexts of adversity in South Africa [6]
- Designing community exercise programmes for older people [7]
- Improving the coordination of cancer care in France [8]

the complex intervention was *inadequately optimised*. For example, many people found it hard to get to the group, and several people in each class did not do the exercises because they found them 'too difficult'. Furthermore, while the yoga teachers put a great deal of effort into the twice-weekly classes and they gave people a tape and a yoga mat to take home, they did not emphasise to participants that they should practise their exercises every day. As we discovered, hardly any of the participants did any exercises at home.

To *optimise* yoga as a complex intervention in diabetes, therefore, we might consider measures such as: (1) getting a doctor or nurse to 'prescribe' it, so that the patient is more motivated to attend every class; (2) working with the yoga teachers to design special exercises for older, under-confident people who cannot follow standard yoga exercises and (3) stipulating more precisely what is expected as 'homework'.

This example shows that when a trial of a complex intervention produces negative results, this does not necessarily prove that all adaptations of this intervention will be ineffective in all settings. Rather, it tends to prompt the researchers to go back to the drawing board and ask how the intervention can be further refined and adapted to make it more likely to work. Note that because our yoga intervention needs more work, we did not go on directly to a full-scale RCT but returned to the development phase to try to refine the intervention.

Box 7.1 shows some examples of recently published complex intervention studies. Not included in that list (or this chapter) are studies of artificial intelligence interventions, which are covered in Chapter 17.

Ten questions to ask about a paper describing a complex intervention

The Medical Research Council (MRC) has published a framework in the *BMJ* for developing and evaluating complex interventions [1]. The questions given later, about how to appraise a paper describing a complex intervention, are based on this MRC framework and other methodological studies [9, 10]. See also the 2017 extension of the CONSORT statement to include non-pharmacological treatments [11].

Question one: What is the problem for which this complex intervention is seen as a possible solution?
It is all too easy to base a complex intervention study on a series of unquestioned assumptions. Teenagers drink too much alcohol and have too much unprotected sex, so surely educational programmes are needed to tell them about the dangers of this behaviour? This does not follow, of course! The problem may be teenage drinking or sexual risk-taking, but the underlying cause of that problem may not be ignorance but (for example) peer pressure and messages from the media. By considering precisely what the problem is, you will be able to look critically at whether the intervention has been (explicitly or inadvertently) designed around an appropriate theory of action (see question 4).

Question two: What was done in the developmental phase of the research to inform the design of the complex intervention?
There are no fixed rules about what should be done in a developmental phase, but the authors should state clearly what they did and justify it. If the developmental phase included qualitative research (this is usually the case), see Chapter 12 for detailed guidance on how to appraise such papers. If a questionnaire was used, see Chapter 14. When you have appraised the empirical work using checklists appropriate to the study design(s), consider how these findings were used to inform the design of the intervention. The design of the intervention will probably need to be informed by both qualitative and quantitative data; how to bring these different sources together is a complex challenge which is covered elsewhere [6].

Question three: What were the core and non-core components of the intervention?
To put this question another way: (1) what are the things that should be standardised so they remain the same wherever the intervention is implemented? And (2) what are the things that should be adapted to context and setting [3]? The authors should state clearly which aspects of the intervention should be standardised and which should be adapted to local contingencies and priorities. An under-standardised complex intervention may lead to a paucity of generalisable findings; an over-standardised one may be unworkable in some settings and hence, overall, an underestimate of the potential effectiveness of the core elements. The decision as to what is 'core' and what is 'non-core' should be made on the basis of the findings of the developmental phase.

Remember to unpack the control intervention in just as much detail as you unpack the experimental one. If the control was 'nothing' (or waiting list), describe what the participants in the control arm of the trial will *not* be receiving compared with those in the intervention arm. More likely, the control group will receive a package that includes (for example) an initial assessment, some review visits, some basic advice and perhaps a leaflet or helpline number.

Defining what the control group is offered will be particularly important if the trial addresses a controversial and expensive new care package. In a trial of telehealth known as the Whole Systems Demonstrator, the findings were interpreted by some commentators as showing that telehealth installed in people's homes leads to significantly lower use of hospital services and improved survival rates (albeit at high cost per case) [12]. However, the intervention group actually received a combination of two interventions: the telehealth equipment *and* regular phone calls from a nurse. The control group received no telehealth equipment – but no phone calls from the nurse either. Perhaps it was the human contact, not the technology, that made the difference. Frustratingly, we cannot know. Arguably, the control group should have received the phone calls too!

Question four: What was the theoretical mechanism of action of the intervention?

The authors of a study on a complex intervention should state explicitly how the intervention is intended to work, including how the different components fit together. This statement is likely to change as the results of the developmental phase are analysed and incorporated into the refinement of the intervention.

It is not always obvious why an intervention works (or why it fails to work), especially if it involves multiple components aimed at different levels (e.g. individual, family and organisation). A few years ago, Trisha's team reviewed the qualitative sections of research trials on school-based feeding programmes for disadvantaged children [13]. In 19 studies, all of which had tested this complex intervention in an RCT (see the linked Cochrane review and meta-analysis [14]), we found a total of six different mechanisms by this intervention may have improved nutritional status, school performance or both: long-term correction of nutritional deficiencies; short-term relief of hunger; the children felt valued and looked after; reduced absenteeism; improved school diet inspired improved home diet and improved literacy in one generation improved earning power and hence reduced the risk of poverty in the next generation.

When critically appraising a paper on a complex intervention, you will need to make a judgement on whether the mechanisms offered by the authors are plausible and adequate. Common sense is a good place to start here, as is discussion among a group of experienced clinicians and service users. You may have to deduce the mechanism of action indirectly if the authors did not state it explicitly. A review a few years ago by Grol and Grimshaw [15] showed that only 27% of studies of implementing evidence included an explicit theory of change.

Question five: What outcome measures were used and were they sensible?
With a complex intervention, a single outcome measure may not reflect all the important effects that the intervention may have. While a trial of a drug against placebo in diabetes would usually have a single primary outcome measure (typically the HbA1c blood test) and perhaps two or three secondary outcome measures (such as body mass index, overall cardiovascular risk and quality of life), a trial of an educational intervention may have multiple outcomes, all of which are important in different ways. In addition to markers of diabetic control, cardiovascular risk and quality of life, it would be important to know whether staff found the educational intervention acceptable and practicable to administer, whether people showed up to the sessions, whether the participants' knowledge changed, whether they changed their self-care behaviour, whether the organisation became more patient-centred, whether calls to a helpline increased or decreased, and so on.

When you have answered questions one to five, you should be able to express a summary so far in terms of population, intervention, comparison and outcome, although this is likely to be less succinct than an equivalent summary for a simple intervention. Now, let's turn to the results section of the paper.

Question six: What were the findings?
Note, from question five, that a complex intervention may have significant impact on one set of outcome measures but no significant impact on other measures. Findings such as these need careful interpretation. Trials of self-management interventions (in which people with chronic illness are taught to manage their condition by altering their lifestyle and titrating their medication against symptoms or home-based tests of disease status) are widely considered to be effective. In fact, such programmes rarely change the underlying course of the disease or make people live longer – they just make people feel more confident in managing their illness [16,17]! Sometimes, however, researchers produce a complex intervention that *does* improve 'hard' outcomes like disease severity. For example, Hilary Pinnock and her team showed that, in relation to self-management interventions for asthma, improvements in both disease severity and quality of life are possible if self-management education is accompanied by two things: addition of a personalised action plan and regular professional

review [18]. If that intervention sounds complex, it is – but that's the reality of changing behaviour.

Question seven: What process evaluation was done and what were the key findings? In particular, to what extent was the intervention implemented as planned ('implementation fidelity')?
A process evaluation is a (mostly) qualitative study carried out in parallel with an RCT, which collects information on the practical challenges faced by front-line staff trying to implement the intervention [1,9,10,19]. In our study of yoga in diabetes, for example, researchers (one of whom was a medical student doing a BSc project) sat in on the yoga classes, interviewed patients and staff, collected the minutes of planning meetings and generally asked the question 'How's it going?' [5]. One key finding from this was the inappropriateness of some of the venues. Only by actually being there when the yoga class was happening could we have discovered that it's impossible to relax and meditate in a public leisure centre with regular announcements over a very loud intercom! Process evaluations should determine whether the intervention was implemented as planned ('fidelity') or if compromises were made (e.g reducing the intensity of contact) [20]. They will also capture the views of participants and staff about how to refine the intervention and/or why it may not be working as planned.

Question eight: If the findings were negative, to what extent can this be explained by implementation failure and/or inadequate optimisation of the intervention?
This question follows on from the process evaluation. In Trisha's review of school-based feeding programmes (see question 4), many studies had negative results and, on reading the various papers, the review team came up with a number of explanations why school-based feeding might *not* improve either growth or school performance [13]. For example, the food offered may not have been consumed, or it provided too little of the key nutrients; the food consumed may have had low bioavailability in undernourished children (e.g. it was not absorbed because their intestines were swollen and damaged); there may have been a compensatory reduction in food intake outside school (e.g. the evening meal was given to another family member if the child was known to have been fed at school); supplementation may have occurred too late in the child's development or the programme may not have been implemented as planned (e.g. in one study, some of the control group were given food supplements because front-line staff felt, probably rightly, that it was unethical to give food to half the hungry children in a class but not the other half).

Question nine: If the findings varied across different subgroups, to what extent have the authors explained this by refining their theory of change?
Did the intervention improve the outcomes in women but not in men? In highly educated affluent people with good Internet access but not in less-educated, less well-off people with poor or no Internet access? In primary care settings but not in secondary care? Or in Manchester but not in Delhi? If so, ask why. This 'why' question is another judgement call, because it's a matter of interpreting findings in context. In general, 'why' questions can't be answered purely by applying a technical algorithm or checklist. Look in the discussion section of the paper and you should find the authors' explanation of why subgroup X benefited but subgroup Y didn't. They should also have offered a refinement of their theory of change that takes account of these differences. For example, the studies of school feeding programmes we reviewed a few years ago showed (overall) statistically greater benefit in younger children, which led the authors of these studies to suggest that there is a critical window of development, after which even nutritionally rich supplements have limited impact on growth or performance [13,14].

Question ten: What further research do the authors believe is needed and is this belief justified?
As you will know if you have read this chapter up to this point, complex interventions are multifaceted, nuanced and impact on multiple different outcomes. Authors who present studies of such interventions have a responsibility to tell us how their study has shaped the overall research field. They should not conclude merely that 'more research is needed' (an inevitable follow-on from any scientific study) but they should indicate where research efforts might best be focused. Indeed, one of the most useful conclusions might be a statement of the areas in which further research is not needed! The authors should state, for example, whether the next stage should be new qualitative research, a new and bigger RCT or further analysis of data already gathered.

Exercises based on this chapter

1. Before you look up any literature, design a complex intervention to promote smoking cessation in pregnant women. Remember that smoking is more prevalent in poor, disadvantaged (e.g. homeless) and some minority ethnic groups (who may not be fluent in English). When you have designed your intervention, do a literature search to find studies of actual interventions. What did the researchers do? What was their theory of change? What did they find – and what explains these findings?

2. Design a complex intervention to improve the quality of education for a clinical group (doctors, nurses, midwives and so on). Think about how you might intervene to change the behaviour of both students and teachers. What is your theory of change? What initial qualitative work might you do to develop your intervention? What would be the core features of your intervention? If you were going to test this intervention in an RCT, what would your control intervention be and what would your process evaluation look like?
3. Think about a non-drug intervention such as education, psychotherapy or patient use of apps. Hunt out some RCTs of interventions you're thinking of using yourself (or recommending to patients). Describe both the 'core' and 'non-core' elements of the intervention. Apply the CONSORT checklist for non-drug interventions to evaluate the study's quality [11].

References

1. Skivington K, Matthews L, Simpson SA, et al. A new framework for developing and evaluating complex interventions: update of Medical Research Council guidance. *BMJ* 2021; **374**, n2061.
2. Greenhalgh T. *How to Implement Evidence-Based Healthcare*. Oxford: Wiley-Blackwell; 2018.
3. Hawe P, Shiell A, Riley T. Complex interventions: how 'out of control' can a randomised controlled trial be? *BMJ* 2004; **328**(7455): 1561–3.
4. O'Cathain A, Croot L, Duncan E, et al. Guidance on how to develop complex interventions to improve health and healthcare. *BMJ Open* 2019; **9**(8): e029954.
5. Skoro-Kondza L, Tai SS, Gadelrab R, et al. Community based yoga classes for type 2 diabetes: an exploratory randomised controlled trial. *BMC Health Services Research* 2009; **9**(1): 33.
6. Burgess RA, Jeske N, Rasool S, et al. Exploring the impact of a complex intervention for women with depression in contexts of adversity: a pilot feasibility study of COURRAGE-plus in South Africa. *International Journal of Social Psychiatry* 2022; **68**(4): 873–80.
7. Bird ML, Mortenson WB, Eng JJ. Evaluation and facilitation of intervention fidelity in community exercise programs through an adaptation of the TIDier framework. *BMC Health Services Research* 2020; **20**: 68.
8. Colombani F, Sibé M, Kret M, et al. EPOCK study protocol: a mixed-methods research program evaluating cancer care coordination nursing occupations in France as a complex intervention. *BMC Health Services Research* 2019; **19**: 483.
9. Noyes J, Booth A, Moore G, et al. Synthesising quantitative and qualitative evidence to inform guidelines on complex interventions: clarifying the purposes, designs and outlining some methods. *BMJ Global Health* 2019; **4**(Suppl 1): e000893.

10. Paparini S, Papoutsi C, Murdoch J, et al. Evaluating complex interventions in context: systematic, meta-narrative review of case study approaches. *BMC Medical Research Methodology* 2021; **21**: 225.
11. Boutron I, Altman DG, Moher D, et al. CONSORT statement for randomized trials of nonpharmacologic treatments: a 2017 update and a CONSORT extension for nonpharmacologic trial abstracts. *Annals of Internal Medicine* 2017;**167**: 40–47Schulz.
12. Steventon A, Bardsley M, Billings J, et al. Effect of telehealth on use of secondary care and mortality: findings from the Whole System Demonstrator cluster randomised trial. *BMJ* 2012; **344**: e3874.
13. Greenhalgh T, Kristjansson E, Robinson V. Realist review to understand the efficacy of school feeding programmes. *BMJ* 2007; **335**: 858–61.
14. Kristjansson EA, Robinson V, Petticrew M, et al. School feeding for improving the physical and psychosocial health of disadvantaged elementary school children. *Cochrane Database of Systematic Reviews* 2007; **(1)**: CD004676.
15. Grol R, Grimshaw J. From best evidence to best practice: effective implementation of change in patients' care. *Lancet* 2003; **362**: 1225–30.
16. Foster G, Taylor S, Eldridge S, et al. Self-management education programmes by lay leaders for people with chronic conditions. *Cochrane Database of Systematic Reviews* 2007; **(4)**: CD005108.
17. Nolte S, Osborne RH. A systematic review of outcomes of chronic disease self-management interventions. *Quality of Life Research* 2013; **22**: 1805–16.
18. Pinnock H, Parke HL, Panagioti M, et al. Systematic meta-review of supported self-management for asthma: a healthcare perspective. *BMC Medicine* 2017; **15**(1): 64.
19. Lewin S, Glenton C, Oxman AD. Use of qualitative methods alongside randomised controlled trials of complex healthcare interventions: methodological study. *BMJ* 2009; **339**: b3496.
20. Hasson H. Systematic evaluation of implementation fidelity of complex interventions in health and social care. *Implementation Science* 2010; **5**: 67.

Chapter 8 **Papers that report diagnostic or screening tests**

Ten suspects in the dock

If you are new to the concept of validating diagnostic tests, and if algebraic explanations ('let's call this value *x*. . .') leave you cold, the following example may help you. Ten suspects are awaiting trial for murder. Only three of them actually committed a murder; the other seven are innocent of any crime. A jury hears each case and finds six of the suspects guilty of murder. Two of the convicted are true murderers. Four suspects are wrongly imprisoned. One murderer walks free.

This information can be expressed in what is known as a *two-by-two table* (Figure 8.1). Note that the 'truth' (i.e. whether or not each suspect *really* committed a murder) is expressed along the horizontal title row, whereas the jury's verdict (which may or may not reflect the truth) is expressed down the vertical title row.

You should be able to see that these figures, if they are typical, reflect a number of features of this particular jury:

- This jury correctly identifies two in every three true murderers.
- It correctly acquits three of every seven innocent people.
- If this jury has found a person guilty, there is still only a one in three chance that the person actually committed the murder.
- If this jury found a person innocent, they have a three in four chance of actually being innocent.
- In 5 cases of every 10, the jury gets the verdict right.

These five features constitute, respectively, the sensitivity, specificity, positive predictive value, negative predictive value and accuracy of this jury's performance. The rest of this chapter considers these five features applied to diagnostic (or screening) tests when compared with a 'true' diagnosis or gold standard. Later in this chapter, we introduce a sixth, slightly more complicated

---

How to Read a Paper: The Basics of Evidence-Based Healthcare, Seventh Edition.
Trisha Greenhalgh and Paul Dijkstra.

		True criminal status	
		Murderer	Not murderer
Jury verdict	'Guilty'	Rightly convicted **2 suspects**	Wrongly convicted **4 suspects**
	'Innocent'	**1 suspect** Wrongly acquitted	**3 suspects** Rightly acquitted

Figure 8.1 2 × 2 table showing outcome of trial for 10 suspects accused of murder.

(but very useful), feature of a diagnostic test – the likelihood ratio. (After you have read the rest of this chapter, look back at this section. You should, by then, be able to work out that the likelihood ratio of a positive jury verdict in the above-mentioned example is 1.17, and that of a negative one 0.78. If you can't, don't worry – many eminent clinicians have no idea what a likelihood ratio is.)

Validating diagnostic tests against a gold standard

Let's consider a urine dipstick test and diabetes, which was the example originally offered in the first edition of this book when urine testing for diabetes was widespread in UK. Urine testing is now out of favour (for good reason) and that's why the example is still a good one to work through. A middle-aged man had been feeling thirsty and had asked his general practitioner (GP) to be tested for diabetes, which runs in his family. An assistant in his GP's surgery had asked him to produce a urine specimen and dipped a special stick in it. The stick stayed green, which meant, apparently, that there was no sugar (glucose) in his urine. This, the assistant had said, meant that he did not have diabetes. Is this possible?

You should be able to explain to the patient that the test result did not necessarily mean this at all, any more than a 'not guilty' verdict *necessarily* means that someone is innocent of murder. According to the World Health Organization (WHO) and UK National Institute for Health and Care Excellence (NICE), we should suspect a diagnosis of type 2 diabetes 'if an adult presents with persistent hyperglycaemia that may be accompanied by clinical features'. Typical symptoms of diabetes include thirst, passing large amounts of urine, blurred vision, tiredness. Persistent hyperglycaemia is defined as HbA1c of 48 mmol/mol (6.5%) or more; fasting plasma glucose level of 7 mmol/l or more; or random plasma glucose of 11.1 mmol/l or more in the presence of symptoms or signs of diabetes (although, in a symptomatic patient, a single HbA1c or fasting plasma glucose level can be used, it is sensible to repeat the tests to confirm the diagnosis of type 2 diabetes) and plasma glucose of 11.1 mmol/l 2 hours after a 75-g oral glucose load (the much-dreaded 'glucose tolerance test', where the participant has to glug down every last drop of a sickly glucose drink and wait 2 hours for a blood test) [1–3]. These values must be achieved on two separate occasions if the person has no symptoms but on only one occasion if they have typical symptoms of diabetes (thirst, passing large amounts of urine, etc.).

These stringent criteria can be termed the *gold standard* for diagnosing diabetes. In other words, if you fulfil the WHO/NICE criteria, you can call yourself diabetic, and if you don't, you can't (although note that official definitions of what is and isn't a disease change regularly, and indeed, every time we produce a new edition of this book we have to see whether the ones we have cited have changed in the light of further evidence). The same cannot be said for dipping a stick into a random urine specimen. For one thing, you might have true diabetes but have a high renal threshold; that is, your kidneys conserve glucose much better than most people's, so your blood glucose level would have to be higher than most people's for any glucose to appear in your urine. Alternatively, you may be an otherwise normal individual with a *low* renal threshold, so glucose leaks into your urine even when there isn't any excess in your blood (this happens, for example, in pregnancy). In fact, as anyone with diabetes will tell you, diabetes is very often associated with a negative test for urine glucose. This is why urine testing, despite the advantages listed in the next paragraph, should generally *not* be used in either diagnosis or monitoring of diabetes [4].

There are, however, many advantages in using a urine dipstick rather than the full-blown glucose tolerance test to check whether someone might have diabetes. The test is inexpensive, convenient, easy to perform, acceptable to most patients and gives an instant, yes/no result. In real life, people like the person in the above example may decline to take an oral glucose tolerance test, especially if they are self-employed and asked to miss a day's work for the test, or even to have a blood test. Even if the patient was prepared to go ahead with it, their GP might decide (rightly or wrongly) that their symptoms did not merit the expense of this relatively sophisticated investigation. We hope you can see that even though the urine test cannot say for sure if someone is diabetic, it has something of a practical edge over the gold standard. That, of course, is why some people still use it, especially in low-resource environments.

To assess objectively just how useful the urine glucose test for diabetes is, we would need to select a sample of people (say, 100) and do two tests on each of them: the urine test (screening test) and a standard oral glucose tolerance test (gold standard). We could then see, for each person, whether the result of the screening test matched the gold standard. Such an exercise is known as a *validation study*. We could express the results of the validation

		Result of gold standard test	
		Disease positive a + c	Disease negative b + d
Result of screening test	Test positive a + b	True positive a	False positive b
	c + d Test negative	c False negative	d True negative

Figure 8.2 2 × 2 table notation for expressing the results of a validation study for a diagnostic or screening test.

Table 8.1 Features of a diagnostic test that can be calculated by comparing it with a gold standard in a validation study

Feature of the test	Alternative name	Question that the feature addresses	Formula (see Figure 8.1)
Sensitivity	True positive rate (positive in disease)	How good is this test at picking up people who have the condition?	*a*/*a* + *c*
Specificity	True negative rate (negative in health)	How good is this test at correctly excluding people without the condition?	*d*/*b* + *d*
Positive predictive value	Post-test probability of a positive test	If a person tests positive, what is the probability that they have the condition?	*a*/*a* + *b*
Negative predictive value (NPV)	Indicates the post-test probability of a negative test[a]	If a person tests negative, what is the probability that they do not have the condition?	*d*/*c* + *d*
Accuracy	–	What proportion of all tests have given the correct result (i.e. true positives and true negatives as a proportion of all results)?	*a* + *d*/*a* + *b* + *c* + *d*
Likelihood ratio of a positive test	–	How much more likely is positive test to be found in a person with, as opposed to without, the condition?	Sensitivity/(1 – specificity)

[a] The post-test probability of a negative test is (1 – NPV).

study in a two-by-two table (also known as a *two-by-two matrix*), as in Figure 8.2, and calculate various features of the test as in Table 8.1, just as we did for the features of the jury above.

If the values for the various features of a test (such as sensitivity and specificity) fell within reasonable limits, we would be able to say that the

		Result of glucose tolerance test	
		Diabetes positive **27 people**	Diabetes negative **973 people**
Result of urine test for glucose	Glucose present **13 people**	True positive **6**	False positive **7**
	987 people Glucose absent	**21** False negative	**966** True negative

Figure 8.3 2 × 2 table showing results of a validation study of urine glucose testing for diabetes against the gold standard of glucose tolerance test. *Source:* based on Andersson et al. [5].

test was *valid* (see question seven below). The validity of urine testing for glucose in diagnosing diabetes was assessed many years ago by Andersson and colleagues [5], whose data we have used in the example in Figure 8.3. The original study was performed on 3268 participants, of whom 67 either refused to produce a specimen or, for some other reason, were not adequately tested. For simplicity's sake, we have ignored these irregularities and expressed the results in terms of a denominator (total number tested) of 1000 participants.

In actual fact, these data came from an epidemiological survey to detect the prevalence of diabetes in a population; the validation of urine testing was a side issue to the main study. If the validation had been the main aim of the study, the participants selected would have included far more diabetic individuals, as question two below shows [5]. If you look up the original paper, you will also find that the gold standard for diagnosing true diabetes was not the oral glucose tolerance test but a more unconventional series of observations. Nevertheless, the example serves its purpose, as it provides us with some figures to put through the equations listed in the last column of Table 8.1. We can calculate the important features of the urine test for diabetes as follows:

- sensitivity = $a/(a + c)$ = 6/27 = 22.2%
- specificity = $d/(b + d)$ = 966/973 = 99.3%
- positive predictive value = $a/(a + b)$ = 6/13 = 46.2%
- negative predictive value = $d/(c + d)$ = 966/987 = 97.9%
- accuracy = $(a + d)/(a + b + c + d)$ = 972/1000 = 97.2%
- likelihood ratio of a positive test = sensitivity/(1 − specificity) = 22.2/0.7 = 32
- likelihood ratio of a negative test = (1 − sensitivity)/specificity = 77.8/99.3 = 0.78.

From these features, you can probably see why we should not share the GP assistant's assurance that the thirsty middle-aged man did not have diabetes. A positive urine glucose test is only 22% sensitive, which means that the test misses nearly four-fifths of people who really do have diabetes. In the presence of classical symptoms and a family history, the patient's baseline odds (pre-test likelihood) of having the condition are pretty high, and they are only reduced to about four-fifths of this (the negative likelihood ratio, 0.78; see section 'Likelihood ratios') after a single negative urine test. In view of his symptoms, this man clearly needs to undergo a more definitive test for diabetes [6]. Note that as the definitions in Table 8.1 show, if the test had been positive the patient would have good reason to be concerned, because even though the test is not very *sensitive* (i.e. it is not good at picking up people with the disease), it is pretty *specific* (i.e. it *is* good at excluding people *without* the disease).

Despite the findings of these studies from over 30 years ago, urine testing to 'exclude diabetes' is still common in some (especially low-resource) settings. But the academic argument has long shifted to the question of whether the HbA1c blood test is sufficiently sensitive and specific to serve as a screening test for diabetes [7] and (in a recent meta-analysis by Trisha's own team) for the intermediate state of 'pre-diabetes' [8]. The arguments have become far more complex as epidemiologists have weighed in with evidence on early (subclinical) microvascular damage, but the essential principles of the 2 × 2 matrix and the questions about false positives and false negatives still apply. In short, the test performs very well but it does require a blood test and the costs are not insignificant.

Students often get mixed up about the sensitivity/specificity dimension of a test and the positive/negative predictive value dimension. As a rule of thumb, the sensitivity or specificity tells you about the test in general, whereas the predictive value tells you about what a particular test result means for the patient in front of you. Hence, sensitivity and specificity are generally used more by epidemiologists and public health specialists whose day-to-day work involves making decisions about populations.

A screening mammogram (breast x-ray) might have an 80% sensitivity and a 90% specificity for detecting breast cancer, which means that the test will pick up 80% of cancers and exclude 90% of women without cancer. But imagine you were a GP or practice nurse and a patient comes to see you for the result of her mammogram. The question she will want answered is (if the test has come back positive), 'What is the chance that I've got cancer?' or (if it has come back negative) 'What is the chance that I can now forget about the possibility of cancer?' Many patients (and far too many health professionals) assume that the negative predictive value of a test is 100% – that is, if the test is 'normal' or 'clear' they think there is no chance of the disease being present – and you only need to read the confessional stories in magazines ('I was told I had cancer but tests later proved the doctors wrong') to find examples of people who have assumed that the positive predictive value of a test is 100%.

Ten questions to ask about a paper that claims to validate a diagnostic or screening test

In preparing these tips, we have drawn on Guyatt *et al.*'s classic chapter 'Evaluating diagnostic tests' [9]. Like many of the checklists in this book, these are no more than pragmatic rules of thumb for the novice critical appraiser. For a much more comprehensive and rigorously developed set of criteria, see the work of the Cochrane Diagnostic Test Accuracy Working Group [10]. Lucas and colleagues have since produced a checklist that is similar but not identical to the questions listed here [11]. If you are interested in comprehensive quality assessment tools of diagnostic and prognostic accuracy studies respectively, you might want to read the QUADAS-2 (A Revised Tool for the Quality Assessment of Diagnostic Accuracy Studies) [12], and QUAPAS (An Adaptation of the QUADAS-2 Tool to Assess Prognostic Accuracy Studies) [13] papers. In addition, the STARD (Standards for Reporting of Diagnostic Accuracy Studies) statement, originally published in 2003 and updated in 2015, was developed 'to improve the completeness and transparency of reports of diagnostic accuracy studies' [14].

Question one: Is this test potentially relevant to my patients and my practice?
This is the 'so what?' question, which epidemiologists call the *utility* of the test. Even if this test were 100% valid, accurate and reliable, would it help me? Would it identify a treatable disorder? If so, would I use it in preference to the test I use now? Could I (or my patients or the taxpayer) afford it? Would my patients consent to it? Would it change the probabilities for competing diagnoses sufficiently for me to alter my treatment plan? If the answers to these questions are all 'no', you may be able to reject the paper without reading further than the abstract or introduction.

Question two: Has the test been compared with a true gold standard?
You need to ask, first, whether the test has been compared with anything at all! Papers have occasionally been published in which nothing has been done except perform the new test on a few dozen participants. This exercise may give a range of possible results for the test, but it certainly does not confirm that the 'high' results indicate that target disorder (the disease or risk state that you are interested in) is present or that the 'low' results indicate that it isn't.

Next, you should verify that the 'gold standard' test used in the survey merits the term. A good way of assessing a gold standard is to use the 'so what?' questions listed earlier. For many conditions, there is no absolute gold standard diagnostic test that will say for certain if it is present or not. Unsurprisingly, these tend to be the very conditions for which new tests are most actively sought! Hence, the authors of such papers may need to develop and justify a combination of criteria against which the new test is to be assessed. One specific point to check is that the test being validated here (or a variant of it) is not being used to contribute to the definition of the gold standard.

Question three: Did this validation study include an appropriate spectrum of participants?

If you validated a new test for cholesterol in 100 healthy male medical students, you would not be able to say how the test would perform in women, children, older people, those with diseases that seriously raise the cholesterol level, or even those who had never been to medical school. Although few people would be naive enough to select quite such a biased sample for their validation study, it is surprisingly common for published studies to omit to define the spectrum of participants tested in terms of age, gender, symptoms and/or disease severity and specific eligibility criteria.

Defining both the range of participants and the spectrum of disease to be included is essential if the values for the different features of the test are to be worth quoting; that is, if they are to be transferable to other settings. A particular diagnostic test may, conceivably, be more sensitive in female participants than in male participants, or in younger rather than in older participants. For the same reasons, the participants on which any test is verified should include those with both mild and severe disease, treated and untreated and those with different but commonly confused conditions.

While the sensitivity and specificity of a test are virtually constant whatever the prevalence of the condition, the positive and negative predictive values are crucially dependent on prevalence. This is why GPs are, often rightly, sceptical of the utility of tests developed exclusively in a secondary care population, where the severity of disease tends to be greater, and why a good *diagnostic* test (generally used when the patient has some symptoms suggestive of the disease in question) is not necessarily a good *screening* test (generally used in people without symptoms, who are drawn from a population with a much lower prevalence of the disease).

Question four: Has work-up (verification) bias been avoided?

This is easy to check. It simply means, 'Did everyone who got the new diagnostic test also get the gold standard, and vice versa?'. We hope you have no problem spotting the potential bias in studies where the gold standard test is only performed on people who have already tested positive for the test being validated. There are, in addition, a number of more subtle aspects of work-up or verification bias that are beyond the scope of this book but which are covered in specialist statistics textbooks [15].

Question five: Has expectation bias been avoided?
Expectation bias occurs when pathologists and others who interpret diagnostic specimens are subconsciously influenced by the knowledge of the particular features of the case (e.g. the presence of chest pain when interpreting an ECG). In the context of validating diagnostic tests against a gold standard, the question means, 'did the people who interpreted one of the tests know what result the other test had shown on each particular participant?'. As we explained in section 'Was assessment "blind"?', all assessments should be 'blind'; that is, the person interpreting the test should not be given any inkling of what the result is expected to be in any particular case.

Question six: Was the test shown to be reproducible both within and between observers?
If the same observer performs the same test on two occasions on a participant whose characteristics have not changed, they will get different results in a proportion of cases. All tests show this feature to some extent, but a test with a reproducibility of 99% is clearly in a different league from one with a reproducibility of 50%. A number of factors that may contribute to the poor reproducibility of a diagnostic test are the technical precision of the equipment, observer variability (e.g. in comparing a colour with a reference chart), arithmetical errors and so on.

Look back again at section 'Was assessment "blind"?' in Chapter 4 to remind yourself of the problem of interobserver agreement. Given the same result to interpret, two people will agree in only a proportion of cases, generally expressed as the kappa score. If the test in question gives results in terms of numbers (such as the serum cholesterol level in millimole per litre), interobserver agreement is hardly an issue. If, however, the test involves reading x-rays (such as the mammogram example in the section 'Was assessment "blind"?' in Chapter 4) or asking a person questions about their drinking habits [16], it is important to confirm that reproducibility between observers is at an acceptable level.

Question seven: What are the features of the test as derived from this validation study?
All these standards could have been met, but the test may still be worthless because the test itself is not valid (i.e. its sensitivity, specificity and other crucial features are too low. That is clearly the case for using urine glucose to

screen for diabetes; see section 'Ten questions to ask about a paper describing a complex intervention' in Chapter 7). After all, if a test has a false-negative rate of nearly 80%, it is more likely to mislead the clinician than assist the diagnosis if the target disorder is actually present.

There are no absolutes for the validity of a screening test, because what counts as acceptable depends on the condition being screened for. Few of us would quibble about a test for colour blindness that was 95% sensitive and 80% specific, but nobody ever died of colour blindness. The Guthrie heel-prick screening test for congenital hypothyroidism, performed on all babies in the UK soon after birth, is over 99% sensitive but has a positive predictive value of only 6% (in other words, it picks up almost all babies with the condition at the expense of a high false-positive rate) [15], and rightly so. It is far more important to pick up every single baby with this treatable condition who would otherwise develop severe mental handicap than to save hundreds of parents the relatively minor stress of a repeat blood test on their baby.

Question eight: Were confidence intervals given for sensitivity, specificity and other features of the test?
As section 'Probability and confidence' explained, a confidence interval, which can be calculated for virtually every numerical aspect of a set of results, expresses the possible range of results within which the true value will lie. Go back to the jury example at the beginning of this chapter. If they had found just one more murderer not guilty, the sensitivity of their verdict would have gone down from 67% to 33%, and the positive predictive value of the verdict from 33% to 20%. This enormous (and quite unacceptable) sensitivity to a single case decision is because we only validated the jury's performance on 10 cases. The confidence intervals for the features of this jury are so wide that our computer programme refuses to calculate them! Remember, the larger the sample size, the narrower the confidence interval, so it is particularly important to look for confidence intervals if the paper you are reading reports a study on a relatively small sample. If you would like the formula for calculating confidence intervals for diagnostic test features, see the excellent textbook *Statistics with Confidence* [16].

Question nine: Has a sensible 'normal range' been derived from these results?
If the test gives non-dichotomous (continuous) results. In other words, if it gives a numerical value rather than a yes/no result, someone will have to say at what value the test result will count as abnormal. Many of us have been there with our own blood pressure reading. We want to know if our result is 'okay' or not, but the doctor insists on giving us a value such as '142/92'.

If 140/90 mmHg were chosen as the cut-off for high blood pressure, we would be placed in the 'abnormal' category, even though our risk of problems from our blood pressure is very little different from that of a person with a blood pressure of 138/88 mmHg. Quite sensibly, many practising doctors and nurses advise their patients, 'Your blood pressure isn't quite right, but it doesn't fall into the danger zone. Come back in three months for another check'. Nevertheless, the clinician must at some stage make the decision that *this* blood pressure needs treating with tablets but *this* one does not. When and how often to repeat a borderline test is often addressed in guidelines; you might, for example, like to look up the detailed guidance and prevailing controversies on how to measure blood pressure [17]. Defining relative and absolute danger zones for a continuous physiological or pathological variable is a complex science, which should take into account the actual likelihood of the adverse outcome that the proposed treatment aims to prevent. This process is made considerably more objective by the use of likelihood ratios (see section below).

Question ten: Has this test been placed in the context of other potential tests in the diagnostic sequence for the condition?
In general, we treat high blood pressure on the basis of the blood pressure reading alone (although as mentioned, guidelines recommend basing management on a series of readings rather than a single value). Compare this with the sequence we use to diagnose stenosis ('hardening') of the coronary arteries. First, we select patients with a typical history of effort angina (chest pain on exercise). Next, we usually do a resting ECG, an exercise ECG, and perhaps a radionuclide scan of the heart to look for areas short of oxygen. Most patients only come to a coronary angiogram (the definitive investigation for coronary artery stenosis) *after* they have produced an abnormal result on these preliminary tests.

If you took 100 people off the street and sent them straight for a coronary angiogram, the test might display very different positive and negative predictive values (and even different sensitivity and specificity) than it did in the sicker population on which it was originally validated. This means that the various aspects of validity of the coronary angiogram as a diagnostic test are virtually meaningless unless these figures are expressed in terms of what they contribute to the overall diagnostic work-up.

Likelihood ratios

Question nine described the problem of defining a normal range for a continuous variable. In such circumstances, it can be preferable to express the test result not as 'normal' or 'abnormal' but in terms of the actual chances of a patient having the target disorder if the test result reaches a particular level. Take, for example, the use of the prostate-specific antigen (PSA) test to screen for prostate cancer. Most men will have some detectable PSA in their blood (say, 0.5 ng/ml), and most of those with advanced prostate cancer will have very high levels of PSA (above about 20 ng/ml). But a PSA level of, say, 7.4 ng/ml may be found either in a perfectly normal man or in someone with early cancer. There simply is not a clean cut-off between normal and abnormal [18].

We can, however, use the results of a validation study of the PSA test against a gold standard for prostate cancer (say, a biopsy) to draw up a whole series of 2 × 2 tables. Each table would use a different definition of an abnormal PSA result to classify patients as 'normal' or 'abnormal'. From these tables, we could generate different likelihood ratios associated with a PSA level above each different cut-off point. Then, when faced with a PSA result in the 'grey zone', we would at least be able to say, 'this test has not proved that the patient has prostate cancer, but it has increased [or decreased] the odds of that diagnosis by a factor of *x*'. In fact, as we mentioned earlier, the PSA test is not a terribly good discriminator between the presence and absence of cancer, whatever cut-off value is used. In other words, there is no value for PSA that gives a particularly high likelihood ratio in cancer detection. The latest advice is to share these uncertainties with the patient and let him decide whether to have the test [18].

Although the likelihood ratio is one of the more complicated aspects of a diagnostic test to calculate, it has enormous practical value, and it is becoming the preferred way of expressing and comparing the usefulness of different tests. The likelihood ratio is a particularly helpful test for ruling a particular diagnosis in or out. For example, if a person enters your consulting room somewhere in the UK with no symptoms at all, you know (on the basis of some rather old epidemiological studies) that they have a 5% chance of having iron-deficiency anaemia, because around one person in 20 in the UK population has this condition. In the language of diagnostic tests, this means that the pre-test probability of anaemia, equivalent to the prevalence of the condition, is 0.05.

Now, if you carry out a diagnostic test for anaemia, the serum ferritin level, the result will usually make the diagnosis of anaemia either more or less likely. A moderately reduced serum ferritin level (between 18 and 45 μg/l) has a likelihood ratio of 3, so the chances of a patient with this result having iron-deficiency anaemia is generally calculated as 0.05 × 3 – or 0.15 (15%). This value is known as the *post-test probability of the serum ferritin test*. (Strictly speaking, likelihood ratios should be used on odds rather than on probabilities, but the simpler method shown here gives a good approximation when the pre-test probability is low. In this example, a pre-test probability of 5% is equal to a pre-test odds of 0.05/0.95 or 0.053; a positive test with a likelihood ratio of 3 gives a post-test odds of 0.158, which is equal to a post-test probability of 14%) [19].

Figure 8.4 shows a nomogram adapted by Sackett and colleagues from an original paper by Fagan [20], for working out post-test probabilities when the

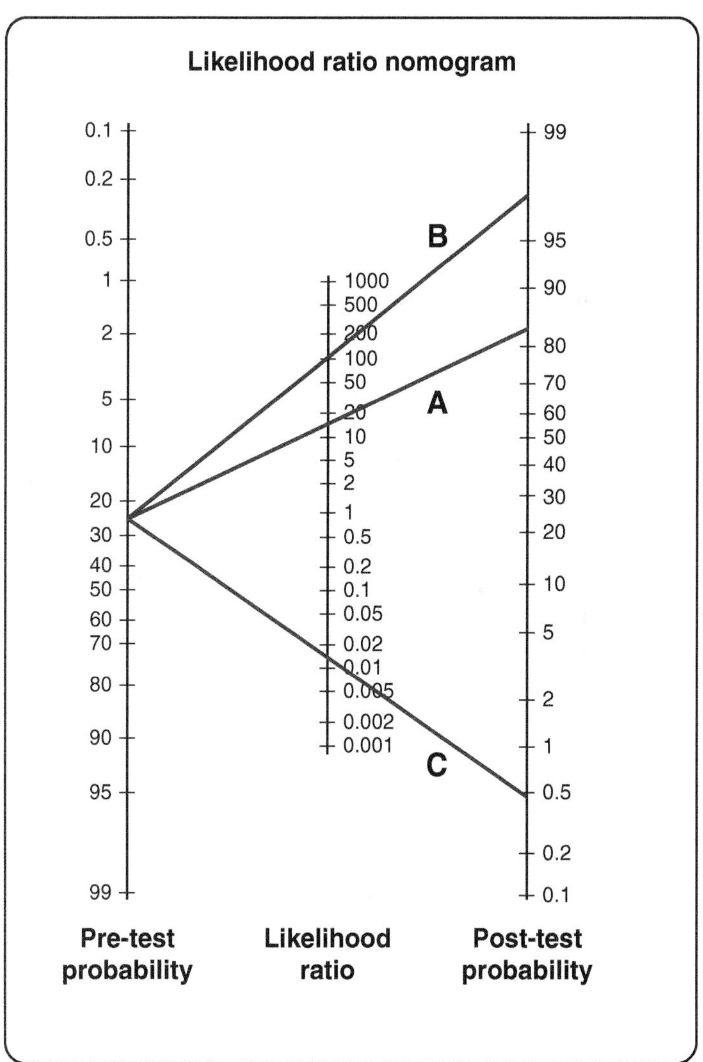

Figure 8.4 Using likelihood ratios to calculating the post-test probability of someone being a smoker.

pre-test probability (prevalence) and likelihood ratio for the test are known. The lines A, B and C, drawn from a pre-test probability of 25% (the prevalence of smoking among British adults) are, respectively, the trajectories through likelihood ratios of 15, 100 and 0.015 – three different (and all somewhat old) tests for detecting whether someone is a smoker. Actually, test C detects whether the person is a *non-smoker*, as a positive result in this test leads to a post-test probability of only 0.5%.

In summary, as we said at the beginning of this chapter, you can go a long way with diagnostic tests without referring to likelihood ratios. We avoided them ourselves for years. But if you put aside an afternoon to get to grips with this aspect of clinical epidemiology, we predict that your time will have been well spent.

Clinical prediction models

In the previous section, we took you through a rather heavy-going example of the PSA test and concluded that there is no single, clear-cut value that reliably distinguishes 'normal' from 'abnormal'. This is why the recommended approach to assessing a man's risk of prostate cancer is a combination of several 'predictors', including the overall clinical assessment and a digital rectal examination [18].

More generally, you can probably see why, in general, clinicians tend to use a combination of several different diagnostic tests (including their clinical examination, blood tests, x-rays, etc.) to build up a picture of what is wrong with the patient. While any one test has a fuzzy boundary between normal and abnormal, combining them may sharpen the diagnostic focus. So, for example, a woman who presents with a breast lump tends to be offered three different tests, none of which is especially useful when used in isolation: fine needle aspiration, x-ray (mammogram) and ultrasound [21].

By following large cohorts of patients with particular symptoms and carefully recording the findings of clinical examinations and diagnostic tests in all of them, we can come up with numerical estimates of the chance of a person having (or going on to develop) disease X in the presence of symptom A, physical sign B, diagnostic test C and so on, or any combination of these. Interest in – and research into – clinical prediction rules has been growing rapidly in recent years, partly because the growth of information technology means that very large numbers of patients can be entered onto online databases by clinicians in different centres.

Clinical prediction models, therefore, play an increasingly important role in contemporary health care and combine several characteristics related to the patient, disease or treatment to predict a diagnostic (estimate an individual's probability of a specific health condition – often a disease – being currently present) or prognostic (predicting a future occurrence of a specific health outcome over a specific time period) outcome [22–24]. Prediction models in healthcare enhance (shared) decision-making, patient outcomes and resource allocation. The *Wells rule* to aid the diagnosis of deep venous thrombosis (DVT) is an example of a diagnostic prediction model [25]. Applying this model successfully decreased the number of unnecessary referrals of low-risk primary care patients suspected of DVT to secondary care. In the mental health field, prognostic models have been developed using routine healthcare data to identify children at risk for mental health conditions [26]. However, implementation of prediction models in clinical practice is easier said than done! See Figure 8.5 for examples of reasons for failed prediction model adoption in clinical practice, reproduced from [27]. The TRIPOD (Transparent Reporting of a multivariable prediction model for Individual Prognosis or Diagnosis) statement is a 22-item checklist aiming to improve the reporting of studies developing, validating, or updating a prediction model, whether for diagnostic or prognostic purposes [24,28].

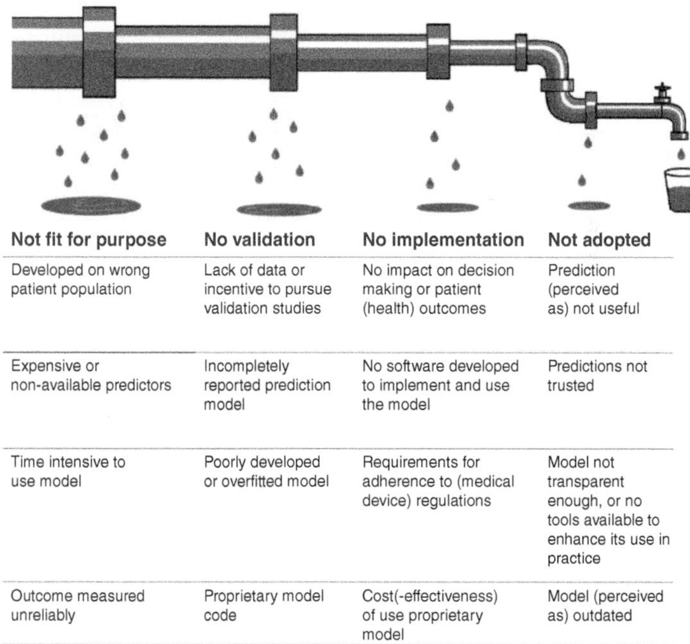

Not fit for purpose	No validation	No implementation	Not adopted
Developed on wrong patient population	Lack of data or incentive to pursue validation studies	No impact on decision making or patient (health) outcomes	Prediction (perceived as) not useful
Expensive or non-available predictors	Incompletely reported prediction model	No software developed to implement and use the model	Predictions not trusted
Time intensive to use model	Poorly developed or overfitted model	Requirements for adherence to (medical device) regulations	Model not transparent enough, or no tools available to enhance its use in practice
Outcome measured unreliably	Proprietary model code	Cost(-effectiveness) of use proprietary model	Model (perceived as) outdated

Figure 8.5 Leaky prognostic model adoption pipeline. Examples of reasons for failed prediction model adoption in clinical practice. *Source:* reproduced from van Royen et al. [27] with permission of the European Respiratory Society.

The PROGRESS (PROGnosis RESearch Strategy) framework classifies prognosis research into four main types of study (see https://www.prognosisresearch.com/progress-framework): (i) overall prognosis research (studies that summarise the average risk of an outcome, such as death, or expected value of an outcome, such as a pain score, among people with the health condition of interest in a particular healthcare setting.) [29]; (ii) prognostic factor research (studies that identify factors whose values or levels are associated with changes in the outcome's risk or expected value.) [30]; (iii) prognostic model research (studies that develop, validate or assess the impact of a prognostic model to predict an individual's outcome risk or expected outcome value using combinations of prognostic factors.) [31]; and, (iv) predictors of treatment effect research (studies that identify how to tailor treatment decisions for individual patients according to whether they are likely to benefit from particular treatments) [32]. If you are interested in prognosis research, you might want to read the excellent book by Richard Riley and colleagues [33].

For examples of how clinical prediction rules can help us work through some of the knottiest diagnostic challenges in health care, see these papers: how to predict whether a head-injured child should be sent for a computed tomography (CT) scan, Maguire et al. [34]; whether someone with early arthritis is developing rheumatoid arthritis, Kuriya et al. [35]; and which combinations of tests best predict whether an acutely ill child has anything serious wrong with him or her, Verbakel et al. [36]. A paper in the JAMA series 'Users' Guides to the Medical Literature' addresses clinical prediction rules [37].

Exercises based on this chapter

1. Think about the last diagnostic test you used on a patient (or, if you prefer, the last one you had yourself). Search the literature for evidence on that test. What is its sensitivity, specificity, positive predictive value and negative predictive value? What is its overall accuracy? Did you interpret the test result as definitive – and have you now changed your mind?
2. Using the results of the previous exercise, design a leaflet or website to explain to patients what your chosen test is and how it might mislead them.
3. Search the literature for a clinical prediction rule on a topic you are interested in. Would you actually use this rule in practice? If not, why not? Why do you think clinicians are not currently using it?
4. Cardiac screening for athletes is a hot topic in sports medicine, and is contested. In Italy, everyone who wants to participate in competitive sports must have their heart screened; do you agree with this? If so, what

are the risks and benefits? Are you concerned about overdiagnosis and over-treatment? Would this type of screening be practical in your setting?

5. You may have self-tested for COVID-19 during the pandemic with a lateral flow test and wondered how accurate such tests are compared with sending a swab to the laboratory for polymerase chain reaction (PCR) testing. Review the paper by Leber et al. 'Comparing the diagnostic accuracy of point-of-care lateral flow antigen testing for SARS-CoV-2 with RT-PCR in primary care (REAP-2)' [38]. What is the sensitivity, specificity, positive predictive value and negative predictive value of the point-of-care lateral flow antigen test? How does the overall accuracy of these two tests compare?

References

1. National Institute for Health and Care Excellence. When should I suspect type 2 diabetes in adults? Clinical Knowledge Summaries. https://cks.nice.org.uk/topics/diabetes-type-2/diagnosis/diagnosis-in-adults (accessed 9 September 2023).
2. World Health Organization. *Definition and Diagnosis of Diabetes Mellitus and Intermediate Hyperglycaemia: Report of a WHO/IDF consultation*. Geneva: WHO; 2006.
3. World Health Organization. *Use of Glycated Haemoglobin (Hba1c) in Diagnosis of Diabetes Mellitus: Abbreviated report of a WHO consultation*. Geneva: WHO; 2011.
4. Wei OY, Teece S. Urine dipsticks in screening for diabetes mellitus. *Emergency Medicine Journal* 2006; **23**: 138.
5. Andersson D k. g., Lundblad E, Svärdsudd K. A model for early diagnosis of type 2 diabetes mellitus in primary health care. *Diabetic Medicine* 1993; **10**: 167–73.
6. Friderichsen B, Maunsbach M. Glycosuric tests should not be employed in population screenings for NIDDM. *Journal of Public Health* 1997; **19**: 55–60.
7. Lu ZX, Walker KZ, O'Dea K, et al. A1C for screening and diagnosis of type 2 diabetes in routine clinical practice. *Diabetes Care* 2010; **33**: 817–19.
8. Barry E, Roberts S, Oke J, et al. Efficacy and effectiveness of screen and treat policies in prevention of type 2 diabetes: systematic review and meta-analysis of screening tests and interventions. *BMJ* 2017; **356**: i6538.
9. Guyatt G, Sackett D, Haynes B. Evaluating diagnostic tests. In: Haynes RB, Sackett DL, Guyatt GH, *et al.*, eds. *Clinical Epidemiology: How to do clinical practice research*. Philadelphia, PA: Lippincott Williams & Wilkins; 2006.
10. Deeks JJ, Bossuyt PM, Leeflang MM, Takwoingi Y (eds). *Cochrane Handbook for Systematic Reviews of Diagnostic Test Accuracy*. Chichester: Wiley; 2023.
11. Lucas NP, Macaskill P, Irwig L, et al. The development of a quality appraisal tool for studies of diagnostic reliability (QAREL). *Journal of Clinical Epidemiology* 2010; **63**: 854–61.

12. Whiting PF, Rutjes AWS, Westwood ME, et al. QUADAS-2: A revised tool for the quality assessment of diagnostic accuracy studies. *Annals of Internal Medicine* 2011; **155**: 529–36.
13. Lee J, Mulder F, Leeflang M, et al. QUAPAS: An adaptation of the QUADAS-2 tool to assess prognostic accuracy studies. *Annals of Internal Medicine* 2022; **175**: 1010–18.
14. Bossuyt PM, Reitsma JB, Bruns DE, et al. STARD 2015: an updated list of essential items for reporting diagnostic accuracy studies. *BMJ* 2015; **351**: h5527.
15. Lu Y, Dendukuri N, Schiller I, *et al.* A Bayesian approach to simultaneously adjusting for verification and reference standard bias in diagnostic test studies. *Statistics in Medicine.* 2010; **29**: 2532–43.
16. Altman DG, Machin D, Bryant TN, et al., eds. *Statistics with Confidence: Cconfidence intervals and statistical guidelines.* 2nd edn. London: BMJ Books; 2011.
17. Stergiou GS, Parati G, McManus RJ, et al. Guidelines for blood pressure measurement: development over 30 years. *Journal of Clinical Hypertension (Greenwich)* 2018; **20**: 1089–91.
18. Qaseem A, Barry MJ, Denberg TD, et al. Screening for prostate cancer: a guidance statement from the Clinical Guidelines Committee of the American College of Physicians. *Annals of Internal Medicine* 2013; **158**: 761–9.
19. Guyatt GH, Patterson C, Ali M, et al. Diagnosis of iron-deficiency anemia in the elderly. *American Journal of Medicine* 1990; **88**: 205–9.
20. Fagan T. Nomogram for Bayes's theorem. *New England Journal of Medicine.* 1975; **293**: 257.
21. National Institute for Health and Care Excellence. *Breast Cancer.* Quality Standard QS12. London: NICE; 2016. https://www.nice.org.uk/Guidance/QS12 (accessed 4 December 2023).
22. Steyerberg EW. Introduction. In: Steyerberg EW, ed. *Clinical Prediction Models: A practical approach to development, validation, and updating.* Cham, Switzerland: Springer; 2019. pp. 1–11.
23. Smeden M van, Reitsma JB, Riley RD, et al. Clinical prediction models: diagnosis versus prognosis. *Journal of Clinical Epidemiology* 2021; **132**: 142–5.
24. Moons KGM, Altman DG, Reitsma JB, et al. Transparent Reporting of a multivariable prediction model for Individual Prognosis Or Diagnosis (TRIPOD): explanation and Eeaboration. *Annals of Internal Medicine* 2015; **162**: W1.
25. Geersing GJ, Zuithoff NPA, Kearon C, et al. Exclusion of deep vein thrombosis using the Wells rule in clinically important subgroups: individual patient data meta-analysis. *BMJ* 2014; **348**: g1340.
26. Koning NR, Büchner FL, Vermeiren RRJM, et al. Identification of children at risk for mental health problems in primary care: development of a prediction model with routine health care data. *eClinicalMedicine* 2019; **15**: 89–97.
27. van Royen FS, Moons KGM, Geersing G-J, et al. Developing, validating, updating and judging the impact of prognostic models for respiratory diseases. *European Respiratory Journal* 2022; **60**: 2200250.

28. Collins GS, Reitsma JB, Altman DG, et al. Transparent reporting of a multivariable prediction model for individual prognosis or diagnosis (TRIPOD): the TRIPOD statement. *BMJ* 2015; **350**: g7594.
29. Hemingway H, Croft P, Perel P, et al. Prognosis research strategy (PROGRESS) 1: a framework for researching clinical outcomes. *BMJ* 2013; **346**: e5595.
30. Riley RD, Hayden JA, Steyerberg EW, et al. Prognosis Research Strategy (PROGRESS) 2: Prognostic Factor Research. *PLOS Medicine* 2013; **10**: e1001380.
31. Steyerberg EW, Moons KGM, van der Windt DA, et al. Prognosis Research Strategy (PROGRESS) 3: prognostic model research. *PLoS Medicine* 2013; **10**: e1001381.
32. Hingorani AD, van der Windt DA, Riley RD, et al. Prognosis research strategy (PROGRESS) 4: stratified medicine research. *BMJ* 2013; **346**: e5793.
33. Riley RD, van der Windt D, Croft P, eds. *Prognosis Research in Healthcare: Concepts, methods, and impact*. Oxford: Oxford University Press; 2019.
34. Maguire JL, Boutis K, Uleryk EM, et al. Should a head-injured child receive a head ct scan? A systematic review of clinical prediction rules. *Pediatrics* 2009; **124**: e145–54.
35. Kuriya B, Cheng CK, Chen HM, et al. Validation of a prediction rule for development of rheumatoid arthritis in patients with early undifferentiated arthritis. *Annals of the Rheumatic Diseases* 2009; **68**: 1482–5.
36. Verbakel JY, Van den Bruel A, Thompson M, et al. How well do clinical prediction rules perform in identifying serious infections in acutely ill children across an international network of ambulatory care datasets? *BMC Medicine* 2013; **11**: 10.
37. Alba AC, Agoritsas T, Walsh M, et al. Discrimination and calibration of clinical prediction models: users' guides to the medical literature. *JAMA* 2017; **318**: 1377–84.
38. Leber W, Lammel O, Siebenhofer A, et al. Comparing the diagnostic accuracy of point-of-care lateral flow antigen testing for SARS-CoV-2 with RT-PCR in primary care (REAP-2). *EClinicalMedicine* 2021; **38**: 101011.

Chapter 9 Papers that summarise other papers (systematic reviews and meta-analyses)

When is a review systematic?

Remember the essays you used to write when you first started college? You would rummage around the Internet (or mooch round the library), browsing through the indexes of books and journals. When you came across a paragraph that looked relevant, you cut and pasted or copied it out, and if anything you found did not fit in with the theory you were proposing, you left it out. This, more or less, constitutes the *journalistic* review – an overview of research and other articles that have not been identified or analysed in a systematic (i.e. standardised and objective) way. Most journalists get paid according to how much they write rather than how much they read or how critically they process it, which explains why most of the 'new scientific breakthroughs' you read in your newspaper today will probably be discredited before the year is out. A common variant of the journalistic review is the invited review, written when an editor asks one of their friends to pen a piece, and summed up by this fabulous title: 'The invited review? Or, my field, from my standpoint, written by me using only my data and my ideas, and citing only my publications' [1]! (We are here critiquing a certain kind of journalism, and doing so to set up an extreme position from which we will then depart. High-quality investigative journalism is an altogether different art – but that is a topic for a different book).

In contrast, a *systematic review* is an overview of primary studies which:

- contains a statement of objectives, sources and methods
- has been conducted in a way that is explicit, transparent and reproducible, and therefore in itself *original research* (Figure 9.1).

The most enduring and reliable systematic reviews, notably those undertaken by the Cochrane Collaboration (discussed later in this chapter) are periodically updated to incorporate new evidence.

How to Read a Paper: The Basics of Evidence-Based Healthcare, Seventh Edition.
Trisha Greenhalgh and Paul Dijkstra.

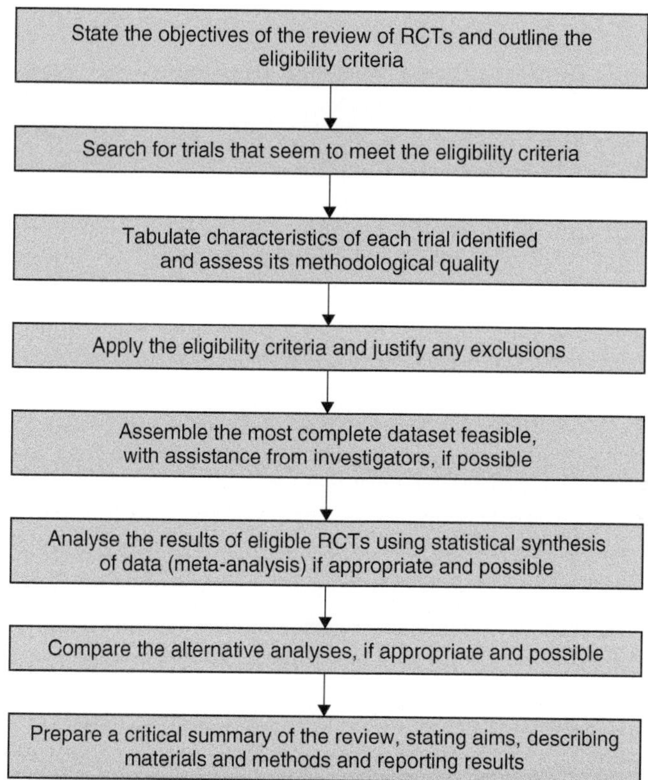

Figure 9.1 Method for a systematic review of randomised controlled trials (RCTs).

As Paul Knipschild observed some years ago, Nobel Prize winner Linus Pauling [2] once published a review, based on selected referencing of the studies that supported his hypothesis, showing that vitamin C cured the common cold. A more objective analysis showed that while one or two studies did indeed suggest an effect, a true estimate based on *all* the available studies suggested that vitamin C had no effect at all on the course of the common cold. Pauling probably did not deliberately intend to deceive his readers, but because his enthusiasm for his espoused cause outweighed his scientific objectivity, he was unaware of the *selection bias* influencing his choice of papers. Evidence shows that if we were to attempt what Pauling did (i.e. hunt through the medical literature for 'evidence' to support our pet theory), we would make an equally idiosyncratic and unscientific job of it [3]. Some advantages of the systematic review are given in Box 9.1.

Experts who have been steeped in a subject for years and know what the answer 'ought' to be were once shown to be significantly less able to produce

Box 9.1 Advantages of systematic reviews [6]

- Explicit methods *limit bias* in identifying and rejecting studies.
- Conclusions are hence more *reliable* and *accurate*.
- Large amounts of *information* can be assimilated quickly by healthcare providers, researchers and policymakers.
- Delay between research discoveries and *implementation* of effective diagnostic and therapeutic strategies is reduced.
- Results of different studies can be formally compared to establish *generalisability* of findings and *consistency* (lack of heterogeneity) of results.
- Reasons for *heterogeneity* (inconsistency in results across studies) can be identified and new hypotheses generated about particular subgroups.
- Quantitative systematic reviews (meta-analyses) increase the *precision* of the overall result (see sections 'Were preliminary statistical questions addressed?' and 'Ten questions to ask about a paper that claims to validate a diagnostic or screening test').

an objective review of the literature in their subject than non-experts [4]. This would have been of little consequence if experts' opinion could be relied upon to be congruent with the results of independent systematic reviews but, at the time, they most certainly couldn't [5]. These condemning studies are still widely quoted by people who would replace all subject experts (such as cardiologists) with search-and-appraisal experts (people who specialise in finding and criticising papers on any subject). But no one in more recent years has replicated the findings. In other words, perhaps we should credit today's experts with more of a tendency to read the systematic reviews in their own topic area. As a general rule, if you want to seek out the best objective evidence of the benefits of (say) different anticoagulants in atrial fibrillation, you should ask someone who is an expert in systematic reviews to work *alongside* an expert in atrial fibrillation.

To be fair to Pauling [2], he did mention a number of trials whose results seriously challenged his theory that vitamin C prevents the common cold. But he described all such trials as 'methodologically flawed'. So were many of the trials that Pauling *did* include in his analysis, but because their results were consistent with Pauling's views, he was, perhaps subconsciously, less critical of weaknesses in their design [7].

We mention this example to illustrate the point that, when undertaking a systematic review, not only must the search for relevant articles be thorough and objective but the criteria used to reject articles as 'flawed' must be explicit and independent of the results of those trials. In other words, you don't discard a trial because all other trials in this area showed something different (see section 'Explaining heterogeneity'); you discard it because, *whatever the results showed*, the trial's objectives or methods did not meet your inclusion criteria and quality standards.

Evaluating systematic reviews: five questions to ask

One of the major developments in evidence-based healthcare since the first edition of this book in 1995 has been the agreement on a standard, structured format for writing up and presenting systematic reviews. The original version of this was called the *QUOROM statement* (equivalent to the CONSORT format for reporting randomised controlled trials discussed in Chapter 6). It was subsequently updated as the Preferred Reporting Items for Systematic Reviews and Meta-Analyses (PRISMA) statement [8], and PRISMA-P for protocols [9]. Following these structured checklists makes systematic reviews and meta-analyses a whole lot easier to find your way around. However, remember that these checklists are designed to guide researchers when they *write* a report of their research; they should not be used uncritically to assess the quality of a published research paper. There is another tool for this task: AMSTAR (A MeaSurement Tool to Assess systematic Reviews) 2, a critical appraisal checklist with 16 items for systematic reviews that include randomised or non-randomised studies of healthcare interventions, or both [10]. If you are keen on systematic review methodology, you may also like to consult the book that systematic reviewers call their 'bible': the *Cochrane Handbook of Systematic Reviews* (but be warned – it's a weighty tome) [11].

Here are some questions based on AMSTAR 2 and PRISMA (greatly shortened and simplified) to ask about any systematic review of quantitative evidence. For qualitative systematic reviews, see Chapter 12.

Question one: What is the important clinical question that the review addressed?

Look back to Chapter 3, in which we explained the importance of defining the question when reading a paper about a clinical trial or other form of primary research. We called this *getting your bearings* because one sure way to be confused about a paper is to fail to ascertain what it is about. The definition of a specific answerable question is, if anything, even more important (and even more frequently omitted!) when preparing an overview of primary studies. If you have ever tried to pull together the findings of a dozen or more clinical papers into an essay, editorial or summary notes for an examination, you will know that it is all too easy to meander into aspects of the topic that you never intended to cover.

The question addressed by a systematic review of quantitative evidence should include components of PICO (population, intervention arm, control arm and outcome), and sometimes a timeframe too (producing the acronym 'PICOT'). The question needs to be defined very precisely, as the reviewer must make a dichotomous (yes/no) decision as to whether each potentially relevant paper will be included or, alternatively, rejected as irrelevant. The question, 'do anticoagulants prevent strokes in patients with atrial fibrillation?' sounds pretty specific, until you start looking through the list of possible studies to include. What kind of anticoagulants? Anticoagulants compared to what? Does 'atrial fibrillation' include both rheumatic and non-rheumatic forms (which are known to be associated with very different risks of stroke)? Does it include intermittent atrial fibrillation? Trisha's grandfather, for example, used to go into this arrhythmia for a few hours on the rare occasions when he drank coffee and would have counted as a 'grey case' in any trial.

Does 'stroke' include both ischaemic stroke (caused by a *blocked* blood vessel in the brain) and haemorrhagic stroke (caused by a *burst* blood vessel)? And, talking of burst blood vessels, shouldn't we be weighing the adverse effects of anticoagulants against their possible benefits? Should the review cover trials on people who have already had a previous stroke or transient ischaemic attack (a mild stroke that gets better within 24 hours) or should it be limited to trials on individuals without these major risk factors for a further stroke? Finally, what about 'high-risk' subpopulations; for example, patients with chronic kidney disease (who are challenging to manage because they are more vulnerable to both thrombotic stroke *and* bleeding complications)? The 'simple' question posed earlier needs to be refined, for example as follows:

> *What is the efficacy, tolerability and safety of different oral anticoagulants, including direct oral anticoagulants and warfarin, in patients with both atrial fibrillation and chronic kidney disease? How do the different anticoagulants compare in this population for prevention of thromboembolic events, bleeding complications, and death from any cause? [12].*

Question two: Was a thorough search carried out of the appropriate database(s) and were other potentially important sources explored?

As Figure 9.1 illustrates, one of the benefits of a systematic review is that, unlike a narrative or journalistic review, the author is required to tell you where the information in it came from and how it was processed. As we explained in Chapter 2, searching the PubMed database for relevant articles is a sophisticated science, and even the best PubMed search will miss important papers. Some additional sources are shown in Box 9.2. The reviewer who seeks a comprehensive set of primary studies must approach the many other databases listed in Chapter 2 (and perhaps others too – ask your librarian).

Box 9.2 Checklist of data sources for a systematic review

- Medline database
- Cochrane Central Register of Controlled Trials (CENTRAL)
- Other medical and paramedical databases
- Non-English language literature
- 'Grey literature' (theses, internal reports, non-peer-reviewed journals, pharmaceutical industry files)
- References (and references of references, etc.) listed in primary sources
- Other unpublished sources known to experts in the field (seek by personal communication)
- Raw data from published trials (seek by personal communication)
- Trial registries (e.g. the US National Institutes of Health List of Registries: https://www.nih.gov/health-information/nih-clinical-research-trials-you/list-registries)

See Chapter 2 for more ideas.

In the search for trials to include in a review, try to avoid linguistic imperialism. As much weight must be given, for example, to the expressions 'Eine Placebo-kontrollierte Doppel-blindstudie' and 'une étude randomisée a double insu face au placebo' as to 'a double-blind RCT' [7], although omission of other-language studies is not, generally, associated with biased results [13]. Furthermore, particularly where a statistical synthesis of results (meta-analysis) is contemplated, it may be necessary to write and ask the authors of the primary studies for data that were not originally included in their published review.

Even when all this has been done, the systematic reviewer's search for material has hardly begun. As Knipschild and colleagues [7] showed when they searched for trials on vitamin C and cold prevention, their electronic databases only gave them 22 of their final total of 61 trials. Another 39 trials were uncovered by hand searching the manual precursor to the Medline database, the *Index Medicus* (14 trials not identified previously), and searching the references of the trials identified in Medline (15 more trials), the references of the references (9 further trials) and the references of the references of the references (one additional trial not identified by any of the previous searches).

Don't be too hard on a reviewer, however, if they have not followed this counsel of perfection to the letter. Knipschild et al.'s additional papers from lesser-known databases added little to the overall synthesis. There is growing evidence that most high-quality studies can be identified by searching a limited number of databases [14] and by 'citation chaining' studies that are seminal in the field [15]. Indeed, growing evidence that exhaustive searching tends to produce diminished returns (not to mention exhausted reviewers) has informed the new science of 'rapid systematic review', defined as 'a form of knowledge synthesis in which components of the systematic review process are simplified or omitted to produce information in a timely manner' [16].

The COVID-19 pandemic exposed several problems with systematic reviews [17], including time to complete a systematic review (on average 67.3 weeks [18]). This was clearly too long to produce timely evidence to guide decision-making in a global emergency. For this reason, the science of *rapid reviews* progressed apace during the pandemic and more than 3000 such reviews were produced on aspects of COVID-19 [19]. Note that a rapid systematic review is not the same as a random, half-hearted review. Like all systematic reviews, rapid reviews must use rigorous and transparent methods but, to achieve an appropriate trade-off with timeliness, they are allowed to leave some stones unturned. The question of how to make these trade-offs without compromising quality is disputed, as illustrated by a paper advocating 'for rapid reviews to be described as what they truly are, restricted reviews or partial systematic reviews' [20]. The Cochrane Collaboration has a methods group devoted to rapid systematic reviews [21].

Question three: Was risk of bias of individual studies assessed and the studies weighted accordingly?

Chapters 3 and 4 and Appendix 1 provide some checklists for assessing whether a paper should be rejected outright on methodological grounds. But given that only around 1% of clinical trials are said to be beyond criticism methodologically [22], the practical question is how to ensure that a 'small but perfectly formed' study is given the weight it deserves in relation to a larger study whose methods are adequate but more open to criticism. As the PRISMA statement emphasises, the key question is the extent to which the methodological flaws are likely to have *biased* the review's findings [8]. The term *quality assessment* refers to the 'measurement of the extent that methodological safeguards against bias have been implemented', while *risk-of-bias assessment* refers to 'bias judgments based on such quality assessment' [23]. You can read more about the differences between quality- and risk-of-bias assessment in Kamper et al. [24] and Büttner et al. [25,26].

Methodological shortcomings that invalidate the results of trials are often generic (i.e. they are independent of the subject matter of the study; see Appendix 1), but there may also be certain methodological features that distinguish between good, medium and poor quality in a particular field. Hence, one of the tasks of a systematic reviewer is to draw up a list of criteria, including both generic and particular aspects of risk of bias, against which to judge each trial. In theory, a composite numerical score could be calculated which would reflect 'overall risk of bias'. In reality, however, care should be taken in developing such scores as there is no gold standard for the 'true' risk of bias of a trial and such composite scores may prove neither valid nor reliable in practice. If you are interested in reading more about the science of developing and applying risk of bias criteria to studies as part of a systematic review, see the latest edition of the *Cochrane Reviewers' Handbook* [11]. A study by Niederer and co-authors illuminates how, in chronic low back pain, the effects of exercise trials at high risk of bias may be overestimated or underestimated [27]. After the authors accounted for risk of bias, they concluded that 'motor control and stabilisation exercises may represent the most effective exercise therapies for chronic low back pain' [27].

Question four: How sensitive are the results to the way the review has been performed?
If you don't understand what this question means, look up the tongue-in-cheek paper by Counsell and colleagues [28] some years ago in the *BMJ*, which 'proved' an entirely spurious relationship between the result of shaking a dice and the outcome of an acute stroke. The authors report a series of artificial dice-rolling experiments in which red, white and green dice, respectively, represented different therapies for acute stroke.

Overall, the 'trials' showed no significant benefit from the three therapies. However, the simulation of a number of perfectly plausible events in the process of meta-analysis, such as the exclusion of several of the 'negative' trials through publication bias (see subsection 'Sources of bias in randomised controlled trials' in Chapter 4), a subgroup analysis that excluded data on red dice therapy (because, on looking back at the results, red dice appeared to be harmful) and other, essentially arbitrary, exclusions on the grounds of 'methodological quality' led to an apparently highly significant benefit of 'dice therapy' in acute stroke.

You cannot, of course, cure anyone of a stroke by rolling a dice, but if these simulated results pertained to a genuine medical controversy (such as which postmenopausal women would be best advised to take hormone replacement therapy or whether breech babies should routinely be delivered by caesarean section), how would you spot these subtle biases? The answer is you need to work through the what-ifs. What if the authors of the systematic review had changed the inclusion criteria? What if they had excluded unpublished studies? What if their 'risk of bias weightings' had been assigned differently? What if trials of higher overall risk of bias had been included (or excluded)? What if all the unaccounted-for patients in a trial were assumed to have died (or been cured)?

An exploration of what-ifs is known as a *sensitivity analysis*. If you find that fiddling with the data like this in various ways makes little or no difference to the review's overall results, you can assume that the review's conclusions are relatively robust. If, however, the key findings disappear when any of the what-ifs changes, the conclusions should be expressed far more cautiously and you should hesitate before changing your practice in the light of them. For more on sensitivity analysis, see the *Cochrane Handbook*.

Question five: Have the numerical results been interpreted with common sense and due regard to the broader aspects of the problem?
As the next section shows, it is easy to be phased by the figures and graphs in a systematic review. But any numerical result, however precise, accurate, 'significant' or otherwise incontrovertible, must be placed in the context of the painfully simple and (often) frustratingly general question that the review addressed. The clinician must decide how (if at all) this numerical result, *whether significant or not*, should influence the care of an individual patient.

A particularly important feature to consider when undertaking or appraising a systematic review is the external validity of included trials (Box 9.3). A trial may be of high methodological quality (and low risk of overall bias) and have a precise and numerically impressive result but it may, for example, have been conducted on participants under the age of 60, and hence may not apply at all to people over 75 for good physiological reasons. The inclusion in systematic reviews of irrelevant studies is guaranteed to lead to absurdities and reduce the credibility of secondary research.

Box 9.3 Assigning weight to trials in a systematic review

Each trial should be evaluated in terms of its:

- *risk of bias* – that is, extent to which the design and conduct are likely to have prevented systematic errors (see section 'Was systematic bias avoided or minimised?');
- *precision* – that is, a measure of the likelihood of random errors (usually depicted as the width of the confidence interval around the result);
- *external validity* – that is, the extent to which the results are generalisable or applicable to a particular target population.

Additional aspects of 'quality' such as scientific importance, clinical importance and literary quality are rightly given great weight by peer reviewers and journal editors, but are less relevant to the systematic reviewer once the question to be addressed has been defined.

Meta-analysis for the non-statistician

If we had to pick one term that exemplifies the fear and loathing felt by so many students, clinicians and consumers towards evidence-based healthcare, that word would be 'meta-analysis'. The meta-analysis, defined as *a statistical synthesis of the numerical results of several trials that all addressed the same question*, is the statisticians' chance to pull a double whammy on you. First, they frighten you with all the statistical tests in the individual papers, and then they use a whole new battery of tests to produce a new set of odds ratios, confidence intervals and values for significance.

As we confessed in Chapter 5, we too tend to go into panic mode at the sight of ratios, square root signs and half-forgotten Greek letters. But before you consign meta-analysis to the set of specialised techniques that you will never understand, remember two things. First, the meta-analyst may wear an anorak but they are *on your side*. A good meta-analysis is often easier for the non-statistician to understand than the stack of primary research papers from which it was derived, for reasons we are about to explain. Second, the underlying statistical principles used for meta-analysis are the same as the ones for any other data analysis – it's just that some of the numbers are bigger.

The first task of the meta-analyst, after following the preliminary steps for systematic review in Figure 9.1, is to decide which of all the various outcome measures chosen by the authors of the primary studies is the best one (or ones) to use in the overall synthesis. In trials of a particular chemotherapy regimen for pancreatic cancer, for example, some authors will have published cumulative mortality figures (i.e. the total number of people who have died to date) at cut-off points of 3 and 12 months, whereas other trials will have published 6-month, 12-month and 5-year cumulative mortality. Some authors will report on time to death, perhaps as hazard ratio or median. The meta-analyst might decide to concentrate on 12-month mortality because this result can be easily extracted from all the papers. They may, however, decide that 3-month mortality is a clinically important end-point, and would need to write to the authors of the remaining trials asking for the raw data from which to calculate these figures.

In addition to crunching the numbers, part of the meta-analyst's job description is to tabulate relevant information on the inclusion criteria, sample size, baseline patient characteristics, withdrawal ('drop-out') rate and results of primary and secondary end-points of all the studies included. If this task has been performed properly, you will be able to compare both the methods and the results of several trials whose authors wrote up their research in different ways. Although such tables are often visually daunting, they save you having to plough through the methods sections of each paper and compare one author's tabulated results with another author's pie chart or histogram.

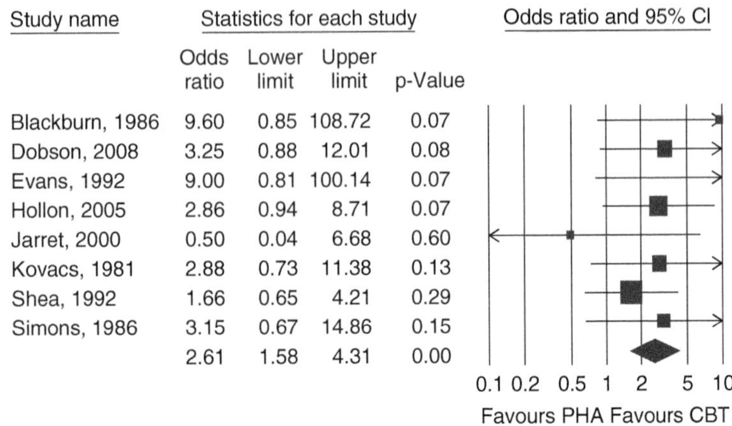

Study name	Odds ratio	Lower limit	Upper limit	p-Value
Blackburn, 1986	9.60	0.85	108.72	0.07
Dobson, 2008	3.25	0.88	12.01	0.08
Evans, 1992	9.00	0.81	100.14	0.07
Hollon, 2005	2.86	0.94	8.71	0.07
Jarret, 2000	0.50	0.04	6.68	0.60
Kovacs, 1981	2.88	0.73	11.38	0.13
Shea, 1992	1.66	0.65	4.21	0.29
Simons, 1986	3.15	0.67	14.86	0.15
	2.61	1.58	4.31	0.00

Figure 9.2 Forest plot showing long-term effects of cognitive behaviour therapy (CBT) compared with no active treatment and discontinuation of pharmacotherapy (PHA). *Source:* Cuijpers et al. [30]. Reproduced with permission from BMJ Publishing Group Ltd. (Nowadays, most Forest plots have only one vertical line, making them easier to interpret.)

These days, the results of meta-analyses tend to be presented in a fairly standard form. This is partly because meta-analysts often use computer software to do the calculations for them (see the latest edition of the Cochrane Reviewers' handbook for an up-to-date menu of options [11]) and most such software packages include a standard graphics tool that presents results as illustrated in Figure 9.2. We have reproduced (with the authors' permission) this pictorial representation (colloquially known as a *forest plot*; the typical plot looks like a forest of lines [29]) of the pooled odds ratios of eight RCTs of therapy for depression. Each of these eight studies had compared a group receiving cognitive behavioural therapy (CBT) with a control group that received no active treatment and in whom pharmacotherapy (PHA, i.e. drug treatment) was discontinued [30]. The primary (main) outcome in this meta-analysis was relapse within 1 year.

The eight trials, each represented by the surname of the first author and the year that paper was published (e.g. 'Blackburn 1986') are listed, one below the other on the left hand side of the figure. The horizontal line corresponding to each trial shows the likelihood of relapse by 1 year in patients randomised to CBT compared with patients randomised to PHA. The 'blob' in the middle of each line is the point estimate of the difference between the groups (the best single estimate of the benefit in improved relapse rate by offering CBT rather than PHA) and the width of the line represents the 95% confidence interval of this estimate (see section 'Have confidence intervals been calculated, and do the authors' conclusions reflect them?'). The key vertical line to look at, known as the *line of no difference*, is the one marking the odds ratio (OR) of 1.0. Note that if the horizontal line for any trial does not cross the line of no difference, there is a 95% chance that there is a 'real' difference between the groups.

As we argued in Chapter 5, if the confidence interval of the result (the horizontal line) *does* cross the line of no difference (i.e. the vertical line at OR = 1.0), that can mean *either* that there is no significant difference between the treatments, *and/or* that the sample size was too small to allow us to be confident about whether there was a beneficial or harmful difference between the treatments. The various individual studies give point estimates of the odds ratio of CBT compared with PHA (of between 0.5 and 9.6), and the confidence intervals of some studies are so wide that they don't even fit on the graph, hence the arrows at their left or right end.

Now, here comes the fun of meta-analysis. Look at the tiny diamond below all the horizontal lines. This represents the *pooled* data from all eight trials (overall OR CBT : PHA = 2.61, meaning that CBT has 2.61 times the odds of preventing relapse compared with PHA), with a new, much narrower, confidence interval of this OR (1.58–4.31). Because the diamond does not overlap the line of no difference, we can say that there is a statistically significant difference between the two treatments in terms of the primary end-point (relapse of depression in the first year). Now, in this example, seven of the eight trials suggested a benefit from CBT, but in none of them was the sample size large enough for that finding to be statistically significant.

Note, however, that this neat little diamond does *not* mean that you should offer CBT to every patient with depression. It has a much more limited meaning – that the *average* patient in the trials presented in this meta-analysis is likely to benefit in terms of the primary outcome (relapse of depression within a year) if they receive CBT instead of PHA. The choice of treatment should, of course, take into account how the patient feels about embarking on a course of CBT (see Chapter 16) and also on the relative merits of this therapy compared to *other* treatments for depression. The paper from which Figure 9.2 is taken also described a second meta-analysis that showed no significant difference between CBT and continuing antidepressant therapy, suggesting, perhaps, that patients who *prefer* not to have CBT may do just as well by continuing to take their tablets [30].

As this example shows, 'non-significant' trials (i.e. ones that, on their own, did not demonstrate a significant difference between treatment and control groups) often make an important contribution to a pooled result in a meta-analysis that *is* statistically significant. The most famous example of this, which the Cochrane Collaboration adopted as its logo (Figure 9.3), is the meta-analysis of seven trials of the effect of giving steroids to mothers who were

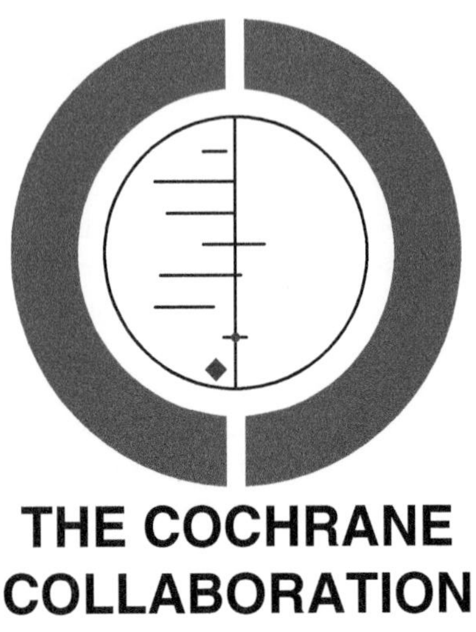

Figure 9.3 Cochrane Collaboration logo.

expected to give birth prematurely [31]. Only two of the seven trials showed a statistically significant benefit (in terms of survival of the infant), but the improvement in precision (i.e. the narrowing of confidence intervals) in the pooled results, shown by the narrower width of the diamond compared with the individual lines, demonstrates the strength of the evidence in favour of this intervention. This meta-analysis showed that infants of steroid-treated mothers were 30–50% less likely to die than infants of mothers in the control group. This example is discussed further in section 'Why are health professionals slow to adopt evidence-based practice?' in relation to changing clinicians' behaviour.

You may have worked out by now that anyone who is thinking about doing a clinical trial of an intervention should first do a systematic review, with a meta-analysis if possible, of all the previous trials on that same intervention. In practice, researchers only occasionally do this [32]. This was graphically illustrated when Dean Fergusson and colleagues of the Ottawa Health Research Institute published a cumulative meta-analysis of all RCTs carried out on the drug aprotinin in perioperative bleeding during cardiac surgery [33]. They lined up the trials in the order they had been published and worked out what a meta-analysis of 'all trials done so far' would have shown (had it been performed at the time). The resulting *cumulative meta-analysis* had shocking news for the research communities. The beneficial effect of aprotinin reached statistical significance after only 12 trials (i.e. back in 1992). But because nobody did a meta-analysis at the time, a further 52 clinical trials were undertaken. All these trials were scientifically unnecessary and hence, strictly speaking, unethical (because half the patients were denied a drug that had been proved to improve outcome). Figure 9.4 illustrates this waste of effort.

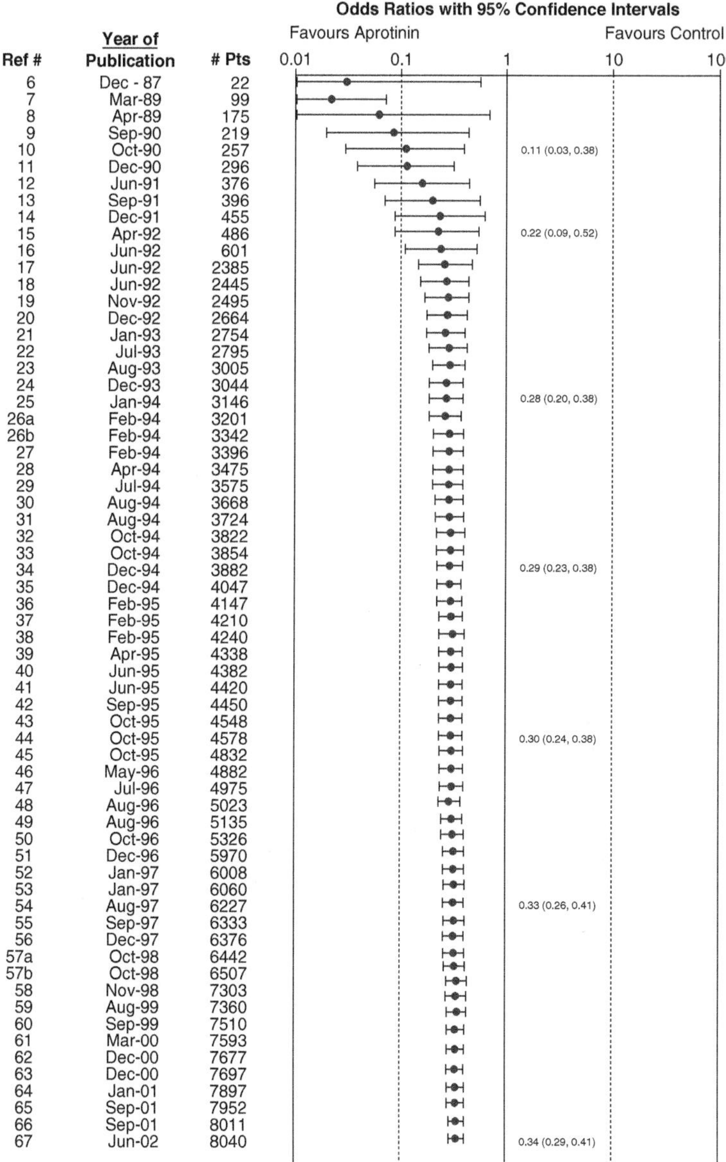

Figure 9.4 Cumulative meta-analysis of randomised controlled trials of aprotinin in cardiac surgery [33]. *Source:* Reproduced from [33] / with permission of Sage Publications.

If you have followed the arguments on meta-analysis of published trial results this far, you might like to read up on the more sophisticated technique of meta-analysis of individual participant data, which provides a more accurate and precise figure for the point estimate of effect [34] and the PRISMA for Individual Participant Data statement [35]. You might also be interested to read up on network meta-analysis: meta-analysis of multiple interventions (instead of the traditional meta-analysis of two interventions at a time) [36].

Explaining heterogeneity

In everyday language, 'homogeneous' means 'of uniform composition' and 'heterogeneous' means 'many different ingredients'. In the language of meta-analysis, homogeneity means that the results of each individual trial are compatible with the results of any of the others. Homogeneity can be estimated at a glance once the trial results have been presented in the format illustrated in Figures 9.2 and 9.5. In Figure 9.2, the lower confidence interval of every trial is below the upper confidence interval of all the others (i.e. the horizontal lines all overlap to some extent). Statistically speaking, the trials could be homogeneous (although not necessarily as the overlap could be minimal). Conversely, in Figure 9.5, there are some trials whose lower confidence interval is above the upper confidence interval of one or more other trials (i.e. some lines do not overlap at all). These trials may be said to be heterogeneous.

You may have spotted by now that declaring a set of trials heterogeneous on the basis of whether their confidence intervals overlap is somewhat arbitrary, as the confidence interval itself is arbitrary (it can be set at 90%, 95%, 99% or indeed any other value). The definitive test involves a slightly more sophisticated statistical manoeuvre than holding a ruler up against the forest plot. Two commonly used statistical manoeuvres are: (1) the I^2; and (2) a variant of the chi-square (χ^2) test (see Chapter 5, Table 5.1), as the question addressed is, 'Is there greater variation between the results of the trials than is compatible with the play of chance?'.

I^2, a value between 0% and 100%, describes the percentage of total variation across studies that is due to heterogeneity rather than chance [37]; larger values indicate higher heterogeneity (25% = low; 50% = moderate; 75% = high). I^2 is simple to calculate and its interpretation is intuitive [37]. I^2 can be calculated and compared across meta-analyses of different sizes, of different types of study and using different types of outcome data (e.g. dichotomous, quantitative or time to event) [37].

The χ^2 statistic for heterogeneity is explained in more detail by Thompson [38,39], who offers the following useful rule of thumb: a χ^2

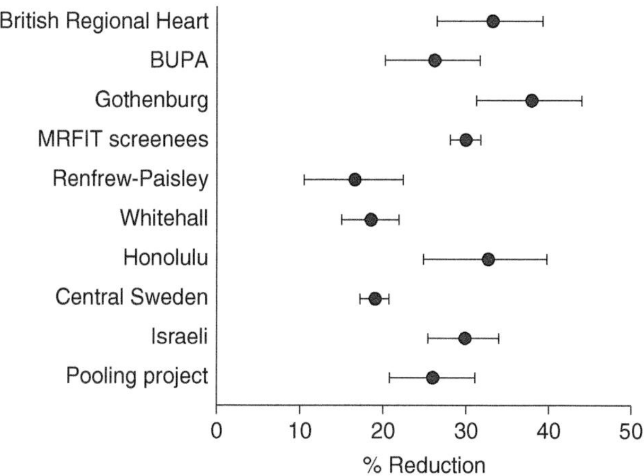

Figure 9.5 Reduction in heart disease risk by cholesterol-lowering strategies. *Source:* Thompson [39]. Reproduced with permission of Wiley.

statistic has, on average, a value equal to its degrees of freedom (in this case, the number of trials in the meta-analysis minus one), so a χ^2 of 7.0 for a set of eight trials would provide no evidence of statistical heterogeneity. In fact, it would not prove that the trials were homogeneous either, particularly because the χ^2 test has low power (see section 'Were preliminary statistical questions addressed?') to detect small but important levels of heterogeneity.

A χ^2 value much greater than the number of trials in a meta-analysis tells us that the trials that contributed to the analysis are different in some important way from one another. There may, for example, be known differences in method (e.g. authors may have used different questionnaires to assess the symptoms of depression) or known clinical differences in the trial participants (e.g. one centre might have been a tertiary referral hospital to which all the sickest patients were referred). There may, however, be unknown or unrecorded differences between the trials which the meta-analyst can only speculate upon until they have extracted further details from the trials' authors. Remember: demonstrating statistical heterogeneity is a mathematical exercise and is the job of the statistician, but *explaining* this heterogeneity (i.e. looking for, and accounting for, *clinical* heterogeneity) is an interpretive exercise and requires imagination, common sense and hands-on clinical or research experience.

Figure 9.5, which is reproduced with permission from Thompson's [39] chapter on the subject, shows the results of 10 trials of cholesterol-lowering strategies. The results are expressed as the percentage reduction in heart disease risk associated with each 0.6 mmol/l reduction in serum cholesterol level. The horizontal lines represent the 95% confidence intervals of each result, and it is clear, even without being told the χ^2 statistic of 127, that the trials are highly heterogeneous.

To simply 'average out' the results of the trials in Figure 9.5 would be very misleading. The meta-analyst must return to their primary sources and ask, 'In what way was trial A different from trial B, and what do trials E, F and H have in common which makes their results cluster at one extreme of the figure?' In this example, a correction for the age of the trial participants reduced χ^2 from 127 to 45. In other words, most of the 'incompatibility' in the results of these trials can be explained by the fact that embarking on a strategy (such as a special diet) that successfully reduces your cholesterol level will be substantially more likely to prevent a heart attack if you are 45 than if you are 85.

This, essentially, is the essence of the grievance of Professor Hans Eysenck [40], who has constructed a vigorous and entertaining critique of the science of meta-analysis. In a world of lumpers and splitters, Eysenck is a splitter, and it offends his sense of the qualitative and the particular (see Chapter 12) to combine the results of studies that were performed on different populations in different places at different times and for different reasons.

Eysenck's reservations about meta-analysis are borne out in the infamously discredited meta-analysis that demonstrated (wrongly) that there was significant benefit to be had from giving intravenous magnesium to heart attack victims. A subsequent megatrial involving 58 000 patients (ISIS-4) failed to find any benefit whatsoever, and the meta-analysts' misleading conclusions were subsequently explained in terms of publication bias, methodological weaknesses in the smaller trials and clinical heterogeneity [41,42]. (Incidentally, for more debate on the pros and cons of meta-analysis versus megatrials, see Hennekens and Demets [43].)

Trisha once took on the question of heterogeneity with Simon Griffin [44], who had published a meta-analysis of primary studies into the management of diabetes by primary health care teams. Although Trisha has a high regard for Simon as a scientist, she felt that he had not been justified in performing a mathematical summation of what she believed were very different studies, which had all addressed slightly different questions. As Trisha said in her commentary on his article, 'four apples and five oranges make four apples and five oranges, not nine apple-oranges' [45]. But Simon numbers himself among the lumpers, and some scholars have argued that he was entirely correct to analyse his data as he did. Debates will no doubt continue between 'lumpers' and 'splitters'.

New approaches to systematic review

This chapter has addressed the most commonly used approach to systematic review: synthesising trials of therapy. If you are comfortable with that, you might like to start exploring the literature on more challenging forms of systematic review, such as diagnostic studies [46,47] and the emerging science of systematic review of qualitative research, for which a brand-new series was published in 2018 in the *Journal of Clinical Epidemiology* [48–53] and the enticing idea of 'living systematic reviews' (a sort of wiki approach in which the review is never declared finished but is placed on the Internet and updated in an ongoing way) [54]. You might be interested in systematic reviews and meta-analysis of prognosis research studies [55,56] or studies on causation [57]. See also our brief mention of rapid systematic reviews under question 4 above, and *Evidence Aid* (https://evidenceaid.org) a not-for-profit organisation that provides summaries of systematic reviews (on topics like earthquakes, health of refugees and asylum seekers, managing mental injuries in disasters, COVID-19, Zika, and Ebola) to decision-makers [58].

Trisha and colleagues have developed new approaches to systematic review, known as realist and meta-narrative review [59,60], which highlight and explore (rather than attempt to 'average out') the fundamental differences between primary studies – an approach that we think is particularly useful for developing systematic reviews in health care policymaking. But these relatively small-print applications are all beyond the basics, and if you are reading this book to get you through a medical exam, you will probably find that they aren't on the syllabus.

If you found yourself sympathising with Professor Eysenck in the previous section, you might like to look at some other theoretical critiques of systematic review. Trisha co-authored a paper arguing for the advantages of narrative review over conventional systematic review, especially when the key task is to illuminate and make sense of the literature on a very broad topic area (as opposed to synthesising data on a very narrow topic) [61]. But we shouldn't throw the baby out with the bath water. The kind of systematic review recommended by the Cochrane Collaboration, in its place, saves lives.

Finally, a few words on using automated tools or artificial intelligence (AI) to assist systematic reviewers. This fast-moving area will no doubt change dramatically between us writing this chapter and you reading it! Using 'systematic review automation tools', a small group of experienced systematic reviewers (with complementary skills and protected time to focus on the systematic review) took 2 weeks to complete a systematic review of the impact of increased fluid intake on recurrence of urinary tract infection (UTI) in individuals at risk for UTIs [62]. However, some of the systematic reviewers of this '2-week systematic review' concurred: 'Not all systematic reviews can be completed in 2 weeks – but many can be (and should be)' [63]. And it seems like, for the majority of systematic review tasks where a systematic review automation tool was used, the time required to complete that task was reduced for novice researchers too, while methodological quality was maintained [64]. When used appropriately, AI tools could also speed up the review process [65]. To facilitate the title and abstract screening process in systematic reviews, an open-source AI tool 'ASReview' was published in 2021 [66] with time-saving potential in simulation studies [67,68]. Active learning models for screening prioritisation could significantly reduce the workload in systematic reviews [67].

Exercises based on this chapter

1. Using the search techniques you read about in Chapter 2, find a systematic review and meta-analysis to answer the following questions. In each case, critically appraise the article(s) you find using the checklist for systematic reviews in Appendix 1 and guided by the questions listed in this chapter.
   a. Does the 'Mediterranean diet' reduce mortality from heart disease?
   b. Should pregnant women with breech presentation be offered planned vaginal delivery or planned elective caesarean section?
   c. Should people with sickle-cell anaemia be given transfusions of normal red blood cells?
2. If you want to learn more about living systematic review and network meta-analysis, have a look at this paper: 'Which treatment is most effective for patients with Achilles tendinopathy? A living systematic review with network meta-analysis of 29 randomised controlled trials' [69]. What is a living systematic review? Discuss why you think this type of systematic review and meta-analysis is appropriate, or not, for the research question: Which treatment is most effective for patients with Achilles tendinopathy?

References

1. Caveman A. The invited review – or, my field, from my standpoint, written by me using only my data and my ideas, and citing only my publications. *Journal of Cell Science* 2000; **113**: 3125–6.
2. Pauling L. *How to live longer and feel better*. New York, NY: WH Freeman; 1986.
3. McAlister FA, Clark HD, van Walraven C, et al. The medical review article revisited: has the science improved? *Annals of Internal Medicine* 1999; **131**: 947–51.
4. Oxman AD, Guyatt GH. The science of reviewing research. *Annals of the New York Academy of Sciences* 1993; **703**: 125–34.
5. Antman EM, Lau J, Kupelnick B, et al. A comparison of results of meta-analyses of randomized control trials and recommendations of clinical experts: treatments for myocardial infarction. *JAMA* 1992; **268**: 240–8.

6. Chalmers I, Altman DG, eds. *Systematic Reviews*. London: BMJ; 1996.
7. Knipschild P. Systematic reviews: some examples. *BMJ* 1994; **309**: 719–21.
8. Moher D, Liberati A, Tetzlaff J, et al. Preferred Reporting Items for Systematic Reviews and Meta-Analyses: The PRISMA statement. *Journal of Clinical Epidemiology* 2009; **62**: 1006–12.
9. Moher D, Shamseer L, Clarke M, et al. Preferred reporting items for systematic review and meta-analysis protocols (PRISMA-P) 2015 statement. *Systematic Reviews* 2015; **4**: 1.
10. Shea BJ, Reeves BC, Wells G, et al. AMSTAR 2: a critical appraisal tool for systematic reviews that include randomised or non-randomised studies of healthcare interventions, or both. *BMJ* 2017; **358**: j4008.
11. Higgins J, Thomas J, Chandler J, et al., eds. *Cochrane Handbook for Systematic Reviews of Interventions*, 2nd edn. Hoboken, NJ: Wiley-Blackwell; 2019.
12. Rhee TM, Lee SR, Choi EK, et al. Efficacy and safety of oral anticoagulants for atrial fibrillation patients with chronic kidney disease: a systematic review and meta-analysis. *Frontiers in Cardiovascular Medicine* 2022 Jun **10**; 9: 885548.
13. Morrison A, Polisena J, Husereau D, et al. The effect of English-language restriction on systematic review-based meta-analyses: a systematic review of empirical studies. *International Journal of Technology Assessment in Health Care* 2012; **28**: 138–44.
14. Hartling L, Featherstone R, Nuspl M, et al. The contribution of databases to the results of systematic reviews: a cross-sectional study. *BMC Medical Research Methodology* 2016; **16**: 127.
15. Greenhalgh T, Peacock R. Effectiveness and efficiency of search methods in systematic reviews of complex evidence: audit of primary sources. *BMJ* 2005; **331**: 1064–5.
16. Tricco AC, Antony J, Zarin W, et al. A scoping review of rapid review methods. *BMC Medicine* 2015; **13**: 224.
17. Evidence-based medicine: how COVID can drive positive change. *Nature* 2021; **593**: 168–168.
18. Borah R, Brown AW, Capers PL, et al. Analysis of the time and workers needed to conduct systematic reviews of medical interventions using data from the PROSPERO registry. *BMJ Open* 2017; **7**: e012545.
19. COVID-19 Evidence Network to support Decision-making. McMaster Health Forum. http://www.mcmasterforum.org/networks/covid-end (accessed 23 November 2023).
20. Munn Z, Pollock D, Barker TH, et al. The dark side of rapid reviews: a retreat from systematic approaches and the need for clear expectations and reporting. *Annals of Internal Medicine* 2023; **176**: 266–7.
21. Garritty C, Stevens A, Gartlehner G, et al. Cochrane Rapid Reviews Methods Group to play a leading role in guiding the production of informed high-quality, timely research evidence syntheses. *Systematic Reviews* 2016; **5**: 184.
22. Pirosca S, Shiely F, Clarke M, et al. Tolerating bad health research: the continuing scandal. *Trials* 2022; **23**: 458.
23. Furuya-Kanamori L, Xu C, Hasan SS, et al. Quality versus risk-of-bias assessment in clinical research. *Journal of Clinical Epidemiology* 2021; **129**: 172–5.

24. Kamper SJ. Risk of bias and study quality assessment: linking evidence to practice. *Journal of Orthopaedic and Sports Physical Therapy* 2020; **50**: 277–9.
25. Büttner F, Winters M, Delahunt E, et al. Identifying the 'incredible'! Part 1: assessing the risk of bias in outcomes included in systematic reviews. *British Journal of Sports Medicine* 2020; **54**: 798–800.
26. Büttner F, Winters M, Delahunt E, et al. Identifying the 'incredible'! Part 2: Spot the difference – a rigorous risk of bias assessment can alter the main findings of a systematic review. *British Journal of Sports Medicine* 2020; **54**: 801–8.
27. Niederer D, Weippert M, Behrens M. What modifies the effect of an exercise treatment for chronic low back pain? A meta-epidemiologic regression analysis of risk of bias and comparative effectiveness. *Journal of Orthopaedic and Sports Physical Therapy* 2022; **52**: 792–802.
28. Counsell CE, Clarke MJ, Slattery J, et al. The miracle of DICE therapy for acute stroke: fact or fictional product of subgroup analysis? *BMJ* 1994; **309**: 1677–81.
29. Lewis S, Clarke M. Forest plots: trying to see the wood and the trees. *BMJ* 2001; **322**: 1479–80.
30. Cuijpers P, Hollon SD, van Straten A, et al. Does cognitive behaviour therapy have an enduring effect that is superior to keeping patients on continuation pharmacotherapy? A meta-analysis. *BMJ Open* 2013; **3**: e002542.
31. Egger M, Higgins JPT, Davey Smith G, eds. *Systematic Reviews in Health Research: Meta-analysis in context*. 3rd edn. Hoboken, NJ: Wiley; 2022.
32. Draborg E, Andreasen J, Nørgaard B, et al. Systematic reviews are rarely used to contextualise new results-a systematic review and meta-analysis of meta-research studies. *Systematic Reviews* 2022; **11**: 189.
33. Fergusson D, Glass KC, Hutton B, et al. Randomized controlled trials of aprotinin in cardiac surgery: could clinical equipoise have stopped the bleeding? *Clinical Trials* 2005; **2**: 218–32.
34. Riley RD, Tierney JF, Stewart LA, eds. *Individual Participant Data Meta-Analysis: A handbook for healthcare research*. Hoboken, NJ: Wiley; 2021.
35. Stewart LA, Clarke M, Rovers M, et al. Preferred Reporting Items for a Systematic Review and Meta-analysis of Individual Participant Data: The PRISMA-IPD statement. *JAMA* 2015; **313**: 1657–65.
36. Hutton B, Salanti G, Caldwell DM, et al. The PRISMA Extension Statement for Reporting of Systematic Reviews Incorporating Network Meta-analyses of Health Care Interventions: checklist and explanations. *Annals of Internal Medicine* 2015; **162**: 777–84.
37. Higgins J, Thompson SG, Deeks JJ, et al. Measuring inconsistency in meta-analyses. *BMJ* 2003; **327**: 557–60.
38. Thompson SG. Why sources of heterogeneity in meta-analysis should be investigated. *BMJ* 1994; **309**: 1351–5.
39. Thompson SG. Why and how sources of heterogeneity should be investigated. In: Egger M, Smith G, Altman DG, eds. *Systematic Reviews in Health Care: Meta-analysis in context*. London: BMJ Books; 2001. pp. 157–75.
40. Eysenck H. Meta-analysis and its problems. *BMJ* 1994; **309**: 789–92.
41. Higgins JPT, Spiegelhalter DJ. Being sceptical about meta-analyses: a Bayesian perspective on magnesium trials in myocardial infarction. *International Journal of Epidemiology* 2002; **31**: 96–104.

42. Egger M, Smith GD. Misleading meta-analysis. *BMJ* 1995; **310**: 752–4.
43. Hennekens CH, Demets D. The need for large-scale randomized evidence without undue emphasis on small trials, meta-analyses, or subgroup analyses. *JAMA* 2009; **302**: 2361–2.
44. Griffin S. Diabetes care in general practice: meta-analysis of randomised control trials. *BMJ* 1998; **317**: 390–6.
45. Greenhalgh T. Commentary: Meta-analysis is a blunt and potentially misleading instrument for analysing models of service delivery. *BMJ* 1998; **317**: 395–6.
46. Deeks JJ, Bossuyt PM, Leeflang MM, Takwoingi Y (eds). *Cochrane Handbook for Systematic Reviews of Diagnostic Test Accuracy*. Chichester: Wiley; 2023.
47. McInnes MDF, Moher D, Thombs BD, et al. Preferred Reporting Items for a Systematic Review and Meta-analysis of Diagnostic Test Accuracy Studies: The PRISMA-DTA statement. *JAMA* 2018; **319**: 388–96.
48. Noyes J, Booth A, Cargo M, et al. Cochrane Qualitative and Implementation Methods Group guidance series-paper 1: introduction. *Journal of Clinical Epidemiology* 2018; **97**: 35–8.
49. Harris JL, Booth A, Cargo M, et al. Cochrane Qualitative and Implementation Methods Group guidance series-paper 2: methods for question formulation, searching, and protocol development for qualitative evidence synthesis. *Journal of Clinical Epidemiology* 2018; **97**: 39–48.
50. Noyes J, Booth A, Flemming K, et al. Cochrane Qualitative and Implementation Methods Group guidance series-paper 3: methods for assessing methodological limitations, data extraction and synthesis, and confidence in synthesized qualitative findings. *Journal of Clinical Epidemiology* 2018; **97**: 49–58.
51. Cargo M, Harris J, Pantoja T, et al. Cochrane Qualitative and Implementation Methods Group guidance series-paper 4: methods for assessing evidence on intervention implementation. *Journal of Clinical Epidemiology* 2018; **97**: 59–69.
52. Harden A, Thomas J, Cargo M, et al. Cochrane Qualitative and Implementation Methods Group guidance series-paper 5: methods for integrating qualitative and implementation evidence within intervention effectiveness reviews. *Journal of Clinical Epidemiology* 2018; **97**: 70–8.
53. Flemming K, Booth A, Hannes K, et al. Cochrane Qualitative and Implementation Methods Group guidance series-paper 6: reporting guidelines for qualitative, implementation, and process evaluation evidence syntheses. *Journal of Clinical Epidemiology* 2018; **97**: 79–85.
54. Elliott JH, Synnot A, Turner T, et al. Living systematic review: 1. Introduction-the why, what, when, and how. *Journal of Clinical Epidemiology* 2017; **91**: 23–30.
55. Riley RD, Moons KGM, Snell KIE, et al. A guide to systematic review and meta-analysis of prognostic factor studies. *BMJ* 2019; **364**: k4597.
56. Damen JAA, Moons KGM, van Smeden M, et al. How to conduct a systematic review and meta-analysis of prognostic model studies. *Clinical Microbiology and Infection* 2023; **29**: 434–40.
57. Khan KS, Ball E, Fox CE, et al. Systematic reviews to evaluate causation: an overview of methods and application. *Evidence-Based Medicine* 2012; **17**: 137–41.
58. Evidence Aid. Evidence Collections Archive. https://evidenceaid.org/evidence (accessed 20 February 2024).

59. Wong G, Greenhalgh T, Westhorp G, et al. RAMESES publication standards: meta-narrative reviews. *BMC Medicine* 2013; **11**: 20.
60. Wong G, Greenhalgh T, Westhorp G, et al. RAMESES publication standards: realist syntheses. *BMC Medicine* 2013; **11**: 21.
61. Greenhalgh T, Thorne S, Malterud K. Time to challenge the spurious hierarchy of systematic over narrative reviews? *European Journal of Clinical Investigation* 2018; **48**.
62. Clark J, Glasziou P, Del Mar C, et al. A full systematic review was completed in 2 weeks using automation tools: a case study. *Journal of Clinicl Epidemiology* 2020; **121**: 81–90.
63. Clark J, Scott AM, Glasziou P. Not all systematic reviews can be completed in 2 weeks: but many can be (and should be). *Journal of Clinical Epidemiology* 2020; **126**: 163.
64. Clark J, McFarlane C, Cleo G, et al. The impact of systematic review automation tools on methodological quality and time taken to complete systematic review tasks: case study. *JMIR Medical Education* 2021; **7**: e24418.
65. van Dijk SHB, Brusse-Keizer MGJ, Bucsán CC, et al. Artificial intelligence in systematic reviews: promising when appropriately used. *BMJ Open* 2023; **13**: e072254.
66. van de Schoot R, de Bruin J, Schram R, et al. An open source machine learning framework for efficient and transparent systematic reviews. *Nature Machine Intelligence* 2021; **3**: 125–33.
67. Ferdinands G, Schram R, de Bruin J, et al. Performance of active learning models for screening prioritization in systematic reviews: a simulation study into the Average Time to Discover relevant records. *Systematic Reviews* 2023; **12**: 100.
68. Ferdinands G. AI-assisted systematic reviewing: selecting studies to compare bayesian versus frequentist SEM for small sample sizes. *Multivariate Behavioral Research* 2021; **56**: 153–4.
69. Vlist AC van der, Winters M, Weir A, et al. Which treatment is most effective for patients with Achilles tendinopathy? A living systematic review with network meta-analysis of 29 randomised controlled trials. *British Journal of Sports Medicine* 2021; **55**: 249–56.

Chapter 10 **Papers that advise you what to do (guidelines)**

The great guidelines debate

Never was the chasm between frontline clinicians and backroom policymakers wider than in their respective attitudes to clinical guidelines. Policymakers (in the broadest sense, including everyone who has a view on how medicine ought to be practised in an ideal world, including politicians, senior managers, clinical directors, academics and teachers) tend to love guidelines. Some frontline clinicians (i.e. people who spend all their time seeing patients) may have a strong aversion to guidelines or, at least, to the kind of guideline that dictates rather than just *advises* what to do in particular circumstances.

Before we carry this controversial topic any further, we need a definition of guidelines, for which the following will suffice:

> *Guidelines are systematically developed statements to assist practitioner decisions about appropriate healthcare for specific clinical circumstances.*

A great paper on evidence-based guidelines (what they are, how they are developed, why we need them and what the controversies are) was written by one of Trisha's ex PhD students, Professor Deborah Swinglehurst [1]. We have drawn on her review in this chapter. One important distinction Deborah makes in her paper is between guidelines (which are usually expressed in terms of general principles and leave room for judgement within broad parameters) and protocols, which she defines as follows: 'Protocols are instructions on what to do in particular circumstances. They are similar to guidelines but include less room for individual judgement, are often produced for less experienced staff, or for use in situations where eventualities are predictable'.

How to Read a Paper: The Basics of Evidence-Based Healthcare, Seventh Edition.
Trisha Greenhalgh and Paul Dijkstra.

Box 10.1 Purpose of guidelines

1 To make evidence-based standards explicit and accessible (but see subsequent text: few guidelines currently in circulation are truly evidence-based).
2 To make decision-making in the clinic and at the bedside easier and more objective.
3 To provide a yardstick for assessing professional performance.
4 To delineate the division of labour (e.g. between GPs and consultants).
5 To educate patients and professionals about current best practice.
6 To improve the cost-effectiveness of health services and reduce waste.
7 To serve as a tool for external control.

The purposes that guidelines serve are given in Box 10.1. Clinician resistance to guidelines has a number of explanations:

- Clinical freedom ('I'm not having anyone telling me how to manage my patients').
- Debates among experts about the quality of evidence ('Well, if they can't agree among themselves . . .').
- Lack of appreciation of evidence by practitioners ('That's all very well, but when I trained we were always taught to hold back on steroids for asthma.').
- Defensive medicine ('I'll check all the tests anyway – belt and braces.').
- Strategic and cost constraints ('We can't afford to replace the equipment.').
- Specific practical constraints ('Where on earth did I put those guidelines?').
- Reluctance of patients to accept procedures ('Mrs Brown insists she needs a cervical smear every year.').
- Competing influences of other non-medical factors ('When we get the new computer system up and running . . .').
- Lack of appropriate, patient-specific feedback on performance ('I seem to be treating this condition OK.').
- Confusion ('The guideline doesn't seem to help me with the problem I'm facing.').

The image of the medical buffoon blundering blithely through the outpatient clinic still diagnosing the same illnesses and prescribing the same drugs they learnt about at medical school 40 years previously and, never having read a paper since, knocks the 'clinical freedom' argument right out of the arena. Such hypothetical situations are grist to the mill of those who would impose 'expert guidelines' on most, if not all, medical practice and hold to account all those who fail to keep in step.

But the counter argument to the excessive use, and particularly the compulsive imposition of clinical guidelines, is a powerful one and it was expressed very eloquently some years ago by the late Professor Sir John Grimley Evans [2]:

> *There is a fear that in the absence of evidence clearly applicable to the case in the hand a clinician might be forced by guidelines to make use of evidence which is only doubtfully relevant, generated perhaps in a different grouping of patients in another country at some other time and using a similar but not identical treatment. This is evidence-biased medicine; it is to use evidence in the manner of the fabled drunkard who searched under the street lamp for his door key because that is where the light was, even though he had dropped the key somewhere else.*

Grimley Evans' fear, which every practising clinician shares but few can articulate, is that politicians and health service managers who have jumped on the evidence-based medicine (EBM) bandwagon will use guidelines to decree the treatment of diseases rather than of patients. They will, it is feared, make judgements about people and their illnesses subservient to published evidence that an intervention is effective 'on average' (this happened to Trisha a few years ago; you can read about it in Greenhalgh [3]. This, and other real and perceived disadvantages of guidelines, are given in Box 10.2 [2]. But if you read the above-mentioned distinction between guidelines and protocols,

Box 10.2 Drawbacks of guidelines (real and perceived)

1 Guidelines may be intellectually suspect and reflect 'expert opinion', which may formalise unsound practice.
2 By reducing medical practice variation, they may standardise to 'average' rather than best practice.
3 They might inhibit innovation and prevent individual cases from being dealt with discretely and sensitively.
4 Guidelines developed at national or regional level may not reflect local needs or have the 'ownership' of local practitioners.
5 Guidelines developed in secondary care may not reflect demographic, clinical or practical differences between this setting and the primary care setting.
6 Guidelines may produce undesirable shifts in the balance of power between different professional groups (e.g. between clinicians and academics, orthopaedic surgeons and physiotherapists, gynaecologists and midwives, or purchasers and providers). Hence, guideline development may be perceived as a political act.
7 Out-of-date guidelines might hold back the implementation of new research evidence.

you will probably have realised that a good guideline wouldn't *force* you to abandon common sense or judgement – it would simply flag up a recommended course of action for you to consider.

Nevertheless, even a perfect guideline can make work for the busy clinician as this quote from an article in the *Lancet* illustrates:

> *We surveyed one [24-hour] acute medical take in our hospital. In a relatively quiet take, we saw 18 patients with a total of 44 diagnoses. The guidelines that the on call physician should have read, remembered and applied correctly for those conditions came to 3679 pages. This number included only NICE [National Institute for Health and Care Excellence], the Royal Colleges and major societies from the last 3 years. If it takes 2 min to read each page, the physician on call will have to spend 122 h reading to keep abreast of the guidelines [4].*

The mushrooming guidelines industry owes its success at least in part to a growing 'accountability culture' that is now (many argue) being set in statute in many countries. In the UK National Health Service, all doctors, nurses, pharmacists and other health professions now have a contractual duty to provide clinical care based on best available research evidence. Officially produced or sanctioned guidelines (e.g. those produced by NICE; www.nice.org.uk) are a way of both supporting and policing that laudable goal. While the medicolegal implications of 'official' guidelines have rarely been tested in the UK, courts in North America have ruled that guideline developers can be held liable for faulty guidelines. A few years ago, a US court refused to accept adherence to an evidence-based guideline (which advised doctors to share the inherent uncertainty associated with prostate-specific antigen (PSA) testing in asymptomatic middle-aged men, and make a shared decision on whether the test was worth doing) as defence by a doctor being sued for missing an early prostate cancer in an unlucky 53-year-old [5]. Partly on the basis of that court case, the guidelines were initially altered (which greatly increased the number of PSA tests done on asymptomatic men, as well as the amount of anxiety and further tests, all with low yield). The author of the original article spent the next 10 years fighting to put the evidence back into the evidence-based guideline; he published a follow-up paper in 2015 to announce that he had 'won' [6].

For a more detailed review of the topic of guideline adherence, see Trisha's book *How to Implement Evidence Based Healthcare*, where she reviews different approaches to influencing clinician behaviour and also different theoretical models of change [7]. The remainder of this chapter addresses what to do with a guideline if you want to evaluate it (i.e. decide on its validity and relevance) with a view to using it in practice.

Ten questions to ask about a clinical guideline

Deborah Swinglehurst [1] rightly points out that all the song and dance about encouraging clinicians to follow guidelines is only justified if the guideline is worth following in the first place. Sadly, not all of them are. She suggests two aspects of a good guideline: (1) the content (e.g. whether it is based on a comprehensive and rigorous systematic review of the evidence); and (2) the process (how the guideline was put together). We would add a third aspect: the presentation of the guideline (how appealing it is to the busy clinician and how easy it is to follow).

Like all published articles, guidelines would be easier to evaluate on all these counts if they were presented in a standardised format. An international standard, the Appraisal of Guidelines for Research and Evaluation (AGREE) instrument, for developing, reporting and presenting guidelines was originally published in 2003 (AGREE) to assess the methodological quality of practice guidelines [8], and revised and updated in 2009 (AGREE II) [9]. The AGREE Reporting Checklist (a tool to improve reporting of clinical practice guidelines) was published in 2016 [10]. Box 10.3 offers a pragmatic checklist, based partly on the work of the AGREE group, for structuring your assessment of a clinical guideline; and Box 10.4 reproduces the revised AGREE II criteria (six domains and 23 items) in full. Because few published guidelines currently follow such a format, you will probably have to scan the

Box 10.3 Outline framework for assessing a clinical guideline

- *Objective*: the primary objective of the guideline, including the health problem and the targeted patients, providers and settings.
- *Options*: the clinical practice options considered in formulating the guideline.
- *Outcomes*: significant health and economic outcomes considered in comparing alternative practices.
- *Evidence*: how and when evidence was gathered, selected and synthesised.
- *Values*: disclosure of how values were assigned to potential outcomes of practice options and who participated in the process.
- *Benefits, harms and costs*: the type and magnitude of benefits, harms and costs expected for patients from guideline implementation.
- *Recommendations*: summary of key recommendations.
- *Validation*: report of any external review, comparison with other guidelines or clinical testing of guideline use.
- *Sponsors and stakeholders*: disclosure of the persons who developed, funded or endorsed the guideline.

Box 10.4 The six domains and 23 items of the AGREE II instrument [9]

Domain 1: Scope and purpose

1 The overall objective(s) of the guideline is(are) specifically described.
2 The health question(s) covered by the guideline is(are) specifically described.
3 The population to whom the guideline is meant to apply are specifically described.

Domain 2: Stakeholder involvement

1 The guideline development group includes individuals from all the relevant professional groups.
2 The views and preferences of the target population have been sought.
3 The target users of the guideline are clearly defined.

Domain 3: Rigour of development

1 Systematic methods were used to search for evidence.
2 The criteria for selecting the evidence are clearly described.
3 The strengths and limitations of the body of evidence are clearly described.
4 The methods used for formulating the recommendations are clearly described.
5 The health benefits, adverse effects and risks have been considered in formulating the recommendations.
6 There is an explicit link between the recommendations and the supporting evidence.
7 The guideline has been externally reviewed by experts prior to its publication.
8 A procedure for updating the guideline is provided.

Domain 4: Clarity and presentation

1 The recommendations are specific and unambiguous.
2 The different options for management of the condition or health issue are clearly presented.
3 Key recommendations are easily identifiable.

Domain 5: Applicability

1 The guideline provides advice or tools to support its implementation.
2 The guideline describes facilitators of, and barriers to, adoption.
3 Potential resource implications of applying the recommendations have been considered.
4 The guideline presents monitoring or auditing criteria.

Domain 6: Editorial independence

1 The views of the funding body have not influenced the content of the guideline.
2 Competing interests of members of the guideline development group have been recorded and addressed.

Source: Reproduced with permission of the Canadian Medical Association.

full text for answers to the questions given here. In preparing this list, we have drawn on many of the other articles referenced in this chapter as well as AGREE II instrument.

Question one: Did the preparation and publication of this guideline involve a significant conflict of interest?
We will resist labouring the point, but a drug company that makes hormone replacement therapy or a research professor whose life's work has been spent perfecting this treatment might be tempted to recommend it for wider indications than the average clinician. Much has been written about the 'medicalisation' of human experience (are energetic children with a short attention span 'hyperactive'; should women with low sex drive be offered 'treatment', etc.). A guideline may be evidence-based but the problem it addresses will have been constructed by a team that views the world in a particular way.

Question two: Is the guideline concerned with an appropriate topic and does it state clearly the target group it applies to?
Key questions in relation to choice of topic, reproduced from an article published a few years ago in the *BMJ* [11], are given in Box 10.5. The Grimley Evans quote on page 153 begs the question 'To whom does this guideline apply?'. If the evidence related to people aged 18–65 with no comorbidity (i.e. with nothing else wrong with them except the disease being considered), it might not apply to your patient. Sometimes this means that you will need to reject it outright but, more commonly, you will have to exercise your judgement in assessing its transferability.

Box 10.5 Key questions on choice of topic for guideline development [11]

- Is the topic high volume, high risk and high cost?
- Are there large or unexplained variations in practice?
- Is the topic important in terms of the process and outcome of patient care?
- Is there potential for improvement?
- Is the investment of time and money likely to be repaid?
- Is the topic likely to hold the interest of team members?
- Is consensus likely?
- Will change benefit patients?
- Can change be implemented?

Source: reproduced with permission of BMJ Publishing Group Ltd.

Question three: Did the guideline development panel include: (1) an expert in the topic area; (2) a specialist in the methods of secondary research (e.g. meta-analyst, health economist) and (3) a person affected by the condition?
If a clinical guideline has been prepared entirely by a panel of internal 'experts', you should, paradoxically, look at it particularly critically as researchers have been shown to be less objective in appraising evidence in their own field of expertise than in someone else's. The involvement of an outsider (an expert in guideline development rather than in the particular clinical topic) to act as arbiter and methodological adviser should make the process more objective. But as Gabbay and his team [12] showed in an elegant qualitative study, the hard-to-measure expertise (what might be called *embodied knowledge*) of frontline clinicians (in this case, GPs) contributed crucially to the development of workable local guidelines. Since then, there has been a lot of research into this somewhat elusive topic (see a systematic review by Trisha's team [13]). But clinical experience and wisdom don't bring the knowledge of what it is like to have the condition in question yourself, and emerging evidence suggests that patients and carers bring a crucial third perspective to the guideline development process [14].

Question four: Have the subjective judgements of the development panel been made explicit and are they justified?
Guideline development is not just a technical process of finding evidence, appraising it and turning it into recommendations. Recommendations also require judgements (relating to personal or social values, ethical principles, etc.). As NICE has stated (www.nice.org.uk), it is right and proper for guideline developers to take account of the 'ethical principles, preferences, culture and aspirations that should underpin the nature and extent of care provided by the National Health Service'. Swinglehurst [1] suggests four subquestions to ask about these subjective judgements.

- What *guiding principles* have been used to decide how effective an intervention must be (compared with its potential harms) before its recommendation is considered?
- What *values* have underpinned the panel's decisions about which guideline developments to prioritise?
- What is the *ethical framework* to which guideline developers are working – in particular relating to matters of distributive justice ('rationing')?
- Where there was disagreement between guideline developers, what *explicit processes* have been used to resolve such disagreements?

Question five: Have all the relevant data been scrutinised and rigorously evaluated?
The academic validity of guidelines depends (among other things) on whether they are supported by high-quality primary research studies and on how strong the evidence from those studies is. At the most basic level, was the literature analysed at all, or are these guidelines simply a statement of the preferred practice of a selected panel of experts (i.e. consensus guidelines)? If the literature was looked at, was a systematic search performed, and if so, did it broadly follow the method described in section 'Evaluating systematic reviews'? Were all papers unearthed by the search included or was an explicit scoring system (such as GRADE [15]) used to reject those of poor methodological quality and give those of high quality the extra weight they deserved?

Up-to-date systematic reviews should ideally be the raw material for guideline development. But in many cases, a search for rigorous and relevant research on which to base guidelines proves fruitless and the authors, unavoidably, resort to 'best available' evidence or expert opinion.

Question six: Has the evidence been properly synthesised and are the guideline's conclusions in keeping with the data on which they are based?
Another key determinant of the validity of a guideline is how the different studies contributing to it have been pulled together (that is, synthesised) in the context of the clinical and policy needs being addressed. For one thing, a systematic review and meta-analysis might have been appropriate and, if the latter, issues of probability and confidence should have been dealt with acceptably.

But systematic reviews don't exist (and never will exist) to cover every eventuality in clinical decision- and policy-making. In many areas, especially complex ones, the opinion of experts is still the best 'evidence' around and, in such cases, guideline developers should adopt rigorous methods to ensure that it is not just the voice of the expert who talks for longest in the meetings that drives the recommendations. Formal guideline development groups usually have an explicit set of methods (see e.g. Hill et al. [16]).

An analysis of three 'evidence-based' guidelines for obstructive sleep apnoea found that they made very different recommendations despite being based on an almost identical set of primary studies. The main reason for the discrepancy was that experts tended to rank studies from their own country more highly [17]!

Question seven: Does the guideline address variations in medical practice and other controversial areas (e.g. optimum care in response to genuine or perceived underfunding)?
It would be foolish to make dogmatic statements about ideal practice without reference to what actually goes on in the real world. There are many instances where some practitioners are marching to an altogether different tune from

the rest of us, and a good guideline should face such realities head on rather than hoping that the misguided minority will fall into step by default.

Another thorny issue that guidelines should tackle head-on is where essential compromises should be made if financial constraints preclude 'ideal' practice. If the ideal, for example, is to offer all patients with significant coronary artery disease a bypass operation (at the time of writing it isn't, but never mind) and the health service can only afford to fund 20% of such procedures, who should be pushed to the front of the queue?

Question eight: Is the guideline clinically relevant, comprehensive and flexible? In other words, is it written from the perspective of the practising doctor, nurse, midwife, physiotherapist and so on, and does it take account of the type of patients they are likely to see, and in what circumstances? Perhaps the most frequent source of trouble here is when guidelines developed in secondary care and intended for use in hospital outpatients (who tend to be at the sicker end of the clinical spectrum) are passed on to the primary healthcare team with the intention of their being used in the primary care setting, where, in general, patients are less ill and may well need fewer investigations and less aggressive management. This issue is discussed in section 'Validating diagnostic tests against a gold standard' in relation to the different utilities of diagnostic and screening tests in different populations.

Guidelines should cover all, or most, clinical eventualities. What if the patient is intolerant of the recommended medication? What if you can't send off all the recommended blood tests? What if the patient is very young, very old or suffers from a coexisting illness? These, after all, are the patients who prompt most of us to reach for our guidelines; while the more 'typical' patient tends to be managed without recourse to written instructions. Bruce Guthrie and his team have done great work to address the challenge of developing guidelines for people with multimorbidity [18]. Be warned, however, that this is to some extent a circle that can't be squared. Glyn Elwyn, Sietse Wieringa and Trisha have written a paper, 'Clinical encounters in the post-guidelines era', which discusses the increasing complexity and uniqueness of many clinical decisions. In such circumstances, selecting and using a guideline will inevitably involve a great deal of situational judgement and negotiation with the patient [19].

Flexibility is a particularly important consideration for national and regional bodies who set themselves up to develop guidelines. As noted earlier, ownership of guidelines by the people who are intended to use them locally is crucial to whether the guidelines are actually used. If there is no free rein for practitioners to adapt them to meet local needs and priorities, a set of guidelines will probably never get taken out of the drawer.

Question nine: Does the guideline take into account what is acceptable to, affordable by and practically possible for patients?
There is an apocryphal story of a physician in the 1940s (a time when no effective medicines for high blood pressure were available), who discovered that restricting the diet of hypertensive patients to plain, boiled, unsalted rice dramatically reduced their blood pressure and also reduced the risk of stroke. The story goes, however, that the diet made the patients so miserable that many of them committed suicide.

This is an extreme example but, within the past few years, we have seen guidelines for treating constipation in the elderly that offered no alternative to the combined insults of large amounts of bran and twice-daily suppositories. Small wonder that the district nurses who were issued with them (for whom we have a good deal of respect) have gone back to giving castor oil.

For a further discussion on how to incorporate the needs and priorities of patients in guideline development, see Boivin et al. [14].

Question ten: Does the guideline include recommendations for its own dissemination, implementation and regular review?
Given the well-documented gap between what is known to be good practice and what actually happens, and the many barriers to the successful implementation of guidelines, it would be in the interests of those who develop guidelines to suggest methods of maximising their use. If this objective were included as standard in the 'Guidelines for good guidelines', the guideline writers' output would probably include fewer ivory tower recommendations and more that are plausible, possible and capable of being explained to patients. Having said that, one very positive development in EBHC since Trisha wrote the first edition of this book is the change in guideline developers' attitudes: they now often take responsibility for linking their outputs to clinicians (and patients) in the real world and for reviewing and updating their recommendations periodically. Nowadays, many guidelines include patient information material, often in several different languages.

Finally, could artificial intelligence (AI) assist in making clinical guidelines more accessible to end users, not only clinicians but also patients? One form of AI, chatbots, could help (see Chapter 17 on AI in healthcare). Paul and his team are investigating how a chatbot based on a custom GPT (generative pretrained transformer) framework and programmed to only use a specific anterior cruciate ligament (ACL) injury rehabilitation guideline [20] to answer end-user questions, could empower clinicians and patients with evidence-based knowledge to make better decisions. This AI tool aims to demystify the potentially complicated ACL rehabilitation guideline by using advanced natural language processing techniques that offer interactive, tailored responses to end-users' ACL rehabilitation questions (ideally in their own language).

Exercises based on this chapter

1. Take a look at the 'Guidance' page of the NICE website (https://www.nice.org.uk/guidance). Alternatively (since links can change after a book is published), put 'NICE guidelines' into Google and work your way to the relevant page. Browse the list of recently added guidelines. You will find that they are typically very long. Look at the recommendations, but also at the underpinning evidence (this may be in appendices). Finally, look at the account of how the guideline was produced. To what extent do you trust it after answering all those questions?
2. Find your way to the TRIP database (www.tripdatabase.com or put 'TRIP database' into Google). Put a topic (say 'PSA testing') into the search engine. Now, on the left-hand side of the screen, find the header 'Guidelines'. You should see a list of different guidelines produced from around the world. Use the questions in this chapter to guide you as you compare and contrast two or more of these guidelines. Can you explain instances when they recommend different courses of action? Is one guideline scientifically better than another or can the differences be explained by differences in setting and application?
3. Take a look at the 'Aspetar clinical practice guideline on rehabilitation after anterior cruciate ligament reconstruction' [20]. Comment on the guideline development process and guideline development group. Do you agree with the limitations stated by the author group? What are your thoughts about the dissemination strategy described by the author group?

References

1. Swinglehurst D. Evidence-based guidelines: The theory and the practice. *Evidence-based Healthcare and Public Health* 2005; **9**: 308–14.
2. Evans JG. Evidence-based and evidence-biased medicine. *Age and Ageing* 1995; **24**: 461–3.
3. Greenhalgh T. Of lamp posts, keys, and fabled drunkards: a perspectival tale of 4 guidelines. *Journal of Evaluation in Clinical Practice* 2018; **24**: 1132–8.
4. Allen D, Harkins K. Too much guidance? *Lancet* 2005; **365**: 1768.
5. Merenstein D. Winners and losers. *JAMA* 2004; **291**: 15–16.
6. Merenstein D. PSA Screening: I Finally Won! *JAMA Internal Medicine* 2015; **175**: 16–17.
7. Greenhalgh T. *How to Implement Evidence-Based Healthcare*. Hoboken, NJ: Wiley-Blackwell; 2018.
8. AGREE Collaboration. Development and validation of an international appraisal instrument for assessing the quality of clinical practice guidelines: the AGREE project. *BMJ Quality and Safety* 2003; **12**: 18–23.

9. Brouwers MC, Kho ME, Browman GP, et al. AGREE II: advancing guideline development, reporting and evaluation in health care. *Canadian Medical Association Journal* 2010; **182**: E839–42.
10. Brouwers MC, Kerkvliet K, Spithoff K. The AGREE Reporting Checklist: a tool to improve reporting of clinical practice guidelines. *BMJ* 2016; **352**: i1152.
11. Thomson R, Lavender M, Madhok R. Fortnightly review: how to ensure that guidelines are effective. *BMJ* 1995; **311**: 237–42.
12. Gabbay J, le May A. Evidence based guidelines or collectively constructed 'mindlines?' Ethnographic study of knowledge management in primary care. *BMJ* 2004; **329**: 1013.
13. Wieringa S, Greenhalgh T. 10 years of mindlines: a systematic review and commentary. *Implementation Science* 2015; **10**: 45.
14. Boivin A, Currie K, Fervers B, et al. Patient and public involvement in clinical guidelines: international experiences and future perspectives. *Quality and Safety in Health Care* 2010; **19**: e22.
15. Guyatt G, Oxman AD, Akl EA, et al. GRADE guidelines: 1. Introduction: GRADE evidence profiles and summary of findings tables. *Journal of Clinical Epidemiology* 2011; **64**: 383–94.
16. Hill J, Bullock I, Alderson P. A summary of the methods that the National Clinical Guideline Centre uses to produce clinical guidelines for the National Institute for Health and Clinical Excellence. *Annals of Internal Medicine* 2011; **154**: 752–7.
17. Aarts MCJ, van der Heijden GJM, Rovers MM, et al. Remarkable differences between three evidence-based guidelines on management of obstructive sleep apnea-hypopnea syndrome. *Laryngoscope* 2013; **123**: 283–91.
18. Guthrie B, Payne K, Alderson P, et al. Adapting clinical guidelines to take account of multimorbidity. *BMJ* 2012; **345**: e6341.
19. Elwyn G, Wieringa S, Greenhalgh T. Clinical encounters in the post-guidelines era. *BMJ* 2016; **353**: i3200.
20. Kotsifaki R, Korakakis V, King E, et al. Aspetar clinical practice guideline on rehabilitation after anterior cruciate ligament reconstruction. *British Journal of Sports Medicine* 2023; **57**: 500–14.

Chapter 11 Papers that estimate what things cost (health economic evaluations)

What is an economic evaluation?

An economic evaluation can be defined as *one that involves the use of analytical techniques to define choices in resource allocation* (i.e. it helps us choose how to spend our money). This chapter draws on two papers in the *BMJ* by Stavros Petrou and Alastair Gray [1,2] and on the Consolidated Health Economic Evaluation Reporting Standards CHEERS [3]. All these sources emphasise the importance of setting the health economic questions about a paper in the context of the overall focus, quality and relevance of the study (see section 'Twelve questions to ask about a health economic evaluation').

First, let's get our heads round some jargon terms in this subject. Back in the 1960s, before the days of dishwashers, Trisha was struck by a TV advertisement in which the pop singer Cliff Richard tried to persuade a housewife that the most expensive brand of washing-up liquid on the market 'actually works out cheaper'. It was, apparently, stronger on stains, softer on the hands and produced more bubbles per penny than 'a typical cheap liquid'. Although she was only nine at the time, she was unconvinced. Which 'typical cheap liquid' was the product being compared with? How much stronger on stains was it? Why should the effectiveness of a washing-up liquid be measured in terms of bubbles produced rather than plates cleaned?

We can use this trivial example to illustrate the four main types of economic evaluation that you will find in the literature (Table 11.1 gives the conventional definitions).

- *Cost-minimisation analysis*: 'Sudso' costs 47 pence per bottle whereas 'Jiffo' costs 63 pence per bottle.
- *Cost-effectiveness analysis*: 'Sudso' gives you 15 extra clean plates per wash than 'Jiffo'.

How to Read a Paper: The Basics of Evidence-Based Healthcare, Seventh Edition.
Trisha Greenhalgh and Paul Dijkstra.

Table 11.1 Types of economic analysis

Type of analysis	Outcome measure	Conditions of use	Example
Cost-minimisation analysis	No outcome measure	Used when the effect of both interventions is known (or may be assumed) to be identical	Comparing the price of a brand name drug with that of its generic equivalent if bioequivalence has been demonstrated
Cost-effectiveness analysis	Natural units (e.g. life-years gained)	Used when the effect of the interventions can be expressed in terms of one main variable	Comparing two preventive treatments for an otherwise fatal condition
Cost–utility analysis	Utility units (e.g. QALYs)	Used when the effect of the interventions on health status has two or more important dimensions (e.g. benefits and adverse effects of drugs)	Comparing the benefits of two treatments for varicose veins in terms of surgical result, cosmetic appearance and risk of serious adverse event (e.g. pulmonary embolus)
Cost–benefit analysis	Monetary units (e.g. estimated cost of loss in productivity)	Used when it is desirable to compare an intervention for this condition with an intervention for a different condition	For a purchasing authority, to decide whether to fund a heart transplantation programme or a stroke rehabilitation ward

- *Cost–utility analysis*: in terms of quality-adjusted homemaker hours (a composite score reflecting time and effort needed to scrub plates clean and hand roughness caused by the liquid), 'Sudso' provides 29 units per pound spent, whereas 'Jiffo' provides 23 units.
- *Cost–benefit analysis*: the net overall cost (reflecting direct cost of the product, indirect cost of time spent washing up and estimated financial value of a clean plate relative to a slightly grubby one) of 'Sudso' per day is 7.17 pence, while that of 'Jiffo' is 9.32 pence.

You should be able to see immediately that the most sensible analysis to use in this example is cost-effectiveness analysis. Cost-minimisation analysis (Table 11.1) is inappropriate as 'Sudso' and 'Jiffo' do not have identical effectiveness. Cost–utility analysis is unnecessary because, in this example, we are interested in very little else apart from the number of plates cleaned per unit of washing-up liquid (i.e. our outcome has only one important dimension). Cost–benefit analysis is, in this example, an over-complicated way of telling you that 'Sudso' cleans more plates per penny.

There are, however, many situations where health professionals and others who purchase healthcare from real cash-limited budgets must choose between interventions for a host of different conditions whose outcomes (e.g. cases of measles prevented, increased mobility after a hip replacement, reduced risk of death from heart attack or likelihood of giving birth to a live baby) cannot be directly compared with one another. One option here is a *cost–consequences analysis*, which presents the results of the economic analysis in a disaggregated form (e.g. take-home babies vs. cases of measles prevented).

Controversy surrounds not just how these kinds of comparisons should be made but also who should make them, and to whom the decision-makers for the 'rationing' of healthcare should be accountable. These essential, fascinating and frustrating questions are beyond the scope of this book, but if you are interested, we recommend a book by Donaldson and Mitton [4].

Health economics studies: two key approaches

Finding out what it costs to obtain a given health benefit can be done in two ways (actually many more, but we will describe the two main ones here): health economic evaluation linked to a randomised controlled trial (RCT) [1] and health economic evaluation linked to simulation modelling [2]. RCTs are covered in Chapters 6 and 7. Models (of which there are many different kinds) can be defined as simplified versions of reality which can provide insights into complex phenomena and test hypothetical future scenarios. For the purposes of this chapter, we are talking about *simulation modelling*, which is explained below. This section explains how to include a health economic evaluation alongside each of these designs.

As you probably know by now, an RCT compares two groups of participants, one of which receives the novel intervention and the other receives either no intervention (or placebo) or 'usual care'. The trial compares differences in efficacy between the two arms; the health economic evaluation compares differences in costs. If the novel intervention is more effective but also more costly, we then need to ask if that extra benefit is 'worth it'. As well as quantitative data on the chosen primary and secondary outcome measures, the researchers must collect the kinds of data that will inform an assessment of costs. These include the amount of time spent on different activities by different members of staff, the costs of drugs or procedures, and measures of the participants' health status (most usually, health-related quality of life). As Petrou and Gray warn, 'Designing a rigorous trial based economic evaluation requires close collaboration between trialists and health economists' [1].

RCTs are expensive and logistically challenging, and they don't always provide a sufficient basis for making policy decisions (such as 'should our national health service introduce a screening programme for disease X?' or 'should healthcare providers be reimbursed for intensively monitoring patients with disease Y?'). This is because a single RCT will not be able to compare all the available options, assess all relevant inputs or go on for enough time to measure and follow differences in economic outcomes. For this reason, many health economic evaluations use a different approach called simulation modelling [2]. In this design, the researchers (using a computer) construct a decision tree whose branches represent the various input options (e.g. screening women over 50 years every 2 years with mammography for breast cancer vs. not screening them) that policymakers might wish to consider along with key outcomes (e.g. development of invasive cancer). The simulation model uses mathematical techniques to estimate the costs and consequences of these different options and their various consequences (e.g. if screening is effective in detecting early breast cancer, the costs of this treatment are likely to be lower than those of treating more advanced cancer detected in unscreened women). In the next sections, we explore how we estimate various kinds of costs.

Costs and benefits of health interventions

A few years ago, Trisha was taken to hospital to have her appendix removed. From the hospital's point of view, the cost of her care included board and lodging for 5 days, a proportion of doctors' and nurses' time, drugs and dressings and investigations (blood tests and a scan). Other *direct costs* (Table 11.2) included the general practitioner's time for attending to her in

Table 11.2 Examples of costs and benefits of health interventions

Costs	Benefits
Direct	*Economic*
'Board and lodging'	Prevention of expensive-to-treat illness
Drugs, dressings, etc	Avoidance of hospital admission
Investigations	Return to paid work
Staff salaries	
Indirect	*Clinical*
Work days lost	Postponement of death or disability
Value of 'unpaid' work	Relief of pain, nausea, breathlessness, etc.
Intangible	Improved vision, hearing, muscular strength, etc.
Pain and suffering	Quality of life
Social stigma	Increased mobility and independence
	Improved wellbeing
	Release from sick role

the middle of the night and the cost of the petrol her husband used when visiting her (not to mention the grapes and flowers).

In addition to this, there were the *indirect* costs of her loss in productivity. She was off work for 3 weeks, and her domestic duties were temporarily divided between various friends, neighbours and a nice young woman from a nanny agency. In addition, there were several *intangible* costs, such as discomfort, loss of independence, the allergic rash developed on the medication and the cosmetically unsightly scar.

As Table 11.2 shows, these direct, indirect and intangible costs constitute one side of the cost–benefit equation. On the benefit side, the operation greatly increased Trisha's chances of staying alive. In addition, she had a nice rest from work, and rather enjoyed all the attention and sympathy. Note that the social 'stigma' of appendicitis is relatively neutral, and indeed the social kudos of (say) a sports injury might even be positive. One would be less likely to view a hospital admission as bringing social benefit if it had been precipitated by, say, an epileptic fit or a psychotic episode, which have negative social stigmata.

In the appendicitis example, few patients would perceive much freedom of choice in deciding to opt for the operation. Most health interventions do not concern definitive procedures for acutely life-threatening diseases. On the contrary, much healthcare these days concerns what are sometimes referred to as 'chronic non-communicable diseases' – incurable, progressive and (depending on how they wax and wane) ranging from inconvenient to downright disabling. Most of us can count on developing at least one such condition (e.g. ischaemic heart disease, high blood pressure, arthritis, chronic bronchitis, cancer, rheumatism, prostatic hypertrophy or diabetes). At some stage, almost all of us will be forced to decide whether having a routine procedure or operation, taking a particular drug or making a compromise in our lifestyle (reducing our alcohol intake or sticking to a cholesterol-lowering diet) is 'worth it'.

It is fine for informed individuals to make choices about their own care by gut reaction ('I'd rather live with my hernia than be cut open', or 'I know about the risk of thrombosis but I want to continue to smoke and stay on the [contraceptive] Pill'). But when the choices are about other people's care, personal values and prejudices are the last thing that should enter the equation. Most of us would want the planners and policymakers to use objective, explicit and defensible criteria when making decisions such as, 'No, Mrs Brown may not have a kidney transplant'.

Measuring the value of health states

One important way of addressing the 'what's it worth?' question for a given health state (such as having poorly controlled diabetes or asthma) is to ask someone in that state how they feel. A number of questionnaires that attempt to measure overall health status, such as the EQ-5D, Nottingham Health

Profile and Short Form 36-question (SF-36) general health questionnaire (widely used in the UK) and the McMaster Health Utilities Index Questionnaire (popular in North America), have been developed. For an overview of these and more tools, see the systematic review by Haraldstad et al. [5]. In some circumstances, disease-specific measures of wellbeing are preferred. For example, answering 'yes' to the question, 'Do you get very concerned about the food you are eating?' might indicate anxiety in someone without diabetes but normal self-care attitudes in someone with diabetes.

The authors of standard instruments (such as the SF-36) for measuring health-related quality of life have often spent years ensuring they are valid (i.e. they measure what we think they are measuring), reliable (they do so every time), and responsive to change (i.e. if an intervention improves or worsens the patient's health, the scale will reflect that). For this reason, you should be highly suspicious of a paper that eschews these standard instruments in favour of the authors' own rough-and-ready scale. Note also that even instruments that have apparently been well validated often do not stand up to rigorous evaluation of their psychometric validity.

Another way of addressing the 'what's it worth?' of particular health states is through *health state preference values* – that is, the value which, in a hypothetical situation, a healthy person would place on a particular deterioration in their health or which a sick person would place on a return to health [6]. There are three main methods of assigning such values:

- *Rating scale measurements*: the respondent is asked to make a mark on a fixed line, labelled, for example, 'perfect health' at one end and 'death' at the other, to indicate where they would place themselves concerning the state in question (e.g. being wheelchair-bound from arthritis of the hip).
- *Time trade-off measurements*: the respondent is asked to consider a particular health state (e.g. infertility) and estimate how many of their remaining years in full health they would sacrifice to be 'cured' of the condition.
- *Standard gamble measurements*: the respondent is asked to consider the choice between living for the rest of their life in a particular health state and taking a 'gamble' (e.g. an operation) with a given odds of success, which would return them to full health if it succeeded but kill them if it failed. The odds are then varied to see at what point the respondent decides the gamble is not worth taking.

Quality-adjusted life-years

The quality-adjusted life-year (QALY) can be calculated by multiplying the preference value for a particular health state with the time the patient is likely to spend in that state. The results of cost–benefit analyses are usually expressed in terms of 'cost per QALY', some examples of which are shown in Table 11.3 [7–12]. The absolute cost per QALY is sometimes less important in decision-making than how much the cost per QALY differs between an old, inexpensive therapy and a new, expensive one. The new drug may be only marginally more effective but many times the price! The value used to compare whether the benefit is 'worth it' is known as the incremental cost-effectiveness ratio or ICER. For example, in the bottom row of Table 11.3, the complex intervention was compared with 'usual care'; the cost per QALY is expressed as an ICER [12]. In this case, it will cost an *additional* £2,642 per QALY if the complex intervention is implemented, compared with people simply attending their (undertrained) doctors for hypertension treatment.

The estimates of cost per QALY in Table 11.3 range from £14 for meticulously following up people after tuberculosis treatment in a deprived setting in South Africa where tuberculosis is prevalent [11] to an upper bound of £143,639 for screening low-risk people in a high-income country for kidney

Table 11.3 Cost per quality-adjusted life year [7–12]

Intervention	Study design	Cost per QALY (£)[a]
Screening the general population for kidney disease (without any risk factors)	Systematic review of simulation models	94,351–143,639
Screening a high-risk population (diabetes) for kidney disease		91–33,950
Screening a high-risk population (minority ethnic group) for kidney disease		19,157
Screening over-65s for atrial fibrillation using a wearable	Simulation modelling	46,402
Pre-exposure prophylaxis in men at high risk of HIV with branded long-acting injectable drug (USA)	Simulation modelling	80,149
Pre-exposure prophylaxis in men at high risk of HIV with generic long-acting injectable drug (USA)		2,966
Intensive versus standard blood pressure control in people with hypertension (UK)	RCT	3,750
Intensive versus standard blood pressure control in people with hypertension (USA)		20,359
Long-term follow-up after tuberculosis treatment in a high-incidence setting (South Africa), calculated as cost per DALY	Simulation modelling	14
Complex intervention to improve management of hypertension in low-income setting (Argentina), including home visits and clinician education, compared with usual care	RCT	2,642

[a] These are mostly 2023 prices, so the absolute values may go out of date, but the relative values will remain striking. Cost estimates have been converted to UK pounds.

disease [7]. Carefully following up ex-tuberculosis patients is highly cost-effective, since promptly detecting and treating recurrence could prevent transmission, saving many more people the suffering and cost of developing tuberculosis. In contrast, screening large numbers of people for a condition they are unlikely to have (and, if they do have it, are not going to pass it on to anyone else) is sometimes not a good use of resources! Costs per QALY are hugely dependent on the cost of the intervention, as the striking example of pre-exposure prophylaxis of HIV from the United States illustrates: switching from an expensive branded drug to a generic version of the same drug reduces the cost per QALY from over £80,000 to under £3,000 [9].

As medical ethicist John Harris has pointed out, QALYs are, like the society which produces them, potentially ageist, sexist, racist and loaded against those with permanent disabilities (because even a complete cure of an unrelated condition would not restore the individual to 'perfect health'). Furthermore, QALYs distort our ethical instincts by focusing our minds on life-years rather than people's lives. A disabled premature infant in need of an intensive care cot will, argues Harris, be allocated more resources than it deserves in comparison with a 50-year-old woman with cancer because the infant, were it to survive, would have so many more life years to quality-adjust [13].

You will find various adaptations of QALYs (such as the disability-adjusted life year or DALY) in the literature [14]; they are all based on the same principle.

Low-value health: choosing wisely

As the population ages and more and more of us live many years with expensive-to-treat chronic illness, many healthcare systems around the world are struggling to make ends meet. While many of us would be willing to pay more taxes to assure the best healthcare for everyone (or higher insurance premiums to get better care for ourselves and our families), there is also the question of how much money we are spending on tests, treatments and follow-up visits that don't do the patient any good (and which might even do harm). When a patient consults with a condition for which the standard management is hard-wired into every doctor's brain, most of us don't routinely consider whether that management is either effective or cost-effective – we just follow the pattern (prescribe, send for tests, refer to specialist and so on).

An international movement called 'Choosing Wisely' is campaigning for the use of evidence-based principles, including questions of efficacy (does it work, and if so how well?) and health economics (how much does it cost?), to inform local and national policy to reduce the use of ineffective and costly healthcare. You may be familiar with some classic examples of treatments that were once considered good practice but are now viewed as unnecessary in most cases (tonsillectomy in children, for example) and a waste of resources. For more on Choosing Wisely, see the papers by Cassel and Guest from the United States [15] and Ross et al. from UK [16].

Twelve questions to ask about a health economic evaluation

The elementary checklist that follows is based largely on the sources mentioned in the first paragraph of this chapter. We strongly recommend that, for a more definitive list, you check out these sources, especially the official recommendations by the CHEERS consortium [3].

Question one: Which health interventions were being compared in what population?
Before you even start looking at the health economic aspects, make sure that you have a clear understanding of what the clinical intervention (and, where relevant, the control intervention) was. Describe what a patient would go through in each arm of the study (what kind of assessment and by whom, which diagnostic tests, what drug(s) or operation, and what kind of follow-up, for how long?). When describing the population, consider whether the sample(s) were drawn from primary or secondary care.

Question two: In what context was the study undertaken?
Consider whether the study was in a high-, middle- or low-income setting, and what kind of health service and system it was conducted in (for example, did people have to pay or co-pay for their care?). You should also consider *when* the primary study was done and if the intervention(s) compared are still relevant today.

Question three: Were the intervention(s) clinically effective?
If the intervention is not *effective*, it can't be *cost-effective*. Note, however, that in a resource-limited healthcare system, it is often sensible to use treatments that are a little less effective when they are a lot less expensive than the best on offer.

Question four: Whose viewpoint were costs and benefits being considered from?
There is no such thing as an economic analysis that is devoid of perspective. The patient generally wants to get better as quickly as possible. From a purely financial perspective (e.g. the Treasury's), the most cost-effective health intervention is probably one that returns all citizens promptly to taxpayer status and, when this status is no longer tenable, causes immediate sudden

death. From the drug company's point of view, it would be difficult to imagine a cost–benefit equation that did not contain one of the company's products and, from a physiotherapist's point of view, the removal of a physiotherapy service would never be cost-effective. Most assume the perspective of the healthcare system itself, although some take into account the hidden costs to the patient and society (e.g. as a result of work days lost). There is no 'right' perspective for an economic evaluation, but the paper should say clearly whose costs and whose benefits have been counted 'in' and 'out'. You might like to look up Carl May's work on 'burden of treatment' – the additional work and hassle that patients take on when encouraged to 'self-manage' their illness [17].

Question five: Did the authors state at the outset how they planned to do the health economic analysis?
Just as a statistical analysis plan for a quantitative study should be stated at the outset, so should a health economic analysis plan. This avoids the temptation to run a different analysis if the results of the first one didn't come out as hoped.

Question six: Were the interventions sensible and workable in the settings where they are likely to be applied?
A research trial that compares one obscure and unaffordable intervention with another will have little impact on medical practice. Remember that standard current practice (which may be 'doing nothing') should usually be one of the alternatives compared. Too many research trials look at intervention packages that would be impossible to implement in the non-research setting (e.g. they assume that general practitioners will own a state-of-the-art computer and agree to follow a protocol, that infinite nurse time is available for the taking of blood tests or that patients will make their personal treatment choices solely on the basis of the trial's primary outcome measure). This is where simulation modelling can add value over RCT-linked health economic studies, since the model can be populated with options that differ from the gold standard intervention that was tested in the trial.

Question seven: What outcomes were measured and were these reasonable?
There will be clinical outcomes (such as survival or cure) and also economic outcomes (such as health status questionnaires or preference values). Ideally, the choice of outcomes will have involved consultation with patients who have the condition. In some health economics modelling studies, extensive work with patient groups will have informed the choice of outcomes and (more generally) the options included in the model.

Question eight: How were costs and benefits measured?

Look back to earlier in this chapter, where we outlined some of the costs associated with Trisha's appendix operation. Now imagine a more complicated example – the rehabilitation of stroke patients into their own homes with attendance at a day centre compared with a standard alternative intervention (rehabilitation in a long-stay hospital). The economic analysis must take into account not just the time of the various professionals involved, the time of the secretaries and administrators who help run the service, and the cost of the food and drugs consumed by the stroke patients but also a fraction of the capital cost of building the day centre and maintaining a transport service to and from it.

There are no hard and fast rules for deciding which costs to include. If calculating 'cost per case' from first principles, remember that someone has to pay for heating, lighting, personnel support and even the accountants' bills of the institution. In general terms, these 'hidden costs' are known as overheads, and generally add an additional 30–60% to the cost of a project. The task of costing things like operations and outpatient visits in the UK is easier than it used to be because these experiences are now bought and sold at a price that reflects (or should reflect) all overheads involved. Be warned, however, that unit costs of health interventions calculated in one country often bear no relation to those of the same intervention elsewhere, even when these costs are expressed as a proportion of gross national product.

Benefits such as earlier return to work for a particular individual can, on the face of it, be measured in terms of the cost of employing that person at his or her usual daily rate. This approach has the unfortunate consequence of valuing the health of well-paid people higher than that of badly paid workers, homemakers or the unemployed, and that of the white majority higher than that of (on average) lower paid minority ethnic groups. In the rare cases when health economists seek to take account of patient-borne costs, it might therefore be preferable to derive the cost of sick days from the average national wage.

In a cost-effectiveness analysis, changes in health status will be expressed in natural units (such as babies taken home or ulcers healed). But just because the units are natural does not automatically make them appropriate. For example, the economic analysis of the treatment of peptic ulcer by two different drugs might measure outcome as 'proportion of ulcers healed after a 6-week course'. Treatments could be compared according to the cost per ulcer healed. However, if the relapse rates on the two drugs were very different, drug A might be falsely deemed 'more cost-effective' than drug B. A better outcome measure here might be 'ulcers which remained healed at one year'.

In cost–benefit analysis, where health status is expressed in utility units, such as QALYs, you would, if you were being really rigorous about evaluating the paper, look back at how the particular utilities used in the analysis were derived. In particular, you will want to know whose health preference values were used – those of patients, doctors, health economists or the government.

Question nine: Were incremental, rather than absolute, benefits considered?
This question is best illustrated by a simple example. Let's say drug X, at £100 per course, cures 10 of every 20 patients. Its new competitor, drug Y, costs £120 per course and cures 11 of 20 patients. The cost per case cured with drug X is £200 (because you spent £2,000 curing 10 people) and the cost per case cured with drug Y is £218 (because you spent £2,400 curing 11 people).

The *incremental* cost of drug Y – that is, the extra cost of curing the extra patient – is NOT £18 but £400, as this is the total amount extra that you have had to pay to achieve an outcome over and above what you would have achieved by giving all patients the cheaper drug. This striking example should be borne in mind the next time a pharmaceutical representative tries to persuade you that their product is 'more effective and only marginally more expensive'.

Question ten: If modelling was used, which model was selected and how was this justified?
You should 'unpack' the model used, examining each of the assumptions made by the modellers. In particular, ask whether the researchers have used similar assumptions about the nature and course of the disease and the effects of treatment to previous studies on the same disease, or whether they are offering a novel model based on different assumptions (which they should justify).

Question eleven: Was the 'here and now' given precedence over the distant future?
'A bird in the hand is worth two in the bush.' In health as well as money terms, we value a benefit today more highly than we value a promise of the same benefit in 5 years' time. When the costs or benefits of an intervention (or lack of the intervention) will occur sometime in the future, their value should be *discounted* to reflect this. The actual amount of discount that should be allowed for future, as opposed to immediate, health benefit, is pretty arbitrary but most analyses use a figure of around 5% per year.

Question twelve: Was a sensitivity analysis performed?
Let's say a cost–benefit analysis comes out as saying that hernia repair by daycase surgery costs £1,500 per QALY, whereas traditional open repair, with

its associated hospital stay, costs £2,100 per QALY. But, when you look at how the calculations were performed, you are surprised at how cheaply the laparoscopic equipment has been costed. If you raise the price of this equipment by 25%, does daycase surgery still come out dramatically cheaper? It may, or it may not.

If adjusting the figures to account for the full range of possible influences gives you a totally different answer, you should not place too much reliance on the bottom-line figures, as the example of pre-exposure prophylaxis of HIV with different drug costs illustrates [9].

Conclusion

We hope that this chapter has shown that the critical appraisal of a health economic evaluation rests as crucially on asking questions such as, 'where did those numbers come from?' and 'have any numbers been left out?' as on checking that the sums themselves were correct. While few papers will fulfil all the criteria listed in the twelve questions above and summarised in Appendix 1, you should, after reading the chapter, be able to distinguish an economic analysis of moderate or good methodological quality from one which slips 'throwaway costings' ('drug X costs less than drug Y; therefore it is more cost-effective') into its results or discussion section.

Exercises based on this chapter

1. Drugs ending in 'ab' are usually monoclonal antibodies (expensive 'designer drugs' aimed at a particular molecule, sometimes nicknamed 'costalotamab'). They sometimes, but not always, have a major effect on disease progression. The economics of such drugs are often dramatic (they cost a lot, but they may also transform patients' lives). Take a look at this paper [18], which describes the evaluation of mepolizumab for severe asthma. Was the drug effective? Was it cost-effective? What assumptions went into the economic model? Why would you not recommend this drug for all cases of asthma?
2. Bullous pemphigoid is a troublesome skin condition affecting older people. Take a look at this cost-effectiveness analysis comparing two different treatments [19]. Go through the twelve questions above and then decide what you would advise a dermatology clinic seeking to develop an evidence-based and cost-effective protocol for managing this condition.
3. Consider the challenging task of helping people with severe mental health conditions to quit smoking. After reading the paper by Li et al. [20], decide first whether attempts to do so are effective and, second, whether they are cost-effective.

References

1. Petrou S, Gray A. Economic evaluation alongside randomised controlled trials: design, conduct, analysis, and reporting. *BMJ* 2011; **342**: d1548.
2. Petrou S, Gray A. Economic evaluation using decision analytical modelling: design, conduct, analysis, and reporting. *BMJ* 2011; **342**: d1766.
3. Husereau D, Drummond M, Augustovski F, et al. Consolidated health economic evaluation reporting standards (CHEERS) 2022 explanation and elaboration: a report of the ISPOR CHEERS II good practices task force. *Value in Health* 2022; **25**(1): 10–31.
4. Donaldson C, Mitton C. *Priority Setting Toolkit: Guide to the use of economics in healthcare decision making*. Oxford: Wiley-Blackwell; 2009.
5. Haraldstad K, Wahl A, Andenæs R, et al. A systematic review of quality of life research in medicine and health sciences. *Quality of Life Research* 2019; **28**: 2641–50.
6. Young T, Yang Y, Brazier JE, et al. The first stage of developing preference-based measures: constructing a health-state classification using Rasch analysis. *Quality of Life Research* 2009; **18**(2): 253–65.
7. Yeo C, Wang H, Ang YG, et al. Cost-effectiveness of screening for chronic kidney disease in the general adult population: a systematic review. *Clinical Kidney Journal* 2023; **17**: sfad137.
8. Chen W, Khurshid S, Singer DE, et al. Cost-effectiveness of screening for atrial fibrillation using wearable devices. *JAMA Health Forum* 2022; **3**: e222419.
9. Neilan AM, Landovitz RJ, Le MH, et al. Cost-effectiveness of long-acting injectable HIV preexposure prophylaxis in the United States: a cost-effectiveness analysis. *Annals of Internal Medicine* 2022; **175**(4): 479–89.
10. Liao CT, Toh HS, Sun L, et al. Cost-effectiveness of intensive vs standard blood pressure control among older patients with hypertension. *JAMA Network Open* 2023; **6**(2): e230708.
11. Marx FM, Cohen T, Menzies NA, et al. Cost-effectiveness of post-treatment follow-up examinations and secondary prevention of tuberculosis in a high-incidence setting: a model-based analysis. *Lancet Global Health* 2020; **8**: e1223–33.
12. Augustovski F, Chaparro M, Palacios A, et al. Cost-effectiveness of a comprehensive approach for hypertension control in low-income settings in Argentina: trial-based analysis of the Hypertension Control Program in Argentina. *Value in Health* 2018; **21**: 1357–64.
13. Harris J. QALYfying the value of life. *Journal of Medical Ethics* 1987; **13**: 117–23.
14. Feng X, Kim DD, Cohen JT, et al. Using QALYs versus DALYs to measure cost-effectiveness: how much does it matter? *International Journal of Technology Assessment in Health Care* 2020; **36**: 96–103.
15. Cassel CK, Guest JA. Choosing wisely: helping physicians and patients make smart decisions about their care. *JAMA* 2012; **307**: 1801–2.
16. Ross J, Santhirapala R, MacEwen C, Coulter A. Helping patients choose wisely. *BMJ* 2018; **361**: k2585.
17. May CR, Eton DT, Boehmer K, et al. Rethinking the patient: using burden of treatment theory to understand the changing dynamics of illness. *BMC Health Services Research* 2014; **14**: 281.

18. Bermejo I, Stevenson M, Cooper K, et al. Mepolizumab for treating severe eosinophilic asthma: an evidence review group perspective of a NICE single technology appraisal. *Pharmacoeconomics* 2018; **36**: 131–44.
19. Mason JM, Chalmers JR, Godec T, et al. Doxycycline compared with prednisolone therapy for patients with bullous pemphigoid: cost-effectiveness analysis of the BLISTER trial. *British Journal of Dermatology* 2018; **178**: 415–23.
20. Li J, Fairhurst C, Peckham E, et al., SCIMITAR+ Collaborative. Cost-effectiveness of a specialist smoking cessation package compared with standard smoking cessation services for people with severe mental illness in England: a trial-based economic evaluation from the SCIMITAR+ study. *Addiction* 2020; **115**: 2113–22.

Chapter 12 **Papers that go beyond numbers (qualitative research)**

What is qualitative research?

When Trisha took up her first research post back in 1986, a work-weary colleague gave this advice: 'Find something to measure, and keep on measuring it until you've got a boxful of data. Then stop measuring and start writing up'.

'But what should I measure?', she asked.

'That', he said cynically, 'doesn't much matter'.

This true example illustrates the limitations of an exclusively quantitative (counting and measuring) perspective in research. Epidemiologist Nick Black once argued that a finding or a result is more likely to be accepted as a fact if it is quantified (expressed in numbers) than if it is not [1]. There is little or no scientific evidence, for example, to support the well-known 'facts' that 1 couple in 10 is infertile or that 1 person in 10 is homosexual, and, of course, the binary categorisations 'fertile/infertile' or 'homosexual/heterosexual' oversimplify reality. Yet, observes Black, all too often we accept uncritically such reductive and often demonstrably incorrect statements so long as they contain at least one number.

Qualitative researchers seek a deeper truth. They aim to 'study things in their natural setting, attempting to make sense of, or interpret, phenomena in terms of the meanings people bring to them', and they use 'a holistic perspective which preserves the complexities of human behaviour' [2].

Interpretive or qualitative research was for years the territory of the social scientists. It is now increasingly recognised as being not just complementary to but, in many cases, a prerequisite for the quantitative research with which most us who trained in the biomedical sciences are more familiar. The view that the two approaches are mutually exclusive has itself become 'unscientific'. These days, young researchers, particularly in the fields of primary care and health services research, are expected to acquire some skills in qualitative

How to Read a Paper: The Basics of Evidence-Based Healthcare, Seventh Edition.
Trisha Greenhalgh and Paul Dijkstra.

research as well as quantitative. Since the first edition of this book was published, qualitative research has become increasingly mainstream within the evidence-based medicine movement, as evidenced by two users' guides to the medical literature [3,4] and a chapter in the *Cochrane Handbook* [5]. There have also been major developments in the science of summarising qualitative studies (see 'Summarising and synthesising qualitative research' later in this chapter) and integrating qualitative and quantitative evidence in the development and evaluation of complex interventions [6].

The late Dr Cecil Helman, an anthropologist as well as a medical doctor, told Trisha the following story to illustrate the qualitative–quantitative dichotomy. A small child runs in from the garden and says, excitedly, 'Mummy, the leaves are falling off the trees'.

'Tell me more', says his mother.

'Well, five leaves fell in the first hour, then ten leaves fell in the second hour …'

That child will become a quantitative researcher.

A second child, when asked 'tell me more', might reply, 'Well, the leaves are big and flat, and mostly yellow or red, and they seem to be falling off some trees but not others. And mummy, why did no leaves fall last month?'

That child will become a qualitative researcher.

Questions such as 'How many parents would consult their general practitioner when their child has a mild temperature?' or 'What proportion of smokers have tried to give up?' clearly need answering through quantitative methods. But questions like 'Why do parents worry so much about their children's temperature?' and 'What stops people giving up smoking?' cannot and should not be answered by leaping in and measuring the first aspect of the problem that we (the outsiders) think might be important. Rather, we need to hang out, listen to what people have to say and explore the ideas and concerns that the individuals themselves come up with. After a while, we may notice a pattern emerging, which may prompt us to make our observations in a different way. We may start with one of the methods shown in Table 12.1, and go on to use a selection of others.

Table 12.2, which is adapted with permission from Nick Mays and Catherine Pope's classic introductory paper 'Qualitative research in health care' [7] summarises (and perhaps overstates) the differences between the qualitative and quantitative approaches to research. In reality, they are increasingly combined in a mixed-methods design [6].

Quantitative researchers generally begin with an idea (usually articulated as a hypothesis), take some measurements to generate data and, by *deduction*, come to a conclusion about what those data mean. Qualitative research is different. Researchers tend to begin with an intention to explore a particular area, collect data (e.g. observations, interviews, documents, even emails can

Table 12.1 Examples of qualitative research methods

Method	Description
Semistructured interview	Interview which seeks to explore people's perspectives on an issue or topic in detail, using the same broad list of prompt questions (known as a *topic guide*) for every interviewee
Narrative or conversational interview	Interview undertaken in a less structured fashion, with the purpose of getting a long story from the interviewee (typically a life story or the story of how an illness has unfolded over time). The interviewer holds back from prompting except to say 'tell me more'
Focus group	A group interview, typically of 3–10 participants, in which the group are encouraged to discuss topics and the researcher captures the group interaction (e.g. laughter, empathy, agreement/disagreement, conflict) as part of the dataset
Ethnography (passive observation)	Systematic watching of behaviour and talk in natural occurring settings (e.g. carefully observing, and making notes on, what goes on in an operating theatre or a music festival)
Ethnography (participant observation)	Observation in which the researcher also occupies a role or part in the setting in addition to observing (e.g. making notes *while* being a member of a working group)
Photo- or video-elicitation	An interview in which a photograph or short video clip is used to prompt reflection and discussion (e.g. showing a doctor a video of a recent consultation they had, and then inviting them to talk about their practice)
Discourse analysis	Detailed study of the words, phrases and formats used in particular social contexts (includes the study of naturally occurring talk as well as written materials such as policy documents or minutes of meetings)

Table 12.2 Qualitative versus quantitative research: the overstated dichotomy

	Qualitative	Quantitative
Question	What is X? (classification)	How many Xs? (enumeration)
Methods	Observation, interview	Experiment, survey
Reasoning	Inductive	Deductive
Sampling method	Theoretical	Statistical
Strength	Validity	Reliability

Source: adapted with permission from Mays and Pope [7].

count as qualitative data) and generate ideas and hypotheses from these data largely through what is known as *inductive reasoning* (as in 'hmm, I wonder what's going on here?') [2]. The strength of quantitative approach lies in its *reliability* (repeatability) – that is, the same measurements should yield the same results time after time. The strength of qualitative research lies in *validity* (closeness to the truth) – that is, good qualitative research, using a selection of data collection methods, really should touch the core of what is going on rather than just skimming the surface.

The validity of qualitative methods is said to be greatly improved by the use of more than one method (Table 12.1) in combination (known as *triangulation*), by the researcher thinking carefully about what is going on and how their own perspective might be influencing the data (known as *reflexivity*) [8], and – some would argue – by more than one researcher analysing the same data independently (known as *inter-rater reliability*). Others say that inter-rater reliability is a concept borrowed from quantitative research and may be misapplied in qualitative studies (for example, if two white male doctors both agree that a non-white female patient in labour has a low pain threshold and is being over-demanding of pain relief, this *could* mean that both are correct, but it could simply mean that they share the same cultural biases and neither of them has ever been in labour).

This is why, when appraising qualitative papers (or doing qualitative research yourself), you need to do more than confirm that the findings were 'checked by someone else'. For one thing, in most qualitative research, one person knows the data far better than anyone else, so the idea that two heads are better than one simply isn't true – a researcher who has been brought in merely to verify 'themes' may rely far more on personal preconceptions and guesswork than the main field worker. For another, with the trend towards more people from biomedical backgrounds doing qualitative research, it is not at all uncommon for two (or even a whole team of) naïve and untrained researchers undertaking interviews, focus groups and ethnography. Since people from similar backgrounds are likely to bring similar biases (see example in previous paragraph), high inter-rater reliability scores among them may be entirely spurious.

Those who are ignorant about qualitative research often believe that it constitutes little more than hanging out and watching leaves fall. It is beyond the scope of this book to take you through the substantial literature on how to (and how not to) proceed when observing, interviewing, leading a focus group and so on. But sophisticated methods for all these techniques certainly exist and, if you are interested, we suggest you try the excellent *BMJ* series by Scott Reeves and colleagues from Canada [9–13], the more up-to-date textbook by Mays and Pope [14] or what is sometimes known as the 'qualitative bible' by Denzin et al. [2]. You will find these books in most academic libraries.

Qualitative methods really come into their own when researching uncharted territory – that is, where the variables of greatest concern are poorly understood, ill-defined and cannot be controlled. In such circumstances, the definitive hypothesis may not be arrived at until the study is well under way. But it is in precisely these circumstances that the qualitative researcher must ensure that they have, at the outset, carefully delineated a particular focus of research and identified some specific questions to try to answer (see Question one in the section below). The methods of qualitative research allow for – indeed, they require – modification of the research question in the light of findings generated along the way – a technique known as *progressive focusing* [2]. (In contrast, sneaking a look at the interim results of a quantitative study is poor science for reasons a statistician will explain to you).

The so-called *iterative* approach (altering the research methods and the hypothesis as you go along) employed by qualitative researchers shows a commendable sensitivity to the richness and variability of the topic. Failure to recognise the legitimacy of this approach has, in the past, led critics to accuse qualitative researchers of continually moving their own goalposts. While these criticisms are often misguided, there is a danger that when qualitative research is undertaken unrigorously by naïve researchers, the 'iterative' approach will slide into confusion. This is one reason why qualitative researchers must allow periods away from their fieldwork for reflection, planning and consultation with colleagues.

Summarising and synthesising qualitative research

Unlike much quantitative research, qualitative research does not aspire to be universally transferable. Researchers who undertake a randomised controlled trial and conclude that the number needed to treat for this drug in this population is 25 are (implicitly) claiming that this effect size will apply, broadly speaking, to the same drug in a different but statistically comparable population. Qualitative researchers who explore the experiences of children in the care system in town X make no claims that cared-for children in town B will talk about the same experiences. It follows that the very notion of a 'systematic review' of qualitative research could be somewhat problematic, at least if the reviewer mechanically follows methods designed for quantitative research.

Qualitative research papers *can* be summarised and drawn together in a single-paper overview, but the key technique here is to describe each primary study in context and give a nuanced account of what each contributed to the understanding of the whole. Often, differences in findings between different primary studies reflect key differences in context. These need to be richly described and explained, not 'averaged out'! In short, whereas the goal of quantitative systematic review is *to summate data*, the goal of qualitative systematic review is to *help us understand.*

The term 'narrative review' used to be used pejoratively to depict a lazy and half-hearted essay that failed to identify many key studies and perhaps cherry-picked the ones that supported the reviewer's prior prejudices. But in recent years, the term 'narrative review' (or sometimes 'narrative systematic review' or 'hermeneutic review') is used to refer to a review that draws mainly on qualitative studies and whose goal is clarification and understanding. A paper by Greenhalgh et al. explains the difference [15].

The science of systematically reviewing qualitative research is expanding rapidly. One exciting development has been the publication of the GRADE-CERQUAL (Grading of Recommendations Assessment, Development and Evaluation – Confidence in the Evidence from Reviews of Qualitative research) criteria for appraising qualitative evidence when undertaking or appraising reviews [16–18]. Some purist qualitative researchers are wary of these checklist-driven tools, but we found them surprisingly useful in a narrative systematic review of gender issues in academic research [19].

The latest edition of the *Cochrane Handbook* includes a chapter on qualitative systematic reviews [20]; further chapters on specific qualitative synthesis techniques are planned.

Nine questions to ask about a qualitative research paper

By its very nature, qualitative research is non-standard, unconfined and dependent on the subjective experience of both the researcher and the researched. It explores what needs to be explored and cuts its cloth accordingly. As implied in the previous section, qualitative research is an in-depth, interpretive task, not a technical procedure. It depends crucially on a competent and experienced researcher exercising the kind of skills and judgements that are difficult, if not impossible, to measure objectively. It is debatable, therefore, whether an all-encompassing critical appraisal checklist along the lines of the *Users' Guides to the Medical Literature* for quantitative research could ever be developed, although valiant attempts have been made [3,4,11,14]. Some people have argued that critical appraisal checklists potentially detract from research quality in qualitative research because they encourage a mechanistic and protocol-driven approach [21].

Our own view, and that of a number of individuals who have attempted or are currently working on this very task, is that such a checklist may not be as exhaustive or as universally applicable as the various guides for appraising quantitative research, but that it is certainly possible to set some ground rules. Perhaps the best attempt to offer guidance (and also the best exposition of the uncertainties and unknowables) has been made by Dixon-Woods and her colleagues [22]. The list that follows has been distilled from the published work cited elsewhere in this chapter, and also from discussions many years ago with Dr Rod Taylor, who produced one of the earliest critical appraisal guides for qualitative papers.

Question one: Did the paper describe an important problem addressed via a clearly formulated question?
In the section 'Three preliminary questions to get your bearings' in Chapter 3, we explained that one of the first things you should look for in any research paper is a statement of why the research was carried out and what specific question it addressed. Qualitative papers are no exception to this rule: there is absolutely no scientific value in interviewing or observing people just for the sake of it. Papers that cannot define their topic of research more closely than 'we decided to interview 20 patients with epilepsy' inspire little confidence that the researchers really knew what they were studying or why. You might be more inclined to read on if the paper stated in its introduction something like, 'Epilepsy is a common and potentially disabling condition, and a significant proportion of patients do not remain seizure-free on medication. Antiepileptic medication is known to have unpleasant adverse effects, and several studies have shown that a high proportion of patients do not take their tablets regularly. We therefore decided to explore patients' beliefs about epilepsy and their perceived reasons for not taking their medication'. The iterative nature of qualitative research is such that the definitive research question may not be clearly focused at the outset of the study, but it should certainly have been formulated by the time the report is written.

Question two: Was a qualitative approach appropriate?
If the objective of the research was to explore, interpret or obtain a deeper understanding of a particular clinical issue, qualitative methods were almost certainly the most appropriate ones to use. If, however, the research aimed to achieve some other goal (such as determining the incidence of a disease or the frequency of an adverse drug reaction, testing a cause-and-effect hypothesis, or showing that one drug has a better risk–benefit ratio than another), qualitative methods are clearly inappropriate. One interesting grey zone is measuring attitudes. Qualitative research can certainly pick up people's attitudes (say, patients' attitudes towards their local health service) but if you want to be able to say something like '90% of people are satisfied with our service', you need a quantitative study design such as a closed-item survey (see Chapter 13).

Question three: How were (a) the setting and (b) the participants selected?
Look back at Table 12.2, which contrasts the statistical sampling methods of quantitative research with theoretical ones of qualitative research. In the earlier chapters, particularly section 'Whom is the study about?' (Chapter 3), we emphasised the importance, in quantitative research, of ensuring that a truly random sample of participants is recruited. A random sample will ensure

that the results reflect, on average, the condition of the population from which that sample was drawn.

In qualitative research, however, we are not interested in an 'on-average' view of a patient population. We want to gain an in-depth understanding of the experience of particular individuals or groups, and we should, therefore, deliberately seek out individuals or groups who fit the bill. If, for example, we wished to study the experience of women when they gave birth in hospital, we would be perfectly justified in going out of our way to find women who had had a range of different birth experiences – an induced delivery, a water birth, an emergency caesarean section, a delivery by a medical student, a late miscarriage, and so on.

We would also wish to select some women who had had entirely specialist care, some who had shared antenatal care between an obstetrician and their general practitioner, and some who had been cared for by community midwives throughout the pregnancy. Of course, all these specifications will give us statistically 'biased' samples, but the goal of qualitative research is not statistical balance but maximum variety.

Watch out for qualitative research where the sample has been selected (or appears to have been selected) purely on the basis of convenience. In the above-mentioned example, taking the first dozen patients to pass through the nearest labour ward would be the easiest way to notch up interviews, but the information obtained may be considerably less helpful.

Question four: What was the researcher's perspective, and has it been taken into account?

Given that qualitative research is necessarily grounded in real-life experience, a paper describing such research should not be 'trashed' simply because the researchers have declared a particular cultural perspective or personal involvement with the participants of the research. Quite the reverse: they should be congratulated for doing that. It is important to recognise that there is no way of abolishing or fully controlling for observer bias in qualitative research. This is most obviously the case when participant observation (Table 12.1) is used, but it is also true for other forms of data collection and of data analysis.

If, for example, the research concerns the experience of adults with asthma living in damp and overcrowded housing and the perceived effect of these surroundings on their health, the data generated by techniques such as focus groups or semistructured interviews are likely to be heavily influenced by what the interviewer believes about this subject and by whether they are employed by the hospital chest clinic, the social work department of the local authority, or an environmental pressure group. But because it is inconceivable that the interviews could have been conducted by someone with no views at all and no ideological or cultural perspective, the most that can be required of the researchers is that they describe in detail where they are coming from so that the results can be interpreted accordingly.

It is for this reason, incidentally, that qualitative researchers generally prefer to write up their work in the first person ('I interviewed the participants' rather than 'the participants were interviewed'), because this makes explicit the role and influence of the researcher. They also prefer the term 'researcher perspective' to 'researcher bias'.

Question five: What methods did the researcher use for collecting data and are they described in enough detail?

Trisha once spent 2 years doing highly quantitative, laboratory-based experimental research in which around 15 hours of every week were spent filling or emptying test tubes. There was a standard way to fill the test tubes, a standard way to spin them in the centrifuge, and even a standard way to wash them up. When she finally published her research, some 900 hours of drudgery was summed up in a single sentence: 'Patients' serum rhubarb levels were measured according to the method described by Bloggs and Bloggs [reference to Bloggs and Bloggs' paper on how to measure serum rhubarb]'.

Trisha now spend quite a lot of her time doing qualitative research and can confirm that it is infinitely more fun. With research colleagues, she has spent some 30 years exploring the beliefs, hopes, fears and attitudes of diabetic patients from the minority ethnic groups in the East End of London (they began with British Bangladeshis and extended the work to other South Asian and, later, other ethnic groups). We had to develop, for example, a valid way of simultaneously translating and transcribing interviews that were conducted in Sylheti, a complex dialect of Bengali that has no written form. We found that participants' attitudes appear to be heavily influenced by the presence in the room of certain of their relatives, so we contrived to interview some patients in both the presence and the absence of these key relatives.

We could go on describing the methods devised to address this particular research topic, but we have probably made our point: the methods section of a qualitative paper often cannot be written in shorthand or dismissed by reference to someone else's research techniques. It may have to be lengthy and discursive because it is telling a unique story without which the results cannot be interpreted. As with the sampling strategy, there are no hard and fast rules about exactly what details should be included in this section of the paper. You should simply ask, 'Have I been given enough information about the methods used?' and, if you have, use your common sense to assess, 'Are these methods a sensible and adequate way of addressing the research question?'

Question six: What methods did the researcher use to analyse the data and what quality control measures were implemented?

The data analysis section of a qualitative research paper is the opportunity for the researcher(s) to demonstrate the difference between sense and nonsense. Having amassed a thick pile of completed interview transcripts or field notes, the genuine qualitative researcher has hardly begun. It is simply not good enough to flick through the text looking for 'interesting quotes' to support a particular theory. The researcher must find a *systematic* way of analysing their data and, in particular, must seek to detect and interpret items of data that appear to contradict or challenge the theories derived from the majority. One of the best short articles on qualitative data analysis was published by Cathy Pope and Sue Ziebland in the *BMJ* a few years ago – look it out if you are new to this field and want to know where to start [23]. If you want the definitive textbook on qualitative research, which describes multiple different approaches to analysis, try the 'qualitative bible', which offers a smorgasbord of approaches [2].

By far the most common way of analysing the kind of qualitative data that are generally collected in biomedical research is thematic analysis. In this, the researchers go through printouts of free text (or do the equivalent on screen), draw up a list of broad themes and allocate coding categories to each. For example, a 'theme' might be patients' knowledge about their illness and within this theme, codes might include 'transmissible causes', 'supernatural causes', 'causes due to own behaviour' and so on. Note that these codes do not correspond to a conventional biomedical taxonomy ('genetic', 'infectious', 'metabolic' and so on), because the point of the research is to explore the interviewees' taxonomy, whether the researcher agrees with it or not. Thematic analysis is often tackled by drawing up a matrix or framework with a new column for each theme and a new row for each 'case' (e.g. an interview transcript) and cutting and pasting relevant segments of text into each box [9]. Thematic analysis can feed into the constant comparative method – in which each new piece of data is compared with the emerging summary of all the previous items, allowing step-by-step refinement of an emerging theory [24].

Chapter 12

Quite commonly these days, qualitative data analysis is performed with the help of a computer programme such as MAXQDA® (VERBI Software, Berlin, Germany), ATLAS-ti® (ATLAS.ti Scientific Software Development, Berlin, Germany) or NVivo® (Lumivero, Denver, CO, USA), which makes it much easier to handle large datasets. The statements made by all the interviewees on a particular topic can be compared with one another, and sophisticated comparisons can be made such as 'did people who made statement A also tend to make statement B?' But, remember, a qualitative computer program does not analyse the data by autopilot, any more than a quantitative program like SPSS® (IBM, Armonk, NY, USA) can tell the researcher which statistical test to apply in each case. While the sentence 'data were analysed using NVivo' might appear impressive, the 'GIGO' rule (garbage in, garbage out) often applies. Excellent qualitative data analysis can occur using the 'VLDRT' (very large dining room table) method, in which printouts of (say) interviews are marked up with felt pens and (say) the constant comparative method is undertaken manually instead of electronically.

It is often difficult when writing up qualitative research to demonstrate how quality control was achieved. As mentioned in the previous section, just because the data have been analysed by more than one researcher does not necessarily assure rigour. Indeed, researchers who never disagree on their subjective judgements (is a particular paragraph in a patient's account really evidence of 'anxiety' or 'disempowerment' or 'trust'?) are probably not thinking hard enough about their own interpretations. The essence of quality in such circumstances is more to do with the level of critical dialogue between the researchers, and in how disagreements were exposed and resolved. In analysing our early research data on the health beliefs of British Bangladeshis with diabetes, for example, three of us looked in turn at a typed interview transcript and assigned codings to particular statements [25]. We then compared our decisions and argued (sometimes heatedly) about our disagreements. Our analysis revealed differences in the interpretation of certain statements that we were unable to fully resolve. For example, we never reached agreement about what the term 'taking exercise' means in this ethnic group. This did not mean that one of us was 'wrong' but that there were inherent ambiguities in the data. Perhaps, for example, this sample of interviewees were themselves confused about what the term exercise meant and the benefits it offered to people with diabetes.

Question seven: Are the results credible and, if so, are they clinically important?

We obviously cannot assess the credibility of qualitative results via the precision and accuracy of measuring devices, nor their significance via confidence intervals and numbers needed to treat. The most important tool to determine whether the results are sensible and believable, and whether they matter in practice, is plain common sense.

One important aspect of the results section to check is whether the authors cite actual data. Claims such as 'general practitioners did not usually recognise the value of annual appraisal' would be more credible if one or two verbatim quotes from the interviewees were reproduced to illustrate them. The results should be independently and objectively verifiable (e.g. by including longer segments of text in an appendix or online resource), and all quotes and examples should be indexed so that they can be traced back to an identifiable interviewee and data source.

Question eight: What conclusions were drawn and are they justified by the results?
A quantitative research paper, presented in standard introduction, methods, research and discussion (or IMRAD) format (see Chapter 3), should clearly distinguish the study's results (usually a set of numbers) from the interpretation of those results. The reader should have no difficulty separating what the researchers *found* from what they think it *means*. In qualitative research, however, such a distinction is rarely possible, as the results are by definition an interpretation of the data. It is therefore necessary, when assessing the validity of qualitative research, to ask whether the interpretation placed on the data accords with common sense and that the researcher's personal, professional and cultural perspective is made explicit so the reader can assess the 'lens' through which the researcher has undertaken the fieldwork, analysis and interpretation. This can be a difficult exercise because the language we use to describe things tends to impugn meanings and motives that the participants themselves may not share. Compare, for example, the two statements, 'three women went to the well to get water' and 'three women met at the well and each was carrying a pitcher'.

It is becoming a cliché that the conclusions of qualitative studies, like those of all research, should be 'grounded in evidence' (i.e. that they should flow from what the researchers found in the field). Mays and Pope [7] suggest three useful questions for determining whether the conclusions of a qualitative study are valid:

- How well does this analysis explain why people behave in the way they do?
- How comprehensible would this explanation be to a thoughtful participant in the setting?
- How well does the explanation cohere with what we already know?

Question nine: Are the findings of the study transferable to other settings?
One of the most common criticisms of qualitative research is that the findings of any qualitative study pertain only to the limited setting in which they were obtained. In fact, this is not necessarily any truer of qualitative research than of quantitative research. Look back at the example of women's birth experiences in question three. A convenience sample of the first dozen women to give birth would provide little more than the collected experiences of these 12 women. A *purposive* sample as described in question three would extend the transferability of the findings to women

having a wide range of birth experience. But by making iterative adjustments to the sampling frame as the research study unfolds, the researchers will be able to develop a theoretical sample and test new theories as they emerge. For example (and note, we are making this example up), the researchers might find that better educated women seem to have more psychologically traumatic experiences than less well educated women. This might lead to a new hypothesis about women's expectations (the better educated the woman, the more she expects a 'perfect birth experience'), which would in turn lead to a change in the purposive sampling strategy (we now want to find extremes of maternal education) and so on. The more the research has been driven by this kind of progressive focusing and iterative data analysis, the more its findings are likely to be transferable beyond the sample itself.

Conclusion

Doctors have traditionally placed a high value on number-based data, which may in reality be misleading, reductionist and irrelevant to the real issues. The increasing popularity of qualitative research in the biomedical sciences has arisen largely because quantitative methods provided either no answers, or the wrong answers, to important questions in both clinical care and service delivery. If you still feel that qualitative research is necessarily second rate by virtue of being a 'soft' science, you should be aware that you are out of step with much mainstream opinion on this topic.

Back in 1993, Catherine Pope and Nicky Britten presented at a conference a paper entitled 'Barriers to qualitative methods in the medical mindset', in which they showed their collection of rejection letters from biomedical journals [26]. The letters revealed a striking ignorance of qualitative methodology on the part of reviewers. In other words, the people who had rejected the papers often appeared to be incapable of distinguishing good qualitative research from bad.

Somewhat ironically, poor-quality qualitative papers now appear regularly in some medical journals, which appear to have undergone an about-face in editorial policy since Pope and Britten's exposure of the 'medical mindset'. We hope, therefore, that the questions listed earlier, and the subsequent references, will assist reviewers in both camps: those who continue to reject qualitative papers for the wrong reasons and those who have climbed on the qualitative bandwagon and are now *accepting* such papers for the wrong reasons! If you're interested in qualitative research, you might like to read the open letter that Trisha and colleagues wrote to the *BMJ* asking them to change their editorial bias against qualitative research [27].

Exercises based on this chapter

1. Search electronically for the paper on attitudes to vaping by Rooke et al. [28]. What was the research question? What kind of sample was selected and why? What qualitative methods were used and what data were collected? What were the findings and how far do you trust them? When you have read Chapter 13, how might you use these qualitative findings to inform the design of a quantitative survey?
2. Take a look at these two papers on diabetes: 'This does my head in' [29] and 'Sociocultural influences on the behaviour of South Asian women with diabetes in pregnancy' [30]. What was the research question in each case? What was the sample and how was it justified? What qualitative methods were used and why? What did you learn about the patient experience of diabetes from these papers that you did not know (and could not have gained) from quantitative studies?

References

1. Black N. Why we need qualitative research. *Journal of Epidemiology and Community Health* 1994; **48**: 425–6.
2. Denzin NK, Lincoln YS, Giardina MD, Cannella GS. *The SAGE Handbook of Qualitative Research*, 6th edn. Sage, London, 2023.
3. Giacomini MK, Cook DJ. Users' guides to the medical literature XXIII. Qualitative research in health care A. Are the results of the study valid? *JAMA* 2000; **284**: 357–62.
4. Giacomini MK, Cook D. Users' guides to the medical literature: XXIII. Qualitative research in health care B. What are the results and how do they help me care for my patients? *JAMA* 2000; **284**: 478–82.
5. Noyes J, Booth A, Cargo M, et al. Chapter 21: Qualitative Evidence. In: Higgins JPT, Green S (eds), *Cochrane Handbook for Systematic Reviews of Interventions* Version 6.3. London: Cochrane Collaboration; 2022.
6. Noyes J, Booth A, Moore G, et al. Synthesising quantitative and qualitative evidence to inform guidelines on complex interventions: clarifying the purposes, designs and outlining some methods. *BMJ Global Health* 2019; **4**(Suppl 1): e000893.
7. Mays N, Pope C. Qualitative research in health care: assessing quality in qualitative research. *BMJ* 2000; **320**: 50.
8. Gilgun JF. Reflexivity and qualitative research. *Current Issues in Qualitative Research* 2010; **1**(2): 1–8.
9. Reeves S, Albert M, Kuper A, et al. Qualitative research: why use theories in qualitative research? *BMJ* 2008; **337**: 631–4.
10. Lingard L, Albert M, Levinson W. Grounded theory, mixed methods, and action research. *BMJ* 2008; **337**: a567.

11. Kuper A, Lingard L, Levinson W. Critically appraising qualitative research. *BMJ* 2008; **337**: a1035.
12. Kuper A, Reeves S, Levinson W. Qualitative research: an introduction to reading and appraising qualitative research. *BMJ* 2008; **337**: 404–7.
13. Reeves S, Kuper A, Hodges BD. Qualitative research methodologies: ethnography. *BMJ* 2008; **337**: a1020.
14. Pope C, Mays N. *Qualitative Research in Health Care*, 5th edn. Chichester: Wiley; 2024.
15. Greenhalgh T, Thorne S, Malterud K. Time to challenge the spurious hierarchy of systematic over narrative reviews? *European Journal of Clinical Investigation* 2018; **48**: e12931.
16. Lewin S, Booth A, Glenton C, et al. Applying GRADE-CERQual to qualitative evidence synthesis findings: introduction to the series. *Implementation Science* 2018; **13**(Suppl 1): 2.
17. Lewin S, Bohren M, Rashidian A, et al. Applying GRADE-CERQual to qualitative evidence synthesis findings. Paper 2: How to make an overall CERQual assessment of confidence and create a summary of qualitative findings table. *Implementation Science* 2018; **13**(Suppl 1):10.
18. Munthe-Kaas H, Bohren MA, Glenton C, et al. Applying GRADE-CERQual to qualitative evidence synthesis findings. Paper 3: How to assess methodological limitations. *Implementation Science* 2018; **13**(Suppl 1): 9.
19. Edmunds LD, Ovseiko PV, Shepperd S, et al. Why do women choose or reject careers in academic medicine? A narrative review of empirical evidence. *Lancet* 2016; **388**: 2948–58.
20. Noyes J, Booth A, Cargo M, et al. Chapter 21: Qualitative evidence. In: *Cochrane Handbook for Systematic Reviews of Interventions*, Version 6.4. Oxford: Cochrane, 2023. URL: https://training.cochrane.org/handbook/current/chapter-21 (accessed 13 June 2024).
21. Barbour RS. Checklists for improving rigour in qualitative research a case of the tail wagging the dog? *BMJ* 2001; **322**: 1115.
22. Dixon-Woods M, Shaw RL, Agarwal S, et al. The problem of appraising qualitative research. *Quality and Safety in Health Care* 2004; **13**(3): 223–5.
23. Pope C, Ziebland S, Mays N. Qualitative research in health care: analysing qualitative data. *BMJ* 2000; **320**: 114.
24. Glaser BG. The constant comparative method of qualitative analysis. *Social Problems* 1965; **12**: 436–45.
25. Greenhalgh T, Helman C, Chowdhury AM. Health beliefs and folk models of diabetes in British Bangladeshis: a qualitative study. *BMJ* 1998; **316**: 978–83.
26. Pope C, Britten N. *The quality of rejection: barriers to qualitative methods in the medical mindset.* Paper presented at BSA Medical Sociology Group annual conference, 1993.
27. Greenhalgh T, Annandale E, Ashcroft R, et al. An open letter to The *BMJ* editors on qualitative research. *BMJ* 2016; **352**: i563.
28. Rooke C, Cunningham-Burley S, Amos A. Smokers' and ex-smokers' understanding of electronic cigarettes: a qualitative study. *Tobacco Control* 2016; **25**(e1): e60–6.

29. Hinder S, Greenhalgh T. 'This does my head in'. Ethnographic study of self-management by people with diabetes. *BMC Health Services Research* 2012; **12**: 83.
30. Greenhalgh T, Clinch M, Afsar N, et al. Socio-cultural influences on the behaviour of South Asian women with diabetes in pregnancy: qualitative study using a multi-level theoretical approach. *BMC Medicine* 2015; **13**: 120.

Chapter 13 Papers that report questionnaire research

The rise and rise of questionnaire research

When and where did you last fill out a questionnaire? They come through the door and appear in our pigeon holes at work. We get them as email attachments and find them in the dentist's waiting room. The kids bring them home from school, and it's not uncommon for one to accompany the bill in a restaurant. Online questionnaires seem to pop up with increasing frequency, asking everything from our political views to our opinions on TV programmes.

This chapter is based on a series of papers that Trisha edited some years ago for the *BMJ*, written by a team led by her colleague Petra Boynton [1–3]. That series has stood the test of time, although, since its publication, questionnaire research has to a large extent gone digital. The principles, however, remain the same. There is probably more bad questionnaire research in the literature than just about any other study design. While you need a laboratory to do bad lab work, and a supply of medicines to do bad pharmaceutical research, all you need to do to produce bad questionnaire research is to write out a list of questions and ask a few people to answer them, either by ticking boxes on a printed sheet or (more commonly these days) entering your responses online.

Questionnaires are often considered as an 'objective' means of collecting information about people's knowledge, beliefs, attitudes and behaviour [4,5]. Do our patients like our opening hours? What do teenagers think of a local anti-drugs campaign and has it changed their attitudes? How much do nurses know about the management of asthma? What proportion of the population view themselves as gay or bisexual? Why don't doctors use computers to their maximum potential? You can probably see from these examples that questionnaires can seek both quantitative data (*x* per cent of people like our services) and qualitative data (people using our services have *xyz* experiences).

How to Read a Paper: The Basics of Evidence-Based Healthcare, Seventh Edition.
Trisha Greenhalgh and Paul Dijkstra.

In other words, questionnaires are not a 'quantitative method' or a 'qualitative method' but a tool for collecting a range of different types of data, depending on the question asked in each item and the format in which responders are expected to answer them.

We've already used the expression 'GIGO' (garbage in, garbage out) in previous chapters to make the point that poorly structured instruments lead to poor quality data, misleading conclusions and woolly recommendations. Nowhere is that more true than in questionnaire research. While clear guidance on the design and reporting of randomised controlled trials (RCTs) and systematic reviews is now widely used (see the discussion about the CONSORT checklist in Chapter 6 and the PRISMA and AMSTAR checklists in Chapter 9), comparable frameworks for questionnaire research have been published in relatively obscure journals and are less widely cited [4–8]. Perhaps for this reason, despite a wealth of detailed guidance in the specialist literature [9,10], elementary methodological errors are common in questionnaire research undertaken by health professionals [1–3].

Before we turn to the critical appraisal, a word about terminology. A questionnaire is designed to measure formally an aspect of human psychology. We sometimes refer to questionnaires as 'instruments'. The questions within a questionnaire are sometimes known as *items*. An item is the smallest unit within the questionnaire that is individually scored. It might comprise a stem ('pick which of the following responses corresponds to your own view') and then five possible options. Or it might be a simple 'yes/no' or 'true/false' response.

Ten questions to ask about a paper describing a questionnaire study

Question one: What was the research question and was the questionnaire appropriate for answering it?

Look back to Chapter 3, where we describe three preliminary questions to get you started in appraising any paper. The first of these was 'What was the research question and why was the study needed?'. This is a particularly good starter question for questionnaire studies, because inexperienced researchers often embark on questionnaire research without clarifying why they are doing it or what they want to find out. In addition, people often decide to use a questionnaire for studies that need a totally different method. Sometimes, a questionnaire will be appropriate but only if used within a mixed-methods study (e.g. to extend and quantify the findings of an initial exploratory phase). Table 13.1 gives some real examples based on papers that Petra Boynton and Trisha collected from the published literature and offered by participants in courses they have run.

Table 13.1 Examples of research questions for which a questionnaire may *not* be the most appropriate design

Broad area of research	Example of research questions	Why is a questionnaire NOT the most appropriate method?	What method(s) should be used instead?
Burden of disease	What is the prevalence of asthma in schoolchildren?	A child may have asthma but the parent does not know it; parents may think incorrectly that their child has asthma; or they may withhold information that is perceived as stigmatising	Cross-sectional survey using standardised diagnostic criteria and/or systematic analysis of medical records
Professional behaviour	How do general practitioners manage low back pain?	What doctors say they do is not the same as what they actually do, especially when they think their practice is being judged by others	Direct observation or video recording of consultations; use of simulated patients; systematic analysis of medical records
Health-related lifestyle	What proportion of people in smoking cessation studies quit successfully?	The proportion of true quitters is less than the proportion who say they have quit. A similar pattern is seen in studies of dietary choices, exercise and other lifestyle factors	'Gold standard' diagnostic test (in this example, urinary or salivary cotinine)
Needs assessment in 'special needs' groups	What are the unmet needs of refugees and asylum seekers for health and social care services?	A questionnaire is likely to reflect the preconceptions of researchers (e.g. it may take existing services and/or the needs of more 'visible' groups as its starting point) and fail to tap into important areas of need	Range of exploratory qualitative methods designed to build up a 'rich picture' of the problem (e.g. semi-structured interviews of users, health professionals and the voluntary sector); focus groups; in-depth studies of critical events

There are many advantages to researchers of using a previously validated and published questionnaire. The research team will save time and resources; they will be able to compare their own findings with those from other studies; they need only give outline details of the instrument when they write up their work; and they will not need to have gone through a thorough validation process for the instrument. Sadly, inexperienced researchers (most typically, students doing a dissertation) tend to forget to look thoroughly in the literature for a suitable 'off the peg' instrument, and such individuals often do not know about formal validation techniques (see below). Even though most such studies will be rejected by journal editors, a worrying proportion find their way into the literature.

Increasingly, health services research uses standard 'off the peg' questionnaires designed explicitly for producing data that can be compared across studies. For example, clinical trials routinely include standard instruments to measure patients' knowledge about a disease [11], satisfaction with services [12] or health-related quality of life [13,14]. The validity of this approach depends crucially on whether the type and range of closed responses (i.e. the list of possible answers that people are asked to select from) reflects the full range of perceptions and feelings that people in all the different potential sampling frames might actually hold.

Question two: Was the questionnaire used in the study valid and reliable?
A valid questionnaire measures what it claims to measure. In reality, many fail to do this. For example, a self-completion questionnaire that seeks to measure people's food intake may be invalid, because in reality it measures what they *say* they have eaten, not what they have *actually* eaten [15]. Similarly, questionnaires asking patients how well they adhere to application-based digital interventions have been shown to differ significantly from their actual level of adherence [16]. An old study showed that doctors' self-reported adherence to guidelines is similarly inflated compared with their actual adherence [17]. Note that an instrument developed in a different time, country or cultural context may not be a valid measure in the group you are studying. Here's a quirky example. The item 'I often attend gay parties' was a valid measure of a person's self-assessed propensity to attend *fun* parties in the UK in the 1950s but the wording has a very different connotation today [1]!

Reliable questionnaires yield consistent results from repeated samples and different researchers over time [9,10]. Differences in the results obtained from a reliable questionnaire come from differences between participants and not from inconsistencies in how the items are understood or how different observers interpret the responses. A standardised questionnaire is one that is written and administered in a strictly set manner, so all participants are asked precisely the same questions in an identical format and responses recorded in a uniform manner. Standardising a measure increases its reliability. If you participated in the UK Census (General Household Survey) in 2021, you may remember being asked a rather mechanical set of questions. This is because the interviewer had been trained to administer the instrument in a highly standardised way, so as to increase reliability. It's often difficult to ascertain from a published paper how hard the researchers tried to achieve standardisation, but they may have quoted inter-rater reliability figures.

Question three: What did the questionnaire look like and was this appropriate for the target population?
When we say 'what did it look like?' we're talking about two things – form and content. Form concerns issues such as how many pages was it, was it visually appealing (or off-putting), how long did it take to fill in, the terminology used, and so on. These are not minor issues! A questionnaire that goes on for 30 pages, includes reams of scientific jargon and contains questions that a respondent might find offensive, will not be properly filled in – and hence the results of a survey will be meaningless [2]. Many questionnaires these days are online, so there are additional design issues to consider (such as whether and how to indicate how far towards completion the respondent has got). Vera Toepoel has written a great book on online survey design [18].

Content is about the actual items. Did the questions make sense and could the participants in the sample understand them? Were any questions ambiguous or overly complicated? Were ambiguous weasel words such as 'frequently', 'regularly', 'commonly', 'usually', 'many', 'some' and 'hardly ever' avoided? Were the items 'open' (respondents can write anything they like) or 'closed' (respondents must pick from a list of options) and, if the latter, were all potential responses represented? Closed-ended designs enable researchers to produce aggregated data quickly but the range of possible answers is set by the researchers, not the respondents, and the richness of responses is therefore much lower [19]. Some respondents (known as *yea-sayers*) tend to agree with statements rather than disagree. For this reason, researchers should not present their items so that 'strongly agree' always links to the same broad attitude. For example, on a patient satisfaction scale, if one question is 'my GP generally tries to help me out', another question should be phrased in the negative (e.g. 'the receptionists are usually *impolite*').

Question four: Were the instructions clear?
If you have ever been asked to fill out a questionnaire and 'got lost' halfway through (or discovered you don't know where to send it once you've filled it

in), you will know that instructions contribute crucially to the validity of the instrument. These include:

- an explanation of what the study is about and what the overall purpose of the research is
- an assurance of anonymity and confidentiality, as well as confirmation that the person can stop completing the questionnaire at any time without having to give a reason
- clear and accurate contact details of whom to approach for further information
- instructions on what they need to send back and a stamped addressed envelope if it is a postal questionnaire
- adequate instructions on how to complete each item, with examples where necessary
- any insert (e.g. leaflet), gift (e.g. book token) or honorarium, if these are part of the protocol.

These aspects of the study are unlikely to be listed in the published paper, but they may be in an appendix, and, if not, you should be able to get the information from the authors.

Question five: Was the questionnaire adequately piloted?
Questionnaires often fail because participants don't understand them, can't complete them, get bored or offended by them or dislike how they look [1–3]. Although friends and colleagues can help check spelling, grammar and layout, they cannot reliably predict the emotional reactions or comprehension difficulties of other groups. For this reason, all questionnaires (whether newly developed or 'off the peg') should be piloted on participants who are representative of the definitive study sample to see, for example, how long people take to complete the instrument, whether any items are misunderstood, or whether people get bored or confused halfway through. Three specific questions to ask are: (i) What were the characteristics of the participants on whom the instrument was piloted? (ii) *How* was the piloting exercise undertaken – what details are given? and (iii) *In what ways* was the definitive instrument changed as a result of piloting?

Question six: What was the sample?
If you have read the previous chapters, you will know that a skewed or non-representative sample will lead to misleading results and unsafe conclusions. When you appraise a questionnaire study, it is important to ask what was the sampling frame for the definitive study (purposive, random and snowball)

and also whether it was sufficiently large and representative. Given here are the main types of sample for a questionnaire study (Table 13.2):

- *Random sample*: a target group is identified and a random selection of people from that group is invited to participate. For example, a computer might be used to select a random one in four sample from a diabetes register.
- *Stratified random sample*: as for a random sample but the target group is first stratified according to a particular characteristic(s), for example, diabetic people on insulin, tablets and diet. Random sampling is carried out separately for these different subgroups.
- *Snowball sample*: a small group of participants is identified and then asked to 'invite a friend' to complete the questionnaire. This group is in turn invited to nominate someone else, and so on.

Table 13.2 Types of sampling frame for questionnaire research

Sample type	How it works	When to use
Opportunity/ convenience	Participants are selected from a group who are available at time of study (e.g. patients attending a GP surgery on a particular morning)	Should be avoided if possible
Random	A target group is identified, and a random selection of people from that group is invited to participate; for example, a computer might be used to select a random one in four sample from a diabetes register	Use in studies where you wish to reflect the average viewpoint of a population
Stratified random	As random sample but the target group is first stratified according to a particular characteristic(s); for example, diabetic people on insulin, tablets and diet. Random sampling is carried out separately for these different subgroups	Use when the target group is likely to have systematic differences by subgroup
Quota	Participants who match the wider population are identified (e.g. into groups such as social class, gender age). Researchers are given a set number within each group to interview (e.g. so many young middle-class women)	For studies where you want to reflect outcomes as closely representative of the wider population as possible. Frequently used in political opinion polls, and so on
Snowball	Participants are recruited, and asked to identify other similar people to take part in the research	Helpful when working with hard-to-reach groups (e.g. lesbian mothers)

- *Opportunity sample*: usually for pragmatic reasons, the first people to appear who meet the criteria are asked to complete the questionnaire. This might happen, for example, in a busy general practice surgery when all patients attending on a particular day are asked to fill out a survey about the convenience of opening hours. But such a sample is clearly biased, as those who find the opening hours inconvenient won't be there in the first place! This example should remind you that opportunity (sometimes known as *convenience*) samples are rarely if ever scientifically justified.
- *Systematically skewed sample*: let's say that you want to assess how satisfied patients are with their general practitioner (GP), and you already know from your pilot study that 80% of people from affluent postcodes will complete the questionnaire but only 60% of those from deprived postcodes will. You could oversample from the latter group to ensure that your dataset reflects the socioeconomic makeup of your practice population. (Ideally, if you did this, you would also have to show that people who refused to fill out the questionnaire did not differ in key characteristics from those who completed it).

It is also important to consider whether the instrument was suitable for all participants and potential participants. In particular, did it take account of the likely range in the sample of physical and intellectual abilities, language and literacy, understanding of numbers or scaling and perceived threat of questions or questioner?

Question seven: How was the questionnaire administered and was the response rate adequate?

The methods section of a paper describing a questionnaire study should include details of three aspects of administration: (i) How was the questionnaire distributed (e.g. by post, face to face or electronically)? (ii) How was the questionnaire completed (e.g. self-completion or researcher-assisted)? (iii) Were the response rates reported fully, including details of participants who were unsuitable for the research or refused to take part? Have any potential response biases been discussed?

The *BMJ* will not usually publish a paper describing a questionnaire survey if fewer than 70% of people approached completed the questionnaire properly. Response rates to surveys sent out online tend to have much lower response rates than those distributed on paper (the average is 44% [20]), since many people delete the email as 'junk mail'. It is not unusual in a mass email distribution to get response rates of 10% or less. The 10% who respond usually differ systematically from the 90% who do not; for example, they are likely to be more interested in the topic and have more spare time!

There have been a number of research studies on how to increase the response rate to a questionnaire study. In summary, the following have all been shown to increase response rates [3, 20, 21]:

- The questionnaire is clearly designed and has a simple layout.
- It offers participants incentives or prizes in return for completion.
- It has been thoroughly piloted and tested.
- Participants are notified about the study in advance, with a personalised invitation.
- The aim of the study and means of completing the questionnaire are clearly explained.
- A researcher is on hand to answer questions and collect the completed questionnaire.
- If using a postal questionnaire, a stamped addressed envelope is included.
- The participants feel they are stakeholders in the study.
- Questions are phrased in a way that holds the participants' attention.
- The questionnaire has clear focus and purpose, and is kept concise.
- The questionnaire is appealing to look at.
- A prize or payment is offered.
- Potential respondents are recruited via peers who have already done the questionnaire.

Another thing to look for in relation to response rates is a table in the paper comparing the characteristics of people who responded with people who were approached but refused to fill out the questionnaire. If there were systematic (as opposed to chance) differences between these groups, the results of the survey will not be generalisable to the population from which the responders were drawn. Responders to surveys conducted in the street, for example, are often older than average (perhaps because they are in less of a hurry!) and less likely to be from an ethnic minority (perhaps because some of the latter are unable to speak the language of the researcher fluently). On the other hand, if the authors of the study have shown that non-responders are pretty similar to responders, you should worry less about generalisability, even if response rates were lower than you would have liked.

Question eight: How were the data analysed?
Analysis of questionnaire data is a sophisticated science. There are some excellent textbooks on social research methods if you are interested in learning the formal techniques [9,10]. If you are just interested in completing a checklist about a published questionnaire study, try considering these aspects of the study. First, broadly what sort of analysis was carried out and was this appropriate? In particular, were the correct statistical tests used for

quantitative responses, and/or was a recognisable method of qualitative analysis (see section 'Measuring costs and benefits of health interventions') used for open-ended questions? It is reassuring (but by no means a flawless test) to learn that one of the paper's authors is a statistician. And as we said in Chapter 5, if the statistical tests used are ones you have never heard of, you should probably smell a rat. The vast majority of questionnaire data can be analysed using commonly used statistical tests such as chi square, Spearman's, Pearson correlation and so on. The most common mistake of all in questionnaire research is to use no statistical tests at all, and you don't need a PhD in statistics to spot that dodge!

You should also check to ensure that there is no evidence of 'data dredging'. In other words, have the authors simply thrown their data into a computer and run hundreds of tests and then dreamt up a plausible hypothesis to go with something that comes out as 'significant'? In the jargon, all analyses should be hypothesis driven; that is, the hypothesis should be thought up first and then the analysis should be performed, not vice versa.

Question nine: What were the main results?

Consider first what the overall findings were, and whether all relevant data were reported. Are quantitative results definitive (statistically significant), and are relevant *non-significant* results also reported? It may be just as important to have discovered, for example, that GPs' self-reported confidence in managing diabetes is *not* correlated to their knowledge about the condition as it would have been to discover that there was a correlation! For this reason, the questionnaire study that only comments on the 'positive' statistical associations is internally biased.

Another important question is have qualitative results been adequately interpreted (e.g. using an explicit theoretical framework) and have any quotes been properly justified and contextualised (rather than 'cherry picked' to spice up the paper)? Look back at Chapter 6 ('Papers that report drug trials and other simple interventions') and remind yourself of the tricks used by unscrupulous marketing people to oversell findings. Check carefully the graphs (especially the zero-intercept on axes) and the data tables.

Question ten: What are the key conclusions?

This is a commonsense question. What do the results actually mean and have the researchers drawn an appropriate link between the data and their conclusions? Have the findings been placed within the wider body of knowledge in the field (especially any similar or contrasting surveys using the same instrument)? Have the authors acknowledged the limitations of their study and couched their discussion in the light of these (e.g. if the sample was small or the response rate low, did they recommend further studies to confirm the preliminary findings)? Finally, are any recommendations fully justified by the findings? For example, if they have performed a small, parochial study, they should not be suggesting changes in national policy as a result! If you are new to critical appraisal, you may find such judgements difficult to make, and the best way to get better is to join in journal club discussions (either face to face or online) where a group of you share your commonsense reactions to a chosen paper.

In conclusion, anyone can write down a list of questions and photocopy it – but this doesn't mean that a set of responses to these questions constitutes research! The development, administration, analysis and reporting of questionnaire studies is at least as challenging as the other research approaches described in other chapters in this book. Questionnaire researchers are a disparate bunch and have not yet agreed on a structured reporting format comparable to CONSORT (RCTs), QUORUM or PRISMA (systematic reviews) and AGREE (guidelines). While a number of suggested structured tools, each designed for slightly different purposes, are now available [4–8], a review of such tools found little consensus and many unanswered questions [6]. We suspect that as such guides come to be standardised and more widely used, papers describing questionnaire research will be more consistent and easier to appraise.

Exercises based on this chapter

1. Collect the next five questionnaires you are asked to fill out. These can be anything from an evaluation form in a restaurant to a student or staff satisfaction questionnaire – or even something that pops up on email. Answer these questions for each. What do you think the purpose of the questionnaire was? What do you think of the sampling frame? Did the questionnaire items cover everything you felt was relevant? Did closed-item questions offer appropriate response options? Was the instrument visually appealing and easily navigable? In what way might flaws in the design have led to biased findings? How would you redesign it?
2. Take a look at the survey of medical and law students' consumption of alcohol and recreational drugs by Bogowicz et al. [22]. Using the list of questions in the previous exercise (or, if you prefer, the more extensive list in the Appendix), critically appraise the paper. How far do you trust the conclusions?
3. Read the paper by Kojima et al., which describes a large survey of rheumatoid arthritis in Japan [23]. What was the research question? What do you think about how the data were collected? What did the study reveal (and what did it fail to reveal) about this disease? To what extent would the findings be transferable to a non-Japanese population?

References

1. Boynton PM, Wood GW, Greenhalgh T. A hands on guide to questionnaire research part three: reaching beyond the white middle classes. *BMJ* 2004; **328**: 1433–6.
2. Boynton PM, Greenhalgh T. A hands on guide to questionnaire research part one: selecting, designing, and developing your questionnaire. *BMJ* 2004; **328**: 1312–15.
3. Boynton PM. A hands on guide to questionnaire research part two: administering, analysing, and reporting your questionnaire. *BMJ* 2004; **328**: 1372–5.
4. Kelley K, Clark B, Brown V, Sitzia J. Good practice in the conduct and reporting of survey research. *International Journal for Quality in Health Care* 2003; **15**: 261–6.
5. Draugalis JR, Coons SJ, Plaza CM. Best practices for survey research reports: a synopsis for authors and reviewers. *American Journal of Pharmaceutical Education* 2008; **72**: 11.
6. Bennett C, Khangura S, Brehaut JC, et al. Reporting guidelines for survey research: an analysis of published guidance and reporting practices. *PLoS Medicine* 2011; **8**(8): e1001069.
7. Eysenbach G. Improving the quality of web surveys: the Checklist for Reporting Results of Internet E-Surveys (CHERRIES). *Journal of Medical Internet Research* 2004; **6**: e34.
8. Burns KE, Duffett M, Kho ME, et al., ACCADEMY Group. A guide for the design and conduct of self-administered surveys of clinicians. *CMAJ* 2008; **179**: 245–52.
9. Robson C. *Real World Research: A resource for users of social research methods in applied settings*. 5th edn. Hoboken, NJ: Wiley; 2023.
10. Clark T, Foster L, Sloan L, et al. *Bryman's Social Research Methods*. 6th edn. Oxford: Oxford University Press; 2021.
11. Mallah N, Rodriguez-Cano R, Figueiras A, Takkouche B. Design, reliability and construct validity of a knowledge, attitude and practice questionnaire on personal use of antibiotics in Spain. *Scientific Reports* 2020; **10**: 20668.
12. Cascella M, Coluccia S, Grizzuti M, et al. Satisfaction with telemedicine for cancer pain management: a model of care and cross-sectional patient satisfaction study. *Current Oncology* 2022; **29**: 5566–78.
13. Phillips D. *Quality of Life: Concept, policy and practice*. London: Routledge; 2012.
14. El-Rabbany M, Blanas N, Sutherland S, et al. Development and evaluation of the clinimetric properties of the Medication-Related Osteonecrosis of the Jaw Quality of Life Questionnaire (MRONJ-QoL). *International Journal of Oral and Maxillofacial Surgery* 2022; **51**: 768–75.
15. Archer E, Marler ML, Lavie CJ. Controversy and debate: memory based methods paper 1: the fatal flaws of food frequency questionnaires and other memory-based dietary assessment methods. *Journal of Clinical Epidemiology* 2018; **104**: P113–24.
16. Flett JA, Fletcher BD, Riordan BC, et al. The peril of self-reported adherence in digital interventions: a brief example. *Internet Interventions* 2019; **18**: 100267.
17. Adams AS, Soumerai SB, Lomas J, et al. Evidence of self-report bias in assessing adherence to guidelines. *International Journal for Quality in Health Care* 1999; **11**: 187–92.
18. Toepoel V. *Doing Surveys Online*. London: Sage; 2015.

19. Houtkoop-Steenstra H. *Interaction and the Standardized Survey Interview: The living questionnaire.* Cambridge: Cambridge University Press; 2000.
20. Wu MJ, Zhao K, Fils-Aime F. Response rates of online surveys in published research: A meta-analysis. *Computers in Human Behavior Reports* 2022; **7**: 100206.
21. Pit SW, Vo T, Pyakurel S. The effectiveness of recruitment strategies on general practitioners' survey response rates: a systematic review. *BMC Medical Research Methodology* 2014; **14**(1): 76.
22. Bogowicz P, Ferguson J, Gilvarry E, et al. Alcohol and other substance use among medical and law students at a UK university: a cross-sectional questionnaire survey. *Postgraduate Medical Journal* 2018; **94**: 131–6.
23. Kojima M, Nakayama T, Tsutani K, et al. Epidemiological characteristics of rheumatoid arthritis in Japan: prevalence estimates using a nationwide population-based questionnaire survey. *Modern Rheumatology* 2020; **30**: 941–7.

Chapter 14 **Papers that report quality improvement case studies**

What are quality improvement studies and how should we research them?

The *BMJ* (www.bmj.com) mainly publishes research articles. Another leading journal, *BMJ Quality and Safety* (http://qualitysafety.bmj.com), mainly publishes descriptions of initiatives to improve the quality and safety of healthcare, often in real-world settings such as hospital wards or general practices [1]. If you are studying for an undergraduate exam, you should ask your tutors whether quality improvement studies are going to feature in your exams, because the material covered here is more often contained in postgraduate courses and you may find that it's not on your syllabus. If that is the case, put this chapter aside for after you've passed – you will certainly need it when you are working full time in the real world!

One key way of improving quality is to implement the findings of research and make care more evidence-based. This is discussed in Trisha's book *How to Implement Evidence-Based Healthcare* [2]. But achieving a high-quality and safe health service requires more than evidence-based practice. Think of the last time you or one of your relatives attended a general practitioner (GP) or was admitted to hospital. No doubt, you wanted to have the most accurate diagnostic tests (Chapter 8), the most efficacious drugs (Chapter 6) or non-drug interventions (Chapter 7), and you also wanted the clinicians to follow evidence-based care plans and guidelines (Chapter 10) based on systematic reviews (Chapter 9). Furthermore, if the providers asked you to help evaluate their service, you would have wanted them to use a valid and reliable questionnaire (Chapter 13).

But did you also care about things like how long you had to wait for an outpatient appointment and/or your operation, the attitudes of staff, the clarity and completeness of the information you were given, the risk of catching an infection (e.g. when staff didn't wash their hands consistently or wear

How to Read a Paper: The Basics of Evidence-Based Healthcare, Seventh Edition.
Trisha Greenhalgh and Paul Dijkstra.

masks) and the general efficiency of the place? If a member of staff made an error, was this openly disclosed to you and an unreserved apology offered? And if this happened, did the organisation have systems in place to learn from what went wrong and ensure that it didn't happen again to someone else? A 'quality' healthcare experience includes all these things and more. The science of quality improvement draws its evidence from many different disciplines including research on manufacturing and air traffic control as well as evidence-based medicine [3–5].

Improving quality and safety in a particular area of healthcare typically involves a complex project lasting at least a few months, with input from different staff members and also from patients and their representatives [6]. The leaders of the project help everyone involved set a goal and work towards it. The fortunes of the project are typically mixed – some things go well, other things not so well, and the initiative is typically written up (if at all) as a story.

For several years now, *BMJ* and *BMJ Quality and Safety* have distinguished research papers (presented as IMRAD: introduction, methods, results and discussion) from quality improvement reports (presented as COMPASEN: context, outline of problem, measures, process, analysis, strategy for change, effects of change, and next steps). In making this distinction, research might be defined as *systematic and focused enquiry seeking truths that are transferable beyond the setting in which they were generated*, while quality improvement might be defined as *real-time, real-world work undertaken by teams who deliver services.*

You might have spotted that there is a large grey zone between these two activities. Some of this grey zone is quality improvement *research*; that is, applied research aimed at building the evidence base on how we should go about quality improvement studies. Quality improvement research embraces a broad range of methods including most of the ones described in the other chapters; see the review by Portela et al. [7] for the many different study types used in improvement research. In particular, the *mixed-method case study* incorporates both quantitative data (e.g. measures of the incidence and prevalence of a particular condition or problem) and qualitative data (e.g. a careful analysis of the themes raised in complaint letters or participant observation of staff going about their duties), all written up in an overarching story about what was done, why, when, by whom and what the consequences were. If the paper is true quality improvement *research*, it should include a conclusion that offers transferable lessons for other teams in other settings [8,9].

Incidentally, while the story ('anecdote') is rightly seen as a weak study design when, say, evaluating the efficacy of a drug, the story *format* ('organisational case study') has unique advantages when the task is to pull together a great deal of complex data and make sense of it, as is the case when an organisation sets out to improve its performance [10].

As you can probably imagine, critical appraisal of quality improvement research is a particularly challenging area. Unlike in randomised trials, there are no hard and fast rules on what the 'best' approach to a quality improvement initiative should be, and subjective judgements may be needed about the methods used and the significance of the findings. But as with all critical appraisal, the more papers you read and appraise, the better you will get.

In preparing the list of questions in the next section, we have drawn heavily on the SQUIRE 2 (Standards for QUality Improvement Reporting Excellence) guidelines, which are the equivalent of Consolidated Standards of Reporting Trials (CONSORT), Preferred Reporting Items for Systematic Reviews and Meta-Analyses (PRISMA) and so on for quality improvement studies [11]. Trisha was peripherally involved in the development of the original version of these guidelines and can confirm that they went through multiple iterations and struggles before appearing in print. This is because of the *inherent* challenges of producing structured checklists for appraising complex, multifaceted studies. To quote from the original paper by the SQUIRE development group ([12], p. 670):

> *Unlike conceptually neat and procedurally unambiguous interventions, such as drugs, tests, and procedures, that directly affect the biology of disease and are the objects of study in most clinical research, improvement is essentially a social process. Improvement is an applied science rather than an academic discipline; its immediate purpose is to change human performance rather than generate new, generalizable knowledge, and it is driven primarily by experiential learning. Like other social processes, improvement is inherently context-dependent . . . . Although traditional experimental and quasiexperimental methods are important for learning whether improvement interventions change behavior, they do not provide appropriate and effective methods for addressing the crucial pragmatic . . . questions [such as] What is it about the mechanism of a particular intervention that works, for whom does it work, and under what circumstances?*

With these caveats in mind, let's see how far we can get with a checklist of questions to help make sense of quality improvement studies.

Ten questions to ask about a paper describing a quality improvement initiative

After we developed the following questions, we applied them to two published quality improvement studies, both of which had some positive features but which might have scored even higher if the SQUIRE 2 guidelines had been published when they were being written up. You might like to track down the papers and follow the examples. One is a study by Verdú et al. [13] from Spain, who wanted to improve the management of deep venous thrombosis (DVT) in hospital patients; and the other is a study by May et al. [14] from the United States, who sought to use academic detailing (which Wikipedia defines as 'non commercially based educational outreach') to improve evidence-based management of chronic illness in a primary care setting.

Question one: What was the context?
'Context' is the local detail of the real-world setting in which the work happened. Most obviously, one of our example studies happened in Spain, the other in the United States. One was in secondary care and the other in primary care. We will not be able to understand how these different initiatives unfolded without some background on the country, the healthcare system and (at a more local level) the particular historical, cultural, economic and micropolitical aspects of our 'case'.

It is helpful, for example, not only to know that May et al.'s academic detailing study was targeted at private general practitioners (GPs) in the United States but also to read their brief description of the particular part of Kentucky where the doctors practised: 'This area has a regional metropolitan demography reflecting a considerable proportion of middle America (population 260,512, median household income US$39,813, 19% non-white, 13% below the poverty line, one city, five rural communities and five historically black rural hamlets)' [14]. So this was an area – 'middle America' – which, overall, was neither especially affluent nor especially deprived, which included both urban and rural areas, and which was ethnically mixed but not dramatically so.

Question two: What was the aim of the study?
It goes without saying that the aim of a quality improvement study is to improve quality! Perhaps the best way of framing this question is 'What was the problem for which the quality improvement initiative was seen as a solution?'

In Verdú et al.'s [13] DVT example, the authors are quite upfront that the aim of their quality improvement initiative was to save money! More specifically, they sought to reduce the time patients spent in hospital ('length of stay'). In the academic detailing example, a 'rep' [UK terminology] or 'detailer' [US terminology] visited doctors to provide unbiased education and, in particular, to provide evidence-based guidelines for the management of diabetes (first visit) and chronic pain (second visit). The aim was to see whether the academic detailing model, which had been shown as long ago as 1983 to improve practice in *research* trials [14], could be made to work in the messier and less predictable environment of real-world middle America.

Question three: What was the mechanism by which the authors hoped to improve quality?
This HOW question is all-important. Look back to Chapter 7 on complex interventions, when we asked (question four) 'What was the theoretical mechanism of action of the intervention?'. This is effectively the same question, although quality improvement initiatives typically have fuzzy boundaries and you should not necessarily expect to identify a clear 'core' to the intervention.

In the DVT care pathway example, the logic behind the initiative was that if they developed an integrated care pathway incorporating all the relevant evidence-based tests and treatments in the right order, stipulating who was responsible for each step and excluding anything for which there was evidence of no benefit, staff would follow it. In consequence, the patient would spend less time in hospital and have fewer unnecessary procedures. Furthermore, sharpening up the pathway would, they hoped, also reduce adverse events (such as haemorrhage).

In the academic detailing example, the 'mechanism' for changing doctors' prescribing behaviour was the principles of interpersonal influence and persuasion on which the pharmaceutical industry has built its marketing strategy (and which we spent much of Chapter 6 warning you about). Personally supplying the guidelines and talking the doctors through them would, it was hoped, increase the chance that they would be followed.

Question four: Was the intended quality improvement initiative evidence-based?
Some measures aimed at improving quality seem like a good idea in theory but actually don't work in practice. One example of this is mergers – that is, joining two small health care organisations (e.g. hospitals) with the aim of achieving efficiency savings, economies of scale, and so on. Fulop's team [15] demonstrated that not only do such savings rarely materialise but merged organisations often encounter new, unanticipated problems. In this example, there is not merely absence of evidence of benefit, there is evidence that the initiative might cause harm!

In the DVT example, there is a systematic review demonstrating that overall, in the research setting, developing and implementing integrated care pathways (also known as critical *care pathways*) *can* reduce costs and length of stay [16]. Similarly, systematic reviews have confirmed the efficacy of academic detailing in research trials [17]. In both of our examples, then, the '*can* it work?' question had been answered and the authors were asking a more specific and contextualised question: '*does* it work here, with *these* people and *this* particular set of constraints and contingencies?' [18].

Question five: How did the authors measure success, and was this method reasonable?
Once, at a conference, Trisha wandered around a poster exhibition in which groups of evidence-based medicine enthusiasts were presenting their attempts to improve the quality of a service. She was impressed by some, but very disheartened to find that, not uncommonly, the authors had not formally measured the success of their initiative at all – or even defined what 'success' would look like!

Our two case examples did better. Verdú et al. [13] evaluated their DVT study in terms of six outcomes: length of hospital stay, cost of the hospital care and what they called care indicators (the proportion of patients whose care actually followed the pathway; the proportion whose length of stay was actually reduced in line with the pathway's recommendations; the rate of adverse events; and the level of patient satisfaction). Taken together, these gave a fair indication of whether the quality improvement initiative was a success. However, it was not perfect; for example, the satisfaction questionnaire would not have shaped up well against the criteria for a good questionnaire study in Chapter 13.

In the academic detailing example, a good measure of the success of the initiative would surely have been the extent to which the doctors followed the guidelines or (even better) some measure of how it impacted on patients' health and wellbeing. But these downstream, patient-relevant outcome measures were not used. Instead, the authors' definition of 'success' was much more modest: they simply wanted their evidence-based detailers to get a regular foot in the door of the private GPs. To that end, their outcome measures included the proportion of doctors in the area who agreed to be visited at all; the duration of the visit (being shown the door after 45 seconds would be a 'failed' visit); whether the doctor agreed to be seen on a second or subsequent occasion; and if so, whether they could readily locate the guidelines supplied at the first visit.

It could be argued that these measures are the equivalent of the 'surrogate endpoints' we discussed in Chapter 6. But given the real-world context (a target group of geographically and professionally isolated private practitioners steeped in pharmaceutical industry advertising, for whom evidence-based practice was not traditionally part of their core business), a 'foot in the door' is a lot better than nothing. Nevertheless, when appraising the paper, we should be clear about the authors' modest definition of success and interpret the conclusions accordingly.

Question six: How much detail was given about the change process, and what insights can be gleaned from this?
The devil of a change effort is often in the nitty-gritty detail. In the DVT care pathway example, the methods section was fairly short. Although many aspects of the paper were commendable, one concern was this briefest of

descriptions of what was actually done to *develop* the pathway: 'After the design of the clinical pathway, we started the study . . .' But *who* designed the pathway and how? Experts in evidence-based practice – or people working at the front line of care? Ideally, it would have been both, but we don't know. Were just the doctors involved, or were nurses, pharmacists, patients and others (such as or the hospital's director of finance) included in the process? Were there arguments about the evidence or did everyone agree on what was needed? The more information about *process* we can find in the paper, the more we can interpret both positive and negative findings.

In the academic detailing example, the methods section is very long and includes details on how the programme of 'detailing' was developed, how the detailers were selected and trained, how the sample of doctors was chosen, how the detailers approached the doctors, what supporting materials were used and how the detailing visits were structured and adapted to the needs and learning styles of different doctors. Whether we agree with their measures of the project's success or not, we can certainly interpret the findings in the light of this detailed information on how they went about it.

The relatively short methods section in the DVT care pathway example may have been a victim of the word length requirements of the journal. Authors summarise their methods to appear succinct, and thereby leave out all the qualitative detail that would allow you to evaluate the process of quality improvement; that is, to build up a 'rich picture' of what the authors actually did. In recognition of this perverse incentive, the authors of the original SQUIRE guidelines issued a plea to editors for 'longer papers' [12]. A well-written quality improvement study might run into a dozen or more pages, and it will generally take you a lot longer to read than, say, a tightly written report on a randomised trial. The increasing tendency for journals to include 'eXtra' (with the 'e' meaning 'online') material in an Internet-accessible format is encouraging, and you should hunt such material down whenever it is available.

Question seven: What were the main findings?

For this question, you need to return to your answer to question five and find the numbers (for quantitative outcomes) or the key themes (for qualitative data), and ask whether and how they were significant. Just as in other study designs, 'significance' in quality improvement case studies is a multifaceted concept. A change in a numerical value may be clinically significant without being statistically significant or vice versa (see Chapter 5) and may also be vulnerable to various biases. For example, in a before-and-after study, time will have moved on between the 'baseline' and 'post-intervention' measures, and a host of confounding variables including the economic climate, public attitudes, availability of particular drugs or procedures, relevant case law and the identity of the chief executive may have changed. Qualitative outcomes may be particularly vulnerable to the Hawthorne effect (staff tend to feel valued and work harder when any change in working conditions aimed at improving performance is introduced, whether it has any intrinsic merits or not) [19].

In the DVT care pathway example, mean length of stay was reduced by 2 days (a difference that was statistically significant), and financial savings were achieved of several hundred euros per patient. Furthermore, 40 of 42 eligible patients were actually cared for using the new care pathway (a further 18 patients with DVT did not meet the inclusion criteria) and 62% of all patients achieved the target reduction in length of stay. Overall, 7 of 60 people experienced adverse events, and in only one of these had the care pathway been followed. These figures, taken together, not only tell us that the initiative achieved the goal of saving money but they also give us a clear indication of the extent to which the intended changes in the process of care were achieved and remind us that many patients with DVT are what are known as exceptions; that is, management by a standardised pathway doesn't suit their needs.

In the academic detailing example, the findings show that of the 130 doctors in the target group, 78% received at least one visit and these people did not differ in demographic characteristics (e.g. age, sex, whether qualified abroad or not) from those who refused a visit. Only one person refused point blank to receive further visits, but getting another visit scheduled often proved challenging, and barriers were 'primarily associated with persuading office staff of the physician's stated intentions for further visits'. In other words, even though the doctor was (allegedly) keen, the detailers had trouble getting past the receptionists; surely a significant qualitative finding about the process of academic detailing, which had not been uncovered in the randomised trial design! Half the doctors could lay their hands on the guidelines at the second visit (and by implication, half couldn't). But the paper also presented some questionable quantitative outcome data such as 'around 90% of practitioners appeared interested in the topics discussed' – an observation which, apart from being entirely subjective, is a Hawthorne effect until proved otherwise. Rather than using the dubious technique of trying to quantify their subjective impressions, perhaps the authors should have either stuck to their primary outcome measure (whether the doctors let them in the door or not) or gone the whole hog and measured compliance with the guidelines.

Question eight: What was the explanation for the success, failure or mixed fortunes of the initiative and was this reasonable?

Once again, conventions on the length of papers in journals may make this section frustratingly short. Ideally, the authors will have considered their findings, revisited the contextual factors you identified in question one, and will have offered a plausible and reasoned explanation for the former in terms of the latter, including a consideration of alternative explanations. More commonly, explanations are brief and speculative.

Why, for example, was it difficult for academic detailers to gain access to doctors for second appointments? According to the authors, the difficulty was because of 'customarily short open-diary times for future appointments and operational factors related to the lack of permanent funding for this service'. But an alternative explanation might have been that the doctor was disinterested but did not wish to be confrontational, so told the receptionists to stall if approached again!

As in this example, evaluating the explanations given in a paper for disappointing outcomes in a quality improvement project is always a judgement call. Nobody is going to be able to give you a checklist that will allow you to say with 100% accuracy, 'this explanation was definitely plausible, whereas that aspect definitely wasn't'. In a quality improvement case study, the authors of the paper will have told a story about what happened and you will have to interpret their story using your knowledge of evidence-based medicine, your knowledge of people and organisations, and your common sense.

The DVT care pathway paper, while offering very positive findings, offers a realistic explanation of them: 'The real impact of clinical pathways on length of stay is difficult to ascertain because these non-randomised, partly retrospective, studies might show significant reductions in hospital stay but cannot prove that the only cause of the reduction is the clinical pathway'. Absolutely!

Question nine: In the light of the findings, what do the authors feel are the next steps in the quality improvement cycle locally?

Quality is not a station you arrive at but a manner of travelling. (If you want a reference for that statement, the best we can offer is Pirsig's *Zen and the Art of Motorcycle Maintenance* [20]). To put it another way, quality improvement is a neverending cycle: when you reach one goal, you set yourself another.

The DVT care pathway team were pleased that they had significantly reduced length of stay, and felt that the way to improve further was to ensure that the care pathway was modified promptly as new evidence and new technologies became available. Another approach, which they did not mention but which would not need to wait for an innovation, might be to apply the care pathway approach to a different medical or surgical condition.

The academic detailing team decided that their next step would be to change the curriculum slightly so that rather than covering two unrelated topics on different topic areas, they would use 'judicious selection of sequential topics allowing subtle reflection of key message elements from previous encounters (e.g. management of diabetes followed by a programme on management of hypertension)'. It is interesting that they did not consider addressing the problem of attrition (42% of doctors did not make themselves available for the second visit).

Question ten: What did the authors claim to be the generalisable lessons for other teams and was this assessment reasonable?
At the beginning of this chapter, we argued that the hallmark of research was generalisable lessons for others. There is nothing wrong with improving quality locally without seeking to generate wider lessons, but if the authors have published their work, they are often claiming that others should follow their approach or, at least, selected aspects of it.

In the DVT care pathway example, the authors make no claims about the transferability of their findings. Their sample size was small, and care pathways have already been shown to shorten hospital stay in other comparable conditions. Their reason for publishing appears to convey the message, 'If we could do it, so can you'!

In the academic detailing example, the potentially transferable finding was said to be that a whole population approach to academic detailing (i.e. seeking access to every GP in a particular geographical area) as opposed to only targeting volunteers, can 'work'. This claim could be true, but because the outcome measures were subjective and not directly relevant to patients, this study fell short of demonstrating it.

Conclusion

In this chapter, we have tried to guide you through how to make judgements about papers on quality improvement studies. As the quote at the end of section 'What are quality improvement studies and how should we research them?' illustrates, such judgements are inherently difficult to make and require you to integrate evidence and information from multiple sources. Hence, while quality improvement studies are often small, local and even somewhat parochial, critically appraising such studies is often more of a headache than appraising a large meta-analysis!

Exercises based on this chapter

1. When people are admitted to mental health inpatient units, their physical health needs may be neglected. Take a look at Green et al's study [21], which describes a quality improvement initiative to implement evidence-based guidelines for physical health in an acute psychiatric unit. Using the ten questions in this chapter, write a critical appraisal of the paper.

2. Critically appraise the paper by Mangla et al. describing the success of an initiative to introduce patient decision aids in orthopaedic care [22]. What do you think the success was due to? To what extent do you think these findings are groundbreaking – and if not, where do your concerns lie?
3. Before you look at this paper, consider what you think the quality improvement challenges are in the management of sickle cell disease, in both high-income and low-income settings. Now, critically appraise the quality improvement study by Alvarez et al. [23] on one aspect of this complex topic. You may also be interested in an excellent linked editorial which takes you through the paper [24].

References

1. Batalden PB, Davidoff F. What is 'quality improvement' and how can it transform healthcare? *Quality and Safety in Health Care* 2007; **16**: 2–3.
2. Greenhalgh T. *How to Implement Evidence-Based Healthcare*. Oxford: Wiley; 2018.
3. Marshall M. Applying quality improvement approaches to health care. *BMJ* 2009; **339**: b3411.
4. Miltner RS, Newsom JH, Mittman BS. The future of quality improvement research. *Implementation Science* 2013; **8**(Suppl 1): S9.
5. Vincent C, Batalden P, Davidoff F. Multidisciplinary centres for safety and quality improvement: learning from climate change science. *BMJ Quality and Safety* 2011; **20**(Suppl 1): i73–8.
6. Alexander JA, Hearld LR. The science of quality improvement implementation: developing capacity to make a difference. *Medical Care* 2011; **49**: S6–20.
7. Portela MC, Pronovost PJ, Woodcock T, et al. How to study improvement interventions: a brief overview of possible study types. *BMJ Quality and Safety* 2015; **24**: 325–36.
8. Casarett D, Karlawish JH, Sugarman J. Determining when quality improvement initiatives should be considered research. *JAMA* 2000; **283**: 2275–80.
9. Lynn J. When does quality improvement count as research? Human subject protection and theories of knowledge. *Quality and Safety in Health Care* 2004; **13**: 67–70.
10. Greenhalgh T, Russell J, Swinglehurst D. Narrative methods in quality improvement research. *Quality and Safety in Health Care* 2005; **14**: 443–9.
11. Ogrinc G, Davies L, Goodman D, et al. SQUIRE 2.0 (Standards for QUality Improvement Reporting Excellence): revised publication guidelines from a detailed consensus process. *BMJ Quality and Safety* 2016; **25**: 986–92.
12. Davidoff F, Batalden P, Stevens D, et al. Publication guidelines for improvement studies in health care: evolution of the SQUIRE Project. *Annals of Internal Medicine* 2008;**149**: 670–6.
13. Verdú A, Maestre A, López P, et al. Clinical pathways as a healthcare tool: design, implementation and assessment of a clinical pathway for lower-extremity deep venous thrombosis. *Quality and Safety in Health Care* 2009;**18**: 314–20.

14. May F, Simpson D, Hart L, et al. Experience with academic detailing services for quality improvement in primary care practice. *Quality and Safety in Health Care* 2009;**18**: 225–31.
15. Fulop N, Protopsaltis G, King A, et al. Changing organisations: a study of the context and processes of mergers of health care providers in England. *Social Science and Medicine* 2005; **60**: 119–30.
16. Rotter T, Kinsman L, James E, et al. Clinical pathways: effects on professional practice, patient outcomes, length of stay and hospital costs. *Cochrane Database of Systematic Reviews* 2010; **(3)**: CD006632.
17. O'Brien M, Rogers S, Jamtvedt G, et al. Educational outreach visits: effects on professional practice and health care outcomes. *Cochrane Database of Systematic Reviews* 2007; **(4)**: CD000409.
18. Haynes B. Can it work? Does it work? Is it worth it? The testing of healthcare interventions is evolving. *BMJ* 1999; **319**: 652–63.
19. Franke RH, Kaul JD. The Hawthorne experiments: first statistical interpretation. *American Sociological Review* 1978; **43**: 623–43.
20. Pirsig R. *Zen and the Art of Motorcycle Maintenance: An enquiry into values.* New York, NY: Bantam Books; 1984.
21. Green S, Beveridge E, Evans L, et al. Implementing guidelines on physical health in the acute mental health setting: a quality improvement approach. *International Journal of Mental Health Systems* 2018; **12**: 1.
22. Mangla M, Cha TD, Dorrwachter JM, et al. Increasing the use of patient decision aids in orthopaedic care: results of a quality improvement project. *BMJ Quality and Safety* 2018; **27**: 347–54.
23. Alvarez OA, Rodriguez-Cortes H, Clay EL, et al. Successful quality improvement project to increase hydroxyurea prescriptions for children with sickle cell anaemia. *BMJ Quality and Safety* 2023; **32**: 608–16.
24. Jacob SA, Yui JC. Moving the needle: using quality improvement to address gaps in sickle cell care. *BMJ Quality and Safety* 2023; 570–2.

Chapter 15 **Papers that describe genetic association studies**

The three eras of human genetic studies (so far)

Beginning even before the discovery of DNA as the genetic code in 1953 – and acknowledging that this chapter is a huge oversimplification of a complex and rapidly developing field – there have been three main eras of genetic studies into human disease.

The first era might be called 'genetics without the genes' – most famously, family tree studies of Mendelian (single mutated gene) disorders. This research consisted of mapping the family trees of people with a particular condition and working out by default whether the condition was dominant or recessive and sex-linked or not. Trisha is a carrier of colour blindness (and the granddaughter, sister and mother of men with this X-linked recessive condition), so became interested in such studies at a young age. But they are of largely historical interest these days, since the inheritance of most single-gene diseases has long been worked out [1]. These early studies did not study the actual genes; they merely inferred the genetic problem from the phenotypes of the humans involved. Examples of single-gene diseases include sickle-cell anaemia (autosomal recessive), polycystic kidney disease (autosomal dominant), Rett syndrome (X-lined dominant), colour blindness (X-linked recessive) and a rare form of azoospermia (Y-linked dominant).

The second era in human genetic research, beginning in the 1980s, was what might be called 'labour-intensive gene mapping'. At that time, mapping actual genes to their chromosomes was a laborious, expensive and painfully slow process involving the use of DNA 'probes' whose biochemical detail, based on the Southern blot technique, is now largely a piece of science history. The first disease to be mapped to a particular place on a particular chromosome was Huntington's disease [2], an autosomal dominant neurodegenerative condition first described in 1872. It was not until 1983

How to Read a Paper: The Basics of Evidence-Based Healthcare, Seventh Edition.
Trisha Greenhalgh and Paul Dijkstra.

that the gene for Huntington's was mapped to a section of chromosome 4 (part of a wider initiative to map the entire human genome [3]) – and it took ten more years of manual DNA probe work to identify the exact mutation in the Huntington's gene.

The labour-intensive era of genetic research often included genetic linkage studies, in which two or more traits carried on the same chromosome were explored in all consenting members of a family, usually with a view to identifying (indirectly) whether someone was likely to be carrying a genetic disease before they showed signs of it [4]. Techniques for single-gene mapping have become much faster and now tend to use the automated polymerase chain reaction (see a genetics textbook for more detail).

The third era in human genetics research, and the one that required us to add this chapter in later editions of the book, began around 2005. It has been characterised by dramatic improvements in the efficiency of gene mapping (the identification of genetic changes), also known as genotyping. Technological advances allowed researchers to study hundreds of genes at once in a cost-effective way. A major focus of such research is the study of genetic *polymorphisms*; that is, the variations in genes that can account for person-to-person differences in a characteristic, such as eye colour, height, susceptibility to disease, severity of disease, or even sensitivity to a particular drug.

With some diseases, a single mutated gene is sufficient to cause disease, as in the examples of Huntington's disease and colour blindness mentioned above. These are conditions you either do or don't have, defined by the presence of one (or a small number of) well-defined mutated genes. However, the inheritance of most conditions is not that simple: it involves *multiple* genes. There is a wide range of different levels of serum cholesterol in the population, for example, and every smoker would react a little differently if they applied a nicotine patch in an attempt to stop smoking. These are both examples of variations in the human phenotype which stem at least partly from *variations* (as opposed to mutations) in our genetic makeup.

If, as is usually the case, these variations are limited to a single genetic locus or allele, they are known as single nucleotide polymorphisms (abbreviated to SNPs and pronounced 'snips'). For example, a particular SNP might replace the nucleotide thymine (T) with the nucleotide cytosine (C) in a certain stretch of DNA. (Remember those bases from your biochemistry class? If not, don't feel the need to memorise them. The point to note is that genes vary in effect because of tiny variations in their molecular structure and/or variations in how much of a protein they make). We all have thousands of SNPs, most of which do us no harm and are not linked to disease. SNPs can occur on the genes themselves, on the linking DNA between genes, and on the bits of DNA that regulate genes.

Researchers in this field want to understand what causes disease and then, additionally, potentially predict disease. One way of doing this is to use SNPs as biological markers, ('biomarkers' for short), helping researchers locate genes that are associated with disease.

Which brings us to the type of study we want to spend most of this chapter talking about: the genome-wide association study (GWAS).

What is a genome-wide association study?

A GWAS is a very large cohort or case–control study which seeks to identify small genomic variations (usually SNPs) that occur more frequently in people with a particular disease or risk state than in those without it [5].

By examining SNPs across the entirety of the genome, GWAS help improve our understanding of why some people develop diseases when others don't. (Remember the advertisement for the heart disease charity in which the thin guy had heart disease while the fat guy escaped it? The former may have had a genetic change that predisposed them to it and had differences in SNPs). GWAS, for example, have identified SNPs related to numerous conditions including Alzheimer's disease, type 2 diabetes, various heart abnormalities, Parkinson's disease and Crohn's disease.

To carry out a GWAS, researchers obtain DNA from each participant (both cases and controls), usually by taking a blood sample or swabbing the inside of the mouth to harvest cells. Each person's complete genome is then purified from the blood or cells, placed on tiny chips ('microarrays') and scanned on automated laboratory machines, allowing it to be quickly assessed for strategically selected SNPs. Typically, a GWAS study involves thousands of participants and hundreds of SNPs measured on each of them, so substantial computer power is needed (not to mention fancy statistics). For this reason, GWAS research tends to be interdisciplinary, involving geneticists, epidemiologists, computer scientists and statisticians as well as clinical specialists.

GWAS are examples of observational studies (see Chapter 3). They take a large sample of people and measure things in them, either comparing people with a disease to controls without the disease (if it's something you either have or don't have, such as sickle-cell disease) or comparing a continuous variable across a population (e.g. cholesterol level, which isn't something you either have or don't have). In both kinds of study, researchers look at the strength of associations between SNPs and the target disease(s) or risk state(s). As Kevin Mitchell points out in his excellent 'Wiring the Brain' blog, 'GWAS are premised on the simple idea that if any of those common variants at any of those millions of SNPs across the genome is associated with an increased risk of disease, then that variant should be more frequent in cases than in controls' [6].

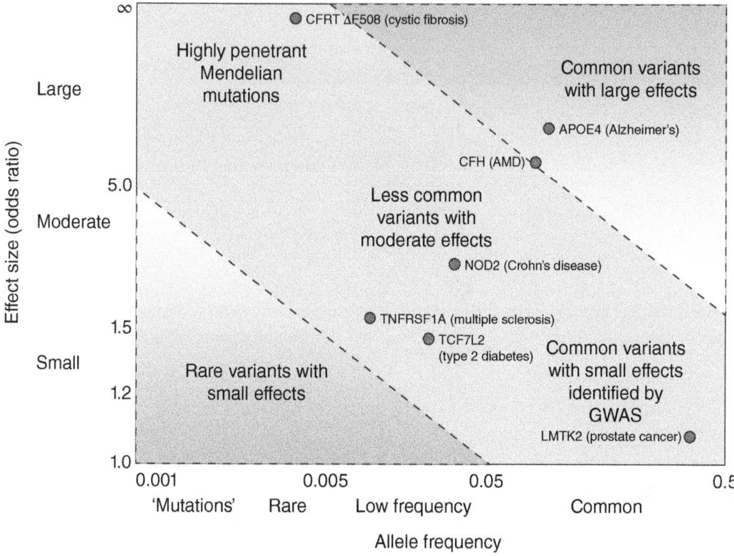

Figure 15.1 Spectrum of disease allele effects revealed by GWAS studies. *Source:* reproduced from Bush et al., 2012, [5] / Public Library of Science/CC-BY-4.0.

GWAS demonstrate the strength of association between gene variants, which can be either common or rare ('allele frequency', the x-axis in Figure 15.1), and diseases, which can be either monogenic (single-gene or Mendelian, e.g. cystic fibrosis) or polygenic (many genes e.g. heart disease). These associations can be strong, weak or in between ('effect size', the y-axis in Figure 15.1). Mendelian diseases involve mutations (very rare variants) and the associated SNPs have a very high effect size. Alzheimer's disease is associated with a common SNP with a large effect size. Most genetic associations discovered to date with implications for human health lie in the zone between the dashed diagonals in Figure 15.1: fairly common SNP variants with small to moderate effect sizes.

If certain SNPs are found to be significantly more frequent in people with the disease compared with people without disease (or people with high levels of a risk factor compared with those with low levels), this does not necessarily mean that these SNPs cause the disease (or even contribute to its cause), since association does not prove causation (see Chapter 3). The associated SNPs may just be tagging along on the same chromosome with the actual causal variants. Because they sit close together on the string of DNA, they get passed on together to the next generation; something geneticists call 'linkage disequilibrium'. An analogy is that a string is always tied to a kite but it's not the string that enables the flight, it's the kite itself. Figure 15.2 illustrates how

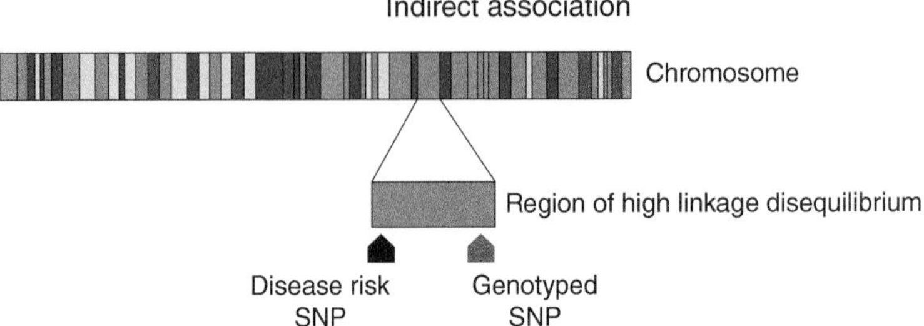

Figure 15.2 Indirect association of a genetic biomarker with a disease.
Source: reproduced from Bush et al., 2012, [5] / Public Library of Science/CC-BY-4.0.

a SNP that is the focus of a GWAS (and is statistically associated with the disease) may not actually be the cause of that disease.

Much work therefore needs to be done to demonstrate the biological plausibility of associations turned up by GWAS. In some but not all cases, such plausibility has indeed been demonstrated. For example, GWAS have implicated skeletal genes in height, immune genes in immune disorders and neurodevelopmental genes in schizophrenia [6].

GWAS studies have their own databases (a bit like the Cochrane Library), which you can search for associations (either proven or disproven); see, for example, dbGaP: the database of genotypes and phenotypes, part of the US National Library of Medicine (https://www.ncbi.nlm.nih.gov/gap). To strengthen the findings of GWAS studies, find more SNPs, since size generates power. And GWAS, like all primary research studies, can be synthesised in systematic reviews and meta-analyses (now there's a new challenge for the methodologists).

One unanswered question widely discussed in genetics circles concerns 'missing heritability'; the fact that despite powerful techniques for demonstrating associations between SNPs and disease, in most diseases genetic variability appears to account for a relatively small percentage of the interindividual phenotypic variation. For example, even if you do carry numerous 'genes for heart disease' (or, more accurately, SNPs that have been associated with heart disease), you may never develop it, and people who lack the incriminating SNPs may nevertheless develop heart disease [7]. As genetics gets more sophisticated, the level of missing heritability for some diseases seems to be falling (although not for all diseases and not as quickly as some researchers hoped).

For a more detailed account of the place of GWAS studies in medicine, see the excellent introduction by Bush and Moore [5] and more recent reviews by Gibson [8] and Bomba et al. [9] explain in more detail why and how thousands of small-effect SNP variants contribute to chronic disease.

Clinical applications of genome-wide association studies

If you have read the previous section with a critical eye, you will be aware that even after a GWAS has shown that a particular SNP makes a person *more likely* to develop a particular condition than someone without that SNP, it does not mean that they *will* develop that condition. Indeed, you will have noted that *most* associations between particular SNPs and disease are weak. It follows that GWAS might be high-tech but this kind of study will always remain an inexact science when applied to the individual. As a hypothetical example, if GWAS studies were to show that left-handed people are, on average, more creative than right-handed people, this does not mean that a particular left-handed individual will be brimming with creative talent.

While we should be circumspect about the potential of genetics to transform all aspects of clinical practice, the genetic revolution is by no means science fiction. One example, you might like to explore is the discovery, through a GWAS, of a rare 'missense' SNP (a substituted piece of DNA that made a piece of the genetic code read as gobbledygook and hence fail to produce a particular protein, PSCK9), which was associated with a reduced risk of heart attack in people who carried it [10]. Lucky for those rare individuals. But here's the bigger story: this GWAS informed a programme of research to try to achieve the same pathway of risk reduction in people *without* the lucky missense SNP, which led to the development of a new class of highly effective low-density lipoprotein (LDL) lowering therapies [11,12]. These drugs were developed primarily for people with familial hypercholesterolaemia whose underlying problem is that they *overproduce* PCSK9, although they also work for anyone with a high LDL level. Drugs such as alirocumab and evolocumab are monoclonal antibodies against PCSK9; a protein whose malign function would never have been discovered if it hadn't been for the GWAS that trawled thousands of SNPs. Ain't science grand?

Another clinical application of GWAS studies is in improving risk scores for diseases so as to target screening and/or preventive measures to those at increased risk. You are probably familiar with risk scores (typically presented as a smartphone application) that ask you to input certain features of your family history and symptoms to predict whether you are at high, medium or low risk of developing a particular disease. 'Under the bonnet' of such applications is a computer algorithm which attaches particular weight to different risk factors. A few years ago, Trisha's PhD student Dougy Noble and Trisha (with some colleagues) looked at risk scores for type 2 diabetes [13]. They found that almost 100 different research teams had played with different weightings on the standard risk factors of age, family history, ethnicity, body mass index, fasting glucose level, cholesterol level and so on, and that quite a few had produced algorithms that weren't bad (although they weren't perfect) at predicting who was going to go on to develop diabetes.

At the time (2011), that team found only a handful of diabetes risk score studies that had included any genetic data. Findings from those studies were consistent and led them to conclude that 'genetic markers added nothing to models over clinical and sociodemographic factors', although they recognised that future research might identify additional genetic variants might improve the predictive power. They were not steeped in the language of genetics, so at the time they did not describe this as a problem of 'missing heritability'. But to genetic epidemiologists, that's exactly what it was, and much research since has focused on hunting out the dozens of SNPs, each of which has a minuscule influence on the overall risk of developing type 2 diabetes.

Depending on your enthusiasm for genetics, this glass is currently either half empty or half full [14]. A 2017 empirical study from Sweden found that adding genetics data only improved the predictability of the risk score for type 2 diabetes by 1% [15], which is considerably less additional data than you would get by factoring in their postcode (a proxy for poverty, which is linked to lifestyle risk factors). On the other hand, Khera and colleagues used the very latest genetic data to identify a subset of 3.5% of the population who have a more than three-fold increase in the risk of type 2 diabetes [16]. These authors suggest that genetic data from GWAS has now reached a stage of maturity that 'polygenic risk scores' for a number of common diseases, type 2 diabetes included, can be used in clinical practice. The same paper identified 8% and 6% of the population at three-fold higher risk of coronary heart disease and atrial fibrillation, respectively.

The glass half empty argument for clinical applicability of genetic association studies says that measuring patients' SNPs rarely gives you more information than examining the patient and taking a good family and social history (e.g. finding that a person has a body mass index of 35, a parent with type 2 diabetes and a personal history of gestational diabetes should give you enough information to recommend a diabetes prevention programme). This argument probably still holds for many common polygenic diseases where the offending SNPs have a weak effect (the bottom right area in Figure 15.1) but there is growing evidence that for rare diseases (e.g. Crohn's), SNPs are better predictors of the condition than a family history [17].

Direct-to-consumer genetic testing

In Chapter 6, we warned of the dangers of direct-to-consumer advertising of drugs. Marketing is based on the science of psychological influence; when it is done well, it works. Because it is now cheap to sequence a genome, private companies are offering whole-genome sequencing to the general public, and

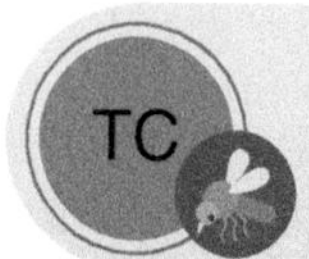

Timothy, based on your genetics and other factors, you are likely to get **fewer** mosquito bites than others.

Figure 15.3 Example of meaningless finding provided by private direct-to-consumer genetics provider.

thousands of people are paying out (currently a few hundred pounds) and sending off a saliva swab to get a report on their risk of developing various diseases (along with various non-disease data such as the proportion of Jewish, or indeed Neanderthal, ancestry in the person's genome).

In many cases, the disease predictions (and reassurances) offered by these packages have been missold, for four reasons. First and foremost, because as we explained above, SNPs typically provide very weak associations, not firm predictions. Second, because many of the predictions provided by such companies about what *might* happen based on genetic associations are less useful that the person's actual knowledge of what *has* happened. Figure 15.3 (reproduced with permission from a colleague Trisha met on social media) shows part of a genetic profile. As Timothy commented, he gets his full share of mosquito bites!

Third, because a focus on genes may distract people away from lifestyle risk factors that are far more powerful predictors of their likelihood of developing disease (smoking, alcohol and lack of exercise spring to mind). And finally, because like any output of a 'big data' study (in this case, a vast amount of data on a single individual), the findings are not self-interpreting. The lay person who (in good faith) sends of their specimen and a few weeks later receives a multipage printout of risk ratios will generally need help to work out what these findings *mean*. If the data are misinterpreted, that individual may become confused, anxious, fatalistic, angry or any combination of the above.

For all these reasons, private 'sequence your genome' services are often viewed as a particularly sinister genre in the wider problem of direct-to-consumer-advertising, and regulatory bodies are (rightly in our view) trying to keep a check on their activities. See the articles by Annas et al. [18] and Zettler et al. [19] for the story of how the US Food and Drug Administration took on the private provider 23andMe, and how that provider's database was recently hacked, with the personal genetic data of 6.9 million people stolen [20].

Mendelian randomisation studies

As Chapter 3 argued, randomised controlled trials are a good design for reducing (and in some senses eliminating) bias. But they are expensive, time-consuming and laborious. Another kind of randomisation happens during cell division in the reproductive cycle: the random allocation of genes, since each egg cell and sperm cell contain half the genetic material of the parent cell. Here's an example. Trisha's two adult sons both have the same parents and were fed similar diets as children, but are very different heights. By chance, one son probably inherited several gene variants for tallness while the other inherited gene variants for average height. They weren't randomised by a researcher to receive more or fewer tallness genes, but Mother Nature allocated those genes unevenly between them. Both sons are healthy, but if the taller son develops a disease (say, prostate cancer) in the future, might this be *because of* his height (or the SNPs he inherited that are linked to tall stature)?

(Genes for) height *causing* disease? We agree, it's not terribly intuitive, but stay with this argument. Epidemiological studies have shown that tall men are slightly but significantly more likely to develop prostate cancer and that there is a 'dose–response' effect (the taller you are, the worse your chances) [21]. But is this because the genes for tallness also cause prostate cancer or because some environmental variable (say, something in the diet) causes both tallness and cancer?

Here's where Mendelian randomisation comes in. Neil Davies and colleagues took a sample of more than 20,000 men with prostate cancer and 20,000 without prostate cancer, and (using GWAS) looked at how genes for height were distributed between them [22]. As expected, taller men had more genes for tallness (though it is worth noting that genes explained only 6.5% of the variance in height). But genes for tallness (as opposed to tallness itself) were *not* more common in the men with prostate cancer. This finding suggests that the link between height and prostate cancer (which is pretty weak anyway, so tall men please don't fret) is due to an unmeasured environmental variable and *not* to a genetically linked mechanism.

The detail of Mendelian randomisation studies is beyond the scope of this book, but they hold the potential to make *some* conventional RCTs unnecessary [23]. If you read only one paper on Mendelian randomisation studies, we recommend Neil Davies and colleagues' paper 'Reading Mendelian randomisation studies: a guide, glossary, and checklist for clinicians' [24]. As they point out, the chief contribution of Mendelian randomisation is to use genetic variation as a natural experiment to investigate whether the relations between risk factors and health outcomes in observational data are causal or caused by an unmeasured confounding variable. These authors warn, however, that Mendelian randomisation depends on a number of assumptions, whose plausibility must be carefully assessed.

Epigenetics: a space to watch

While much is written about epigenetics, its clinical relevance is currently speculative, so this section is intentionally short.

If genetics is the study of genes, epigenetics is the study of how genes interact with the environment. Your genome, as you will remember from your Crick and Watson, is made of DNA (and, derivatively, RNA). Your *epigenome* is made up of chemical compounds and proteins that can attach to DNA and produce actions such as turning genes on or off, thereby controlling the production of proteins in particular cells.

The only epigenetic change to DNA that has been reliably documented to date is methylation. Methylated DNA (mDNA) is said to mediate the influence of environmental risk factors on the development of disease. Potentially, we could study environmental influences in terms of how effectively they lead to DNA methylation, and perhaps we can produce interventions to block such methylation even in the presence of environmental pressure. Hopeful review articles predict another revolution in the role of (epi)genetics in clinical care along these lines [25, 26], and a critical appraisal checklist for epigenetic studies has been published [27].

One area where methylation potentially holds promise for the future is oncology. When a cell flips from being a peaceful neighbour, turns into a cancer and grows out of country, spreading across the body, it is possible to detect differences in methylation. A cancer's DNA is methylated in very different areas to a normal cell's DNA. This observation is now used in the very core of a new blood test to diagnose cancer. The *Galleri test* is the world's first test to potentially pick up 50 types of cancer through the identification of abnormally mDNA in a single blood draw. The manufacturers even believe that the methylation pattern can tell you what type of cancer it is (breast or pancreatic, for example). At the time of writing, the UK is running the world's biggest study of 140,000 people to assess sensitivity and specificity of this test, with the results expected by 2025. A blog by cancer geneticist Dr Lennard Lee gives more details [28].

Despite this and other potentially revolutionary tests on the horizon, epigenetics also has its sceptics, who point out that the mismatch between the claims about what epigenetics *could* achieve and what it actually *has* achieved to date is wide [29,30]. Perhaps most troubling is the assumption that the study of societal and environmental influences on disease can and should be reduced to (or even primarily centred on) the study of molecular changes to DNA. Even if this is what *mediates* the complex influences of environment on human illness, that does not necessarily mean that interventions should be targeted at the molecular level.

In 2017, Trisha reviewed a book by David Wastell (a sceptical neuroscientist) and Sue White (a social scientist) on the epigenetics of childhood disadvantage [31]. The book is worth reading as it tells two stories: the epigenetics of neurodevelopmental problems in disadvantaged children and the 'social science of science' (how studies of the social determinants of health have been overlooked as research funding is instead poured into the study of DNA methylation). Should we develop better ways of interfering with the methylation of DNA in the brains of children raised in extreme poverty or should we channel resources into reducing poverty and its impact on young children? Read the book and decide for yourself.

Ten questions to ask about a genetic association study

Because this is an introductory textbook (and because we are not geneticists), we have not included a fully comprehensive checklist for exhaustively evaluating a GWAS or Mendelian randomisation study. For more definitive checklists, see three articles in the Users' Guides to the Medical Literature [32–34], Sohani et al.'s Q-Genie tool for genetic association studies [35], Iglesias et al.'s checklist for appraising genetic risk prediction studies [36], Little et al.'s guidelines for reporting genetic association studies [37] and Davies et al.'s review paper on Mendelian randomisation [24]. For some elementary questions based on those papers to get you started, try the ones below.

Question one: What was the research question (and to what extent was it hypothesis driven)?
Genetics studies these days rely on 'big data' – many observations on large numbers of participants (see Chapter 17). When the volume of data is large and computers make it relatively easy to test large numbers of statistical associations, researchers may be tempted to 'data dredge' (i.e. to look for any significant associations *before* considering specific hypotheses or biological mechanisms). This is poor science, since the more associations you test, the more likely some will come out statistically significant by chance.

For these reasons, before you dive straight into the dataset of a large genetic study, read the introductory section to assess the background to the study and the scientific plausibility of the associations that were being explored.

Question two: What was the population studied and was that appropriate?
The vast majority of GWAS research to date has focused on white European and North American populations. Populations whose ancestors are traced to Africa, the Middle East or South Asia, for example, have different genetic makeup (and, more specifically, they will differ in the frequency of risk alleles), so associations established to date may not apply to those populations. Questioning the ethnic representativeness of a population or sample is particularly important when considering diseases (e.g. type 2 diabetes) which are highly patterned by ethnicity.

Question three: Did the genome-wide association study meet the established methodological quality criteria for a cohort or case–control study?

Putting the high-tech genetics component aside, much of what we wrote in Chapter 4 about methodological quality and Chapter 5 about statistics applies to GWAS and similar studies.

In a case–control study, for example, cases should have the same characteristics as the controls except for the condition being studied. Comparing 'cases' recruited from hospital clinics with 'controls' recruited from a community database, for example, will tend to inflate the association. Ethnicity differences between cases and controls can also produce significant biases (see question four).

The study also needs to be adequately powered, of course. Because most SNP associations for common diseases are weak, GWAS usually need to be very large to establish statistically significant associations. In general, the bigger the study, the more likely the GWAS is to identify true SNPs, rather than SNPs that could have arisen through random chance. A decent size for a GWAS study is 10,000 people or more. You should find a power calculation (or at least, a justification of the sample size) somewhere in the methods section.

Because genetic association studies are characterised by multiple comparisons, there is a substantial risk of finding significant associations by chance (type 1 error). It is important to note how the authors have tried to deal with this, both statistically (e.g. using an arbitrary p cut-off value, say $p < 0.001$ rather than $p < 0.05$ or using a formal correction factor for multiple comparisons) and interpretively (e.g. for every association found, try to produce a plausible explanation and mechanism [see Chapter 18]; if one cannot be produced, be circumspect about its significance).

Question four: Were the alleles of interest distributed as expected in the population?

This is really a question about sampling bias (where what is being 'sampled' is the genes). You may or may not remember from your biology lessons something called the Hardy–Weinberg equilibrium (sometimes abbreviated HWE). This means that if a condition has two alleles (classically depicted *A* and *a*), and if everyone in the population selects their mates at random, there will be a particular distribution of phenotypes in that population. Of course, people don't mate at random, which introduces a potential bias in the findings of a genetic association study. Distortions to Hardy–Weinberg equilibrium occur, for example, through inbreeding, migration, new mutations and selection (e.g. if one allele leads to reduced fertility).

Question five: Were phenotypes defined precisely and using standardised criteria?
A particular problem in genetic association studies is unclear definitions of the phenotypic characteristics that are being explored. Whereas the phenotypic manifestations of Mendelian diseases like sickle-cell anaemia or cystic fibrosis are usually readily distinguished, those of polygenic conditions are continuous with 'normal' (and may also be distorted by treatment effects). A clear and consistent definition of what counts as a phenotypic variant is essential.

Question six: How technically robust was the genetic analysis?
As you might imagine, laboratory testing of genetic microarrays is a sophisticated science, and not every laboratory is good at it. This is not the place to go into detail of the precise quality standards, but it is worth noting that poor laboratory standards can lead to two kinds of error. If genotypes are systematically misclassified in one direction or other, this will positively or negatively affect associations depending on the direction of misclassification. If the misclassifications occur non-systematically, this will bias association toward the null.

Question seven: Are the findings consistent with other studies?
It is still fairly early days in building the evidence base in genetic association studies. Some published studies are methodologically poor, and some apparently robust studies have yet to be replicated. If the study you are appraising seems to contradict other evidence in the literature, treat the study cautiously (as you would for any other study design). An interesting trend here is the tendency to insularity by geographical region (European, North American and Asian GWAS scientists tend to collaborate with other scientists from the same region, but not those from different regions). Different findings across these cohorts may be due to scientific flaws in some GWAS studies, but the possibility that some SNPs are seen only in certain ethnic and racial groups should be borne in mind.

Question eight: How large and how precise are the associations?
If you have read the earlier chapters in this book, you already know that a 'statistically significant' finding is not necessarily clinically significant. This maxim is particularly relevant to a genetic study with a sample size of several thousand. Do I care if my risk of developing colon cancer is 1.05 times the population average, even if that is statistically significant? But I might care if my risk is ten times the average.

Question nine: Are the conclusions justified by the findings?
Some genetic epidemiologists are circumspect by nature; others are wont to overegg the significance of their findings. More importantly perhaps, press releases and articles in the lay press based on genetic studies may vastly

overinterpret the clinical significance of the findings. As John Attia and colleagues set out in their users' guides to the medical literature on genetic association studies, even genuinely positive results will initially tend to overestimate the significance of a genetic association (as they put it, 'The phenomenon, sometimes referred to as the winner's curse, arises because overestimates are more likely to cross threshold *P* values for declaring an association' (page 305) [34].

When you study the conclusions of a genetic association study, consider whether the authors have considered this 'winner's curse' explanation for their findings.

Question ten: What (if any) are the implications for patient care in my practice? This is the commonsense, so-what question, and in our view it is relatively under-explored for a lot of conditions that are now said to be 'genetic' in origin. As the example of risk scores for type 2 diabetes above illustrates, the findings from genetic association studies, even when statistically significant, sometimes add little or nothing to the predictive power of standard clinical variables such as fasting blood glucose, body mass index and a simple family history.

When considering whether to offer the patient genetic testing for a particular allele, the clinician also needs to take account of the effect the news might have on the patient if the test is positive (or indeed, if the results come back equivocal).

There is also the question of whether and how the genetic information would change the patient's management. If we are treating a 55-year-old person who is overweight, a smoker and has a strong family history of type 2 diabetes, are we going to change our clinical advice based on the results of genetic profiling? In a few clinical situations, we might do genetic testing to identify a rare variant with strong effect where the management would be influenced (e.g. referral to specialist clinic or selection of a particular drug), but for common variants with small effects, clinical management is rarely influenced.

An additional question, which takes us to the subject of Chapter 18, is: Did the authors then try to find *mechanistic* evidence to support their GWAS findings in laboratory studies such as cell culture or animal models? If SNPs identified GWAS studies are then confirmed in another model, then you can feel a lot more confident in their findings.

In conclusion, genetic association studies remain a contested area which some describe as a rapidly advancing field and others dismiss as overhyped. At the time of writing, clinical practice for most conditions has not changed dramatically as a result of these studies (although, apparently, the question banks in multiple-choice exams have). But here is a study to watch. The largest and most ambitious national research programme, using microarrays to identify SNPs, is now well underway in the UK. 'Our Future Health' will identify all the SNPs in 5 million members of the UK public, and will then link all these SNPs to their electronic health records in the National Health Service. If successful, it will enable the world to perform the biggest GWAS studies known to man, and time will tell if it is the single greatest project for genetic association studies, or the biggest white elephant a country has ever invested in. Follow the trial on the Our Future Health website (https://ourfuturehealth.org.uk/our-research-mission/how-our-future-health-works).

Exercises based on this chapter

1. Take a look at three articles describing polygenic risk scores for breast cancer [38], type 1 diabetes [39] and statin benefit in cardiovascular disease [40]. Would you submit to genetic testing to see if you were at higher than average risk of these conditions? If so, why (and if not, why not)? If you were found to be at higher risk on the basis of your genetic profile, what would you do to try to alter your outcome?
2. Low vitamin D levels have been associated with colon cancer. Get hold of the full text of the paper entitled 'Exploring causality in the association between circulating 25-hydroxyvitamin D and colorectal cancer risk: a large Mendelian randomisation study' [41]. Read the paper with a critical eye, asking yourself why the authors consider that they have demonstrated that the relation between vitamin D levels and colon cancer is an association rather than a true causal link. What reasons can you think of for this association?

References

1. McKusick VA. *Mendelian Inheritance in Man: A catalog of human genes and genetic disorders*. Baltimore, MD: Johns Hopkins University Press; 1998.
2. Chial H. Huntington's disease: the discovery of the Huntingtin gene. *Nature Education* 2008; **1**: 71.
3. Watson JD. The human genome project: past, present, and future. *Science* 1990; **248**: 44–9.
4. Teare MD, Barrett JH. Genetic linkage studies. *Lancet* 2005; **366**: 1036-44.
5. Bush WS, Moore JH. Genome-wide association studies. *PloS Computational Biology* 2012; **8**: e1002822.
6. Mitchell K: *What do GWAS signals mean? [blog post] Wiring the Brain, 22* November 2015. http://www.wiringthebrain.com/2015/11/what-do-gwas-signals-mean.html?spref=tw (accessed 29 August 2018).
7. Manolio TA, Collins FS, Cox NJ, et al. Finding the missing heritability of complex diseases. *Nature* 2009; **461**: 747.

8. Gibson G. Population genetics and GWAS: A primer. *PloS Biology* 2018; **16**: e2005485.
9. Bomba L, Walter K, Soranzo N: The impact of rare and low-frequency genetic variants in common disease. *Genome Biology* 2017; **18**: 77.
10. Kathiresan S: A PCSK9 missense variant associated with a reduced risk of early-onset myocardial infarction. *New England Journal of Medicine* 2008; **358**: 2299–300.
11. Sabatine MS, Giugliano RP, Keech AC, et al. Evolocumab and clinical outcomes in patients with cardiovascular disease. *New England Journal of Medicine* 2017; **376**: 1713–22.
12. Reiss AB, Shah N, Muhieddine D, et al. PCSK9 in cholesterol metabolism: from bench to bedside. *Clinical Science* 2018; **132**: 1135–53.
13. Noble D, Mathur R, Dent T, et al. Risk models and scores for type 2 diabetes: systematic review. *BMJ* 2011; **343**: d7163.
14. Vassy JL, Meigs JB. Is genetic testing useful to predict type 2 diabetes? *Best Practice and Research Clinical Endocrinology and Metabolism* 2012; **26**: 189–201.
15. Zarkoob H, Lewinsky S, Almgren P, et al. Utilization of genetic data can improve the prediction of type 2 diabetes incidence in a Swedish cohort. *PloS One* 2017; **12**: e0180180.
16. Khera AV, Chaffin M, Aragam KG, et al. Genome-wide polygenic scores for common diseases identify individuals with risk equivalent to monogenic mutations. *Nature Genetics* 2018; **50**: 1219–24.
17. Do CB, Hinds DA, Francke U, Eriksson N. Comparison of family history and SNPs for predicting risk of complex disease. *PloS Genetics* 2012; **8**: e1002973.
18. Annas GJ, Elias S. 23andMe and the FDA. *New England Journal of Medicine* 2014; **370**: 985–8.
19. Zettler PJ, Sherkow JS, Greely HT. 23andMe, the Food and Drug Administration, and the future of genetic testing. *JAMA Internal Medicine* 2014; **174**: 493–4.
20. Franceschi-Bicchierai L. 23 and Me confirms hackers stole ancestry data on 6.9 million users [blog post]. *TechCrunch* 4 December 2023 https://techcrunch.com/2023/12/04/23andme-confirms-hackers-stole-ancestry-data-on-6-9-million-users/?guce_referrer=aHR0cHM6Ly93d3cuZ29vZ2xlLmNvbS8&guce_referrer_sig=AQAAAJ4zdZ0d5ofFe_518ZO4dMZyLkjacKnRskFEw6vbYrsRLz-NypOsd-csvCyzfkAU9zMhxA9M4-BrgUVyXr2VWd (accessed 13 March 2024).
21. Zuccolo L, Harris R, Gunnell D, et al. Height and prostate cancer risk: a large nested case-control study (ProtecT) and meta-analysis. *Cancer Epidemiology and Prevention Biomarkers* 2008; **17**: 2325–36.
22. Davies NM, Gaunt TR, Lewis SJ, et al. The effects of height and BMI on prostate cancer incidence and mortality: a Mendelian randomization study in 20,848 cases and 20,214 controls from the PRACTICAL consortium. *Cancer Causes and Control* 2015; **26**: 1603–16.
23. Taubes G. Researchers find a way to mimic clinical trials using genetics [blog post]. *MIT Technology Review* 28 August 2018 https://www.technologyreview.com/s/611713/researchers-find-way-to-mimic-clinical-trials-using-genetics (accessed 13 May 2024).

24. Davies NM, Holmes MV, Smith GD. Reading Mendelian randomisation studies: a guide, glossary, and checklist for clinicians. *BMJ* 2018; **362**: k601.
25. Relton CL, Smith GD. Epigenetic epidemiology of common complex disease: prospects for prediction, prevention, and treatment. *PloS Medicine* 2010; **7**: e1000356.
26. Teschendorff AE, Relton CL. Statistical and integrative system-level analysis of DNA methylation data. *Nature Reviews Genetics* 2018; **19**: 129.
27. Riancho J, Del Real A, Riancho JA. How to interpret epigenetic association studies: a guide for clinicians. *BoneKEy Reports* 2016; **5**: 797.
28. Lee L. A moment to celebrate in our potentially revolutionary cancer blood tests trial [blog post]. *NHS England Blog* 18 July 2022. https://www.england.nhs.uk/blog/a-moment-to-celebrate-in-our-potentially-revolutionary-cancer-blood-tests-trial (accessed 13 March 2024).
29. Ptashne M: Epigenetics: core misconcept. *Proceedings of the National Academy of Sciences* 2013; **110**: 7101–3.
30. Bird A. Perceptions of epigenetics. *Nature* 2007; **447**: 396.
31. Wastell D, White S. *Blinded by Science: The social implications of epigenetics.* London: Policy Press; 2017.
32. Attia J, Ioannidis JP, Thakkinstian A, et al. How to use an article about genetic association. A: Background concepts. *JAMA* 2009; **301**: 74–81.
33. Attia J, Ioannidis JP, Thakkinstian A, et al. How to use an article about genetic association. B: Are the results of the study valid? *JAMA* 2009; **301**: 191–7.
34. Attia J, Ioannidis JP, Thakkinstian A, et al. How to use an article about genetic association. C: What are the results and will they help me in caring for my patients? *JAMA* 2009; **301**: 304–8.
35. Sohani ZN, Meyre D, de Souza RJ, et al. Assessing the quality of published genetic association studies in meta-analyses: the quality of genetic studies (Q-Genie) tool. *BMC Genetics* 2015; **16**: 50.
36. Iglesias AI, Mihaescu R, Ioannidis JP, et al. Scientific reporting is suboptimal for aspects that characterize genetic risk prediction studies: a review of published articles based on the Genetic RIsk Prediction Studies statement. *Journal of Clinical Epidemiology* 2014; **67**: 487–99.
37. Little J, Higgins JP, Ioannidis JP, et al. STrengthening the REporting of Genetic Association Studies (STREGA): an extension of the STROBE statement. *Human Genetics* 2009; **125**: 131–51.
38. Mavaddat N, Pharoah PD, Michailidou K, et al. Prediction of breast cancer risk based on profiling with common genetic variants. *Journal of the National Cancer Institute* 2015; **107**: djv036.
39. Patel KA, Oram RA, Flanagan SE, et al. Type 1 diabetes genetic risk score: a novel tool to discriminate monogenic and type 1 diabetes. *Diabetes* 2016; **65**: 2094–9.
40. Natarajan P, Young R, Stitziel NO, et al. Polygenic risk score identifies subgroup with higher burden of atherosclerosis and greater relative benefit from statin therapy in the primary prevention setting. *Circulation* 2017; **135**: 2091–101.
41. He Y, Timofeeva M, Farrington SM, et al. Exploring causality in the association between circulating 25-hydroxyvitamin D and colorectal cancer risk: a large Mendelian randomisation study. *BMC Medicine* 2018; **16**: 142.

Chapter 16 **Applying evidence with patients**

The patient perspective

There is no such thing as *the* patient perspective, and that is precisely the point of this chapter. At times in our lives, often more frequently the older we get, we are all patients. Some of us are also health professionals, but when the decision relates to *our* health, *our* medication, *our* operation, the adverse effects that *we* may or may not experience with a particular treatment, we look on that decision differently from when we make the same kind of decision in our professional role.

As you will know by now if you have read the earlier chapters of this book, evidence-based healthcare (EBHC) is mainly about using some kind of population average – an odds ratio, a number needed to treat, an estimate of mean effect size, and so on – to inform decisions. But very few of us will behave exactly like the point average on the graph: some will be more susceptible to benefit and some more susceptible to harm from a particular intervention (see Chapter 15 for some genetic reasons for this, but there are also personal, social and cultural reasons). And few of us will value a particular outcome to the same extent as a group average on (say) a standard gamble question (see Chapter 11).

The individual unique experience of being ill (or indeed being 'at risk' or classified as such) can be expressed in narrative terms: that is, a story can be told about it. And everyone's story is different. The 'same' set of symptoms or piece of news will have a host of different meanings depending on who is experiencing them and what else is going on in their lives. The exercise of taking a history from a patient is an attempt to 'tame' this unique set of personal experiences and put it into a more or less standard format to align with the protocols for assessing, treating and preventing disease. Indeed, England's first professor of general practice, Marshall Marinker, once said

How to Read a Paper: The Basics of Evidence-Based Healthcare, Seventh Edition.
Trisha Greenhalgh and Paul Dijkstra.

that the role of medicine is to distinguish the clear message of the disease from the interfering noise of the patient as a person.

As Trisha has written elsewhere, an 'evidence-based' perspective on *disease* and the patient's unique perspective on their *illness* ('narrative-based medicine', if you like) are not at all incompatible [1].

It is worth going back to the original definition of evidence-based medicine (EBM) proposed by Sackett and colleagues. This definition is reproduced in full, although only the first sentence is generally quoted:

> *Evidence based medicine is the conscientious, explicit, and judicious use of current best evidence in making decisions about the care of individual patients. The practice of evidence based medicine means integrating individual clinical expertise with the best available external clinical evidence from systematic research. By individual clinical expertise we mean the proficiency and judgment that individual clinicians acquire through clinical experience and clinical practice. Increased expertise is reflected in many ways, but especially in more effective and efficient diagnosis and in the more thoughtful identification and compassionate use of individual patients' predicaments, rights, and preferences in making clinical decisions about their care. By best available external clinical evidence we mean clinically relevant research, often from the basic sciences of medicine, but especially from patient centred clinical research into the accuracy and precision of diagnostic tests (including the clinical examination), the power of prognostic markers, and the efficacy and safety of therapeutic, rehabilitative, and preventive regimens (p. 71) [2].*

Thus, while the original protagonists of EBM are sometimes wrongly depicted as having airbrushed the poor patient out of the script, they were actually very careful to depict EBM/EBHC as being contingent on patient choice (and also dependent on clinical judgement, but that's a subject for another day). The 'best' treatment is not necessarily the one shown to be most efficacious in randomised controlled trials but the one that fits a particular set of individual circumstances and aligns with the patient's preferences and priorities.

The 'evidence-based' approach is sometimes stereotypically depicted by the clinician who feels, for example, that every patient with a high cholesterol level should take a statin because trials have shown these drugs, on average, prevent significant numbers of cardiovascular events in people at a certain level of risk, whether or not the patients say they don't want to take tablets, can't face the adverse effects or don't feel that attending for regular blood tests to monitor the impact is worth the inconvenience.

Almost all research in the EBM tradition between 1990 and 2010 focused on the epidemiological component and sought to build an evidence base of randomised controlled trials and other 'methodologically robust' research designs. Later, a tradition of 'evidence-based patient choice' emerged in which the patient's right to choose the option most appropriate and acceptable to them was formalised and systematically studied [3]. The third component of EBM referred to in the above quote – individual clinical judgement – has not been extensively theorised by scholars within the EBM tradition, but if interested, see Greenhalgh [4].

Patient-reported outcome measures

Before we get into how to involve patients in individualising the decisions of EBHC, we need to introduce an approach for selecting the outcome measures used in clinical trials: patient-reported outcome measures or PROMs. Here's a definition:

> *PROMs are the tools we use to gain insight from the perspective of the patient into how aspects of their health and the impact the disease and its treatment are perceived to be having on their lifestyle and subsequently their quality of life (QoL). They are typically self-completed questionnaires, which can be completed by a patient or individual about themselves, or by others on their behalf [5].*

By 'outcome measure' we mean the aspect of health or illness that researchers (perhaps in consultation with patients) choose to measure to demonstrate (say) whether a treatment has been effective. Death is an outcome measure. So is blood pressure (although it's a surrogate measure; see Chapter 6). So is the chance of leaving hospital with a live baby when you go into hospital in labour. So is the ability to walk upstairs or make a cup of tea on your own. The point is that in any study the researchers have to define what it is they are trying to influence.

PROMs are not individualised measures. On the contrary, they are still a form of population average but, unlike most outcome measures, they are an average of what matters most to patients rather than an average of what researchers or clinicians felt they ought to measure. The way to develop a PROM is to undertake an extensive phase of qualitative research (see Chapter 12) with a representative sample of people who have the condition you are interested in, analyse the qualitative data and then use it to design a survey instrument ('questionnaire', see Chapter 13) that captures all the key features of what patients are concerned about [6].

PROMs were first popularised by a team in Oxford led by Ray Fitzpatrick, who used the concept to develop measures for assessing the success of hip and knee replacement surgery [7]. They are now used fairly routinely in many clinical topics in the wider field of 'outcomes research'; a review by Kate Churruca and colleagues summarises the evidence on PROMs and discusses the pros and cons of generic PROMS such as the EQ-5D tool (which you can use for any condition) versus disease-specific PROMS [8]. The *Journal of the American Medical Association* has published a set of standards for PROMs [9]. PROMs are important for all conditions, but they may be particularly important for those which do not have a biomarker (e.g. blood test) that reliably monitors its progress. We can diagnose and monitor diabetes using the HbA1c test, for example, but at the time of writing there is no equivalent biomarker for diagnosing and monitoring long covid, although there are PROMs [10].

Shared decision-making

Important though PROMs are, they only tell us what patients, on average, value most, not what the patient in front of us values most. To find that out, as we said back in Chapter 1, you would have to ask the patient. And there is now a science and a methodology for 'asking the patient' [3,11].

The science of shared decision-making began in the late 1990s as a quirky interest of some keen academic GPs, notably Glyn Elwyn and Adrian Edwards [12]. The idea is based on the notion of the patient as a rational chooser, able and willing (perhaps with support) to join in the deliberation over options and make an informed choice.

One challenge is maintaining equipoise; that is, holding back on what you feel the course of action should be and setting out the different options with the pros and cons presented objectively, so the patients can make their own decisions [13]. Box 16.1 lists the competencies that clinicians need to practise shared decision-making with their patients.

The various instruments and tools to support shared decision-making have evolved over the years. At the very least, a decision aid would have a way of making the rather dry information of EBHC more accessible to a non-expert, for example by turning numerical data into diagrams and pictures. An example, shown in Figure 16.1, uses colours and simple icons to convey quantitative estimates of risk [14,15]. The ways of measuring the extent to which patients have been involved in a decision have also evolved [16].

Coulter and Collins [17] have produced an excellent guide called *Making Shared Decision-Making a Reality*, which sets out the characteristics of a really good decision aid (Box 16.2).

Increasingly commonly, decision aids are available online, allowing the patient to click through different steps in the decision algorithm (with or

Box 16.1 Competencies for shared decision-making

Define the problem – clear specification of the problem that requires a decision.

Portray equipoise – that professionals may not have a clear preference about which treatment option is the best in the context.

Portray options – one or more treatment options and the option of no treatment if relevant.

Provide information in preferred format – identify patients' preferences if they are to be useful to the decision-making process.

Check understanding – of the range of options and information provided about them.

Explore ideas, concerns and expectations about the clinical condition, possible treatment options and outcomes.

Checking role preference – that patients accept the process and identify their decision-making role preference.

Decision-making – involving the patient to the extent they desire to be involved.

Deferment if necessary – reviewing treatment needs and preferences after time for further consideration, including with friends or family members, if the patient requires.

Review arrangements – a specified time period to review the decision.

Source: Adapted from Elwyn et al. [13].

without support from a health professional). The best way to get your head round shared decision-making tools is to take a look at a few and, if possible, put them to use in practice. The English National Health Service has a website with links to tools for sharing decisions, from abdominal aortic aneurysm repair to stroke prevention in atrial fibrillation (see https://www.england.nhs.uk/personalisedcare/shared-decision-making/decision-support-tools). A similar (and more comprehensive) range of decision tools is available from the Ottawa Hospital in Canada (http://decisionaid.ohri.ca/AZinvent.php).

Dr Julian Treadwell, a GP and ex-PhD student of Trisha's, developed a website called GP Evidence (https://gpevidence.org), which provides decision tools for general practitioners. Each clinical condition has an infographic similar to the one in Figure 16.1, with green smiley faces and red sad ones, to use in conversations with patients. The website is intended for clinicians but it is publicly accessible so there is no reason why patients shouldn't take a peek at it themselves.

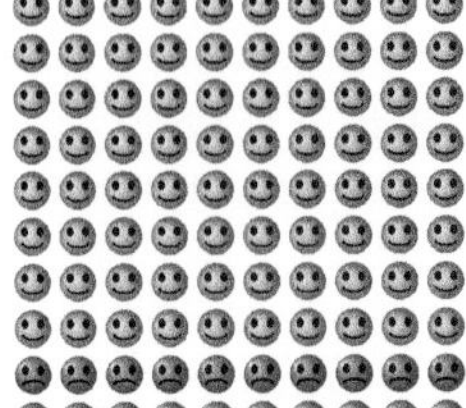

1. What is my risk of having a heart attack in the next 10 years?
The risk for 100 people like you who DO NOT take statins
NO STATIN
80 people DO NOT have a heart attack (grey, happy)
20 people DO have a heart attack (grey, sad)
The risk for 100 people like you who DO take statins
YES STATIN
80 people still DO NOT have a heart attack (grey, happy)
5 people AVOIDED heart attack (white, happy)
15 people still DO have a heart attack (grey, sad)
95 people experienced NO BENEFIT from taking statins
Had a heart attack
Avoided a heart attack
Didn't have a heart attack
2. What are the downsides of taking statins (cholesterol pill)?
• Statins need to be taken every day for a long time (maybe forever)
• Statins cost money (to you or your drug plan)
• Common side effects: nausea, diarrhoea, constipation (most patients can tolerate)
• Muscle aching/stiffness: 5 in 100 patients (some need to stop statins because of this)
• Liver blood test goes up (no pain, no permanent liver damage): 2 in 100 patients (some need to stop statins because of this)
• Muscle and kidney damage: 1 in 20 000 patients requires patients to stop statins)
3. What do you want to do now?
☐ Take (or continue to take) statins
☐ Not take (or stop taking) statins
☐ Prefer to decide at some other time

Figure 16.1 Example of a decision aid: choosing statin in a diabetes patient with a 20% risk of myocardial infarction. *Source:* adapted from Stiggelbout et al. [15].

> **Box 16.2 Characteristics of a good decision aid**
>
> Decision aids are different from traditional patient information materials because they do not tell people what to do. Instead, they set out the facts and help people to deliberate about the options. They usually contain:
>
> - a description of the condition and symptoms;
> - the likely prognosis with and without treatment;
> - the treatment and self-management support options and outcome probabilities;
> - what's known from the evidence and not known (uncertainties);
> - illustrations to help people understand what it would be like to experience some of the most frequent side effects or complications of the treatment options (often using patient interviews);
> - a means of helping people clarify their preferences;
> - references and sources of further information;
> - the authors' credentials, funding source and declarations of conflict of interest.
>
> *Source:* Adapted from Coulter and Collins [17].

Option grids

These days, most health professionals are (allegedly) keen to share decisions with patients in principle, but qualitative and questionnaire research has shown that they perceive a number of barriers to doing so in practice, including time constraints, lack of applicability of the decision support model to the unique predicament of a particular patient, a perception that they are already sharing decisions in routine consultation talk, and because they feel that patients do not wish to be involved in this way [19].

The reality of a typical general practice consultation, for example, is a long way from the objective reality of a formal decision algorithm. When a patient attends with symptoms suggestive of (say) sciatica, the doctor has 10 minutes to make progress. Typically, they will examine the patient, order some tests and then have a rather blurry conversation about how (on the one hand) the patient's symptoms might resolve with physiotherapy but (on the other hand) they might like to see a specialist because some cases will need an operation. The patient typically expresses a vague preference for either conservative or interventionist management, and the doctor (respecting the 'empowered' views) goes along with the patient's preference.

If the doctor is committed to evidence-based shared decision-making, they may try using a more structured approach; for example, by logging on to an online algorithm or by using pie charts or preprogrammed spreadsheets to elicit numerical scores of how much the patient values particular procedures and outcomes vis à vis one another. But, very often, such tools will have been tried once or twice and then abandoned as technocratic, time-consuming, overly quantitative and oddly disengaged from the unique personal illness narrative that fills the consultation.

The good news is that our colleagues working in the field of shared decision-making have recently acknowledged that the perfect may be the enemy of the good. Most discussions about management options in clinical practice do not require – and may even be thrown off kilter by – an exhaustive analysis of probabilities, risks and preference scores. What most people want is a brief but balanced list of the options, setting out the costs and benefits of each and including an answer to the question 'what would happen if I went down this route?'.

Enter the option grid (see the examples in My Health Decisions: https://www.ebsco.com/health-care/products/my-health-decisions), which is the product of a collaborative initiative between patients, doctors and academics [19]. An option grid is usually a one-page table covering a single topic. The grids list the different options as columns (COVID-19 vaccine options, for example), with each row answering a different question (such as 'Should I get a booster?', 'How soon would I feel better?' and 'How would this treatment

Chapter 16

affect my ability to work?'). An example relating to the question of whether to have the PSA (prostate specific antigen) test for prostate cancer is shown in Figure 16.2.

Option grids are developed in a similar way to PROMs, but there is often more of a focus on involvement of the multidisciplinary clinical team, as in the example of an option grid for head and neck cancer management from Elwyn et al. [20]. The distinguishing feature of the option grid approach is that it promotes and supports what has been termed *option talk*; that is, the discussions and deliberations around the different options. The grids are, in effect, analogue rather than digital in design.

The information in an option grid is presented in a format that allows both reflection and dialogue. The grid can be printed off (or the patient can be given the URL) and invited to go away and consider the options before returning for a further consultation. And unlike the previous generation of shared decision-making tools, neither the patient nor the clinician needs to be a geek to use them.

n-of-1 trials and other individualised approaches

The last approach to involving patients that we want to introduce in this chapter is the *n*-of-1 trial. This is a very simple design in which each participant receives, in randomly allocated order, both the intervention and the control treatment [21].

An example is probably the best way to explain this approach. Back in 1994, some Australian general practitioners wanted to address the clinical issue of which painkiller to use in osteoarthritis [22]. Some patients, they felt, did fine on paracetamol (which has relatively few adverse effects), while others did not respond so well to paracetamol but obtained great relief from a non-steroidal anti-inflammatory drug (NSAID). In the normal clinical setting, one might try paracetamol first and move to the NSAID if the patient did not respond. But supposing there was a strong placebo effect? The patient might conceivably have limited confidence in paracetamol because it is such a commonplace drug, whereas an NSAID in a fancy package might be subconsciously favoured.

The idea of the *n*-of-1 trial is that all treatments are anonymised, prepared in identical formulations and packaging, and just labelled 'A', 'B' and so on. The participants do not know which drug they are taking, hence their response is not influenced by whether they 'believe in' the treatment. To add to scientific rigour, the drugs may be taken in sequence such as ABAB or AABB, with 'washout' periods in between.

March and colleagues' *n*-of-1 trial of paracetamol versus NSAIDs did confirm the clinical hunch that some patients did markedly better on the NSAID but many did equally well on paracetamol. Importantly, unlike a standard optiongrid

Prostate Specific Antigen (PSA) Test: *Yes or No?*

The prostate-specific antigen (PSA) test looks for signs of prostate cancer in your blood. Use this decision aid to help you and your healthcare team decide whether or not to have a PSA test. Men usually consider this test when they are between 55 and 69 years old. Men of black race may have different risks.

Patient questions	Having a PSA test	Not having a PSA test
What does the test involve?	This blood test measures the level of prostate specific antigen (PSA) in your blood. Discuss costs.	No blood test is done.
Does a high PSA level mean I have cancer?	High PSA levels can be due to many reasons, including infection. To check for cancer, you will likely have a sample taken from your prostate gland (a prostate biopsy).	You will not know your PSA level.
Does a normal PSA test mean I do not have cancer?	No, about 15 out of 100 men (15%) with a normal PSA level will have prostate cancer sometime in the next 15 years.	You will not know your PSA level.
How many men will die from prostate cancer?	Up to 6 out of 1,000 men (0.6%) will die from prostate cancer sometime in the next 15 years.	Up to 7 out of 1,000 men (0.7%) will die from prostate cancer sometime in the next 15 years.
What are the benefits?	Benefits are uncertain. You may be the 1 man in 1,000 (0.1%) who avoids death from prostate cancer.	You will avoid biopsies, having prostate cancer treatment, and the risks that come with having treatment.
What are the risks?	If your PSA level is high, you will likely have an outpatient prostate biopsy. About 3 out of 100 men (3%) will have a cancer that causes worry, but is unlikely to cause problems. Biopsies and treatments have risks.	You could be the 1 man in 1,000 (0.1%) who might have avoided death from prostate cancer sometime in the next 15 years.
What are the risks of a prostate biopsy?	Most men have pain or bleeding for a few days after a biopsy. Out of 100 men: • 9 (9%) have infection including 1 (1%) needing emergency care • 7 (7%) have serious bleeding • 3 (3%) have problems peeing • 3 (3%) stay in the hospital for a problem after a biopsy	You will avoid the risks of having a prostate biopsy.
What are the risks (if testing leads to treatment of prostate cancer)?	Out of 100 men treated for prostate cancer: • more than 60 (60%) will have problems with erections • about 20 (20%) will leak pee	Out of 100 men not treated for prostate cancer: • up to 47 (47%) will have problems with erections • about 10 (10%) will leak pee

Figure 16.2 Example of an option grid. *Source:* reproduced with permission of Glyn Elwyn.

randomised trial, the *n*-of-1 design allowed the researchers to identify which patients were in each category. But the withdrawal rate from the trial was high, partly because when participants found a medication that worked, they just wanted to keep taking it rather than swap to the alternative!

But despite its conceptual elegance and a distant promise of linking to the 'personalised medicine' paradigm in which every patient will have their tests and treatment options individualised to their particular genome, physiome, microbiome and so on, the *n*-of-1 trial has not caught on widely in either research or clinical practice. A review article by Lillie and colleagues [23] suggests why. Such trials are labour intensive to carry out, requiring a high degree of individual personalisation and large amounts of data for every participant. 'Washout' periods raise practical and ethical problems (does one have to endure one's arthritis with no pain relief for several weeks to serve the scientific endeavour?). Combining the findings from different participants raises statistical challenges. And the (conceptually simple) science of *n*-of-1 trials has begun to get muddled up with the much more complex and uncertain science of personalised medicine.

In short, the *n*-of-1 trial is a useful design (and one you may be asked about in exams!), but it is not the panacea it was once predicted to be. If you do an *n*-of-1 trial yourself, don't forget to consult the CENT (CONSORT Extension for N-of-1 trials) publication guidelines when writing it up [24].

A (somewhat untested) alternative approach to individualising treatment regimens has been proposed by Moore and colleagues [25] in relation to pain relief. Their basic argument is that we should 'expect failure' (because the number needed to treat for many interventions is more than 2, statistically speaking any individual is more likely *not* to benefit than benefit) but 'pursue success' (because the 'average' for any intervention response masks a subgroup of responders who will do very well on that intervention). They propose a process of guided trial and error, systematically trying one intervention followed by another, until the one that works effectively for *this* patient is identified. Many front-line clinicians would probably agree with this strategy!

Exercises based on this chapter

1. Hallux valgus (usually known as bunion) surgery is widely undertaken but produces mixed results, with up to one-third of patients wishing they'd never had it done. Search the PubMed database for the paper by Schrier et al., which reports a systematic review of outcome measures for hallux valgus surgery [26]. List all the different outcome measures and explore how they were developed. How many of these measures are actually based on outcomes that patients themselves value? Which outcome measure would you want to use if you had this operation? Why?

2. Take a look at the paper by Macfarlane and Greenhalgh (which, in the interests of full disclosure, was written by Trisha's son Al Macfarlane, at the time a newly qualified doctor, with some help from mum) [27]. Al was interested in the recent introduction of a 'ban' on prescribing the anti-epileptic drug sodium valproate in women who are (or could become) pregnant. The 'ban' was not absolute, since it was recognised that, in certain difficult cases, valproate might be the only drug that would control the woman's epilepsy or mental health condition. Al and Trish felt that since valproate has both benefits and potential harms, shared decision-making using an option grid should be used to weigh up the pros and cons. When you have read the evidence in the paper, look carefully at our option grid. Do you think this grid will help or hinder productive conversations between women and their doctors? Do you agree that the woman has a right (and perhaps a duty) to join in the decision?
3. Hunt out the review article by Marwick et al. [28], which searched over 4000 studies and found a mere six *n*-of-1 trials in patients with schizophrenia. What were the main flaws identified in those studies? Why did the authors think so few *n*-of-1 studies had been undertaken? Can you find any more such studies published since the review came out (hint: use citation chaining by putting the title into Google Scholar and identifying the studies that cited it)?

References

1. Greenhalgh T. Narrative based medicine: narrative based medicine in an evidence based world. *BMJ* 1999; **318**: 323.
2. Sackett DL, Rosenberg WM, Gray JM, et al. Evidence based medicine: what it is and what it isn't. *BMJ* 1996; **312**: 71–2.
3. Edwards A, Elwyn G. *Shared Decision-Making in Health Care: Achieving evidence-based patient choice.* New York, NY: Oxford University Press; 2009.
4. Greenhalgh T. Uncertainty and clinical method. In: Sommers LS, Lauiner J (eds). *Clinical Uncertainty in Primary Care.* Berlin: Springer Nature; 2013. pp. 23–45.
5. Meadows KA. Patient-reported outcome measures: an overview. *British Journal of Community Nursing* 2011; **16**: 146–51.
6. Ader DN. Developing the patient-reported outcomes measurement information system (PROMIS). *Medical Care* 2007; **45**(5): S1–2.
7. Dawson J, Fitzpatrick R, Murray D, et al. Questionnaire on the perceptions of patients about total knee replacement. *Journal of Bone and Joint Surgery* 1998; **80**: 63–9.
8. Churruca K, Pomare C, Ellis LA, et al. Patient-reported outcome measures (PROMs): a review of generic and condition-specific measures and a discussion of trends and issues. *Health Expectations* 2021; **24**: 1015–24.
9. Basch E. Standards for patient-reported outcome-based performance measures standards for patient-reported outcome-based performance measures view-point. *JAMA* 2013; **310**: 139–40.

10. Sivan M, Wright S, Hughes S, Calvert M. Using condition specific patient reported outcome measures for long covid. *BMJ* 2022; **376**: o257.
11. Makoul G, Clayman ML. An integrative model of shared decision making in medical encounters. *Patient Education and Counseling* 2006; **60**: 301–12.
12. Elwyn G, Edwards A, Kinnersley P. Shared decision-making in primary care: the neglected second half of the consultation. *British Journal of General Practice* 1999; **49**: 477–82.
13. Elwyn G, Edwards A, Kinnersley P, et al. Shared decision making and the concept of equipoise: the competences of involving patients in healthcare choices. *British Journal of General Practice* 2000; **50**: 892–9.
14. Edwards A, Elwyn G, Mulley A. Explaining risks: turning numerical data into meaningful pictures. *BMJ* 2002; **324**: 827.
15. Stiggelbout A, Weijden T, Wit MD, et al. Shared decision making: really putting patients at the centre of healthcare. *BMJ* 2012; **344**: e256.
16. Elwyn G, Hutchings H, Edwards A, et al. The OPTION scale: measuring the extent that clinicians involve patients in decision-making tasks. *Health Expectations* 2005; **8**: 34–42.
17. Coulter A, Collins A. *Making Shared Decision-Making a Reality. No decision about me, without me*. London: King's Fund; 2011.
18. Elwyn G, Rix A, Holt T, et al. Why do clinicians not refer patients to online decision support tools? Interviews with front line clinics in the NHS. *BMJ Open* 2012; **2**(6): e001530.
19. Elwyn G, Lloyd A, Joseph-Williams N, et al. Option grids: shared decision making made easier. *Patient Education and Counseling* 2013; **90**: 207–12.
20. Elwyn G, Lloyd A, Williams NJ, et al. Shared decision-making in a multidisciplinary head and neck cancer team: a case study of developing option grids. *International Journal of Person Centered Medicine* 2012; **2**: 421–6.
21. Mirza RD, Punja S, Vohra S, Guyatt G. The history and development of N-of-1 trials. *Journal of the Royal Society of Medicine* 2017; **110**: 330–40.
22. March L, Irwig L, Schwarz J, et al. *n*-of-1 trials comparing a non-steroidal anti-inflammatory drug with paracetamol in osteoarthritis. *BMJ* 1994; **309**: 1041–6.
23. Lillie EO, Patay B, Diamant J, et al. The *n*-of-1 clinical trial: the ultimate strategy for individualizing medicine? *Personalized Medicine* 2011; **8**: 161–73.
24. Vohra S, Shamseer L, Sampson M, et al.; CENT group. CONSORT extension for reporting *N*-of-1 trials (CENT) 2015 statement. *BMJ* **2015**; 350: h1738.
25. Moore A, Derry S, Eccleston C, et al. Expect analgesic failure; pursue analgesic success. *BMJ* 2013; **346**: f2690.
26. Schrier JC, Palmen LN, Verheyen CC, et al. Patient-reported outcome measures in hallux valgus surgery. A review of literature. *Foot and Ankle Surgery* 2015; **21**: 11–15.
27. Macfarlane A, Greenhalgh T. Sodium valproate in pregnancy: what are the risks and should we use a shared decision-making approach? *BMC Pregnancy and Childbirth* 2018; **18**: 200.
28. Marwick KF, Stevenson AJ, Davies C, Lawrie SM. Application of n-of-1 treatment trials in schizophrenia: systematic review. *British Journal of Psychiatry* 2018; **213**: 398–403 (erratum in *British Journal of Psychiatry* 2018; 213: 502).

Chapter 17 Papers on artificial intelligence in healthcare

Introduction

As we write this (in early 2024), we are on the cusp of an artificial intelligence (AI) revolution in healthcare. The 6th edition of this book, published in 2019, contained nothing at all on AI. The next edition is likely to contain a great deal more. Right now, there is much excitement about the *potential* for AI, and also warnings about the downsides and risks, but very little empirical evidence. But new studies are appearing at a dizzying rate, and nobody was surprised when the generative AI product ChatGPT (explained later in this chapter) was chosen as *The Economist*'s word of the year for 2023: 'This was the year of AI, and not any kind but generative AI, which can churn out text and images with only simple prompts' [1].

Realising the problem of keeping up to date with the explosion of AI in healthcare research (around 9000 articles in the first 10 weeks of 2024 searching 'artificial intelligence' in PubMed), a group of researchers from Kings College, London created an interactive dashboard (the Global Clinical Artificial Intelligence Dashboard: https://aiforhealth.app) 'to track themes, development maturity, and global equity in clinical artificial intelligence research' [2]. When we wrote this book, the dashboard already contained thousands of articles, mostly describing AI models in early stages of development, but also some that the authors described as 'mature'. You might like to check back at that and other dashboards to pick up on new developments.

For a balanced introduction to AI in healthcare, we recommend Peter Lee and colleagues' book *The AI Revolution in Healthcare* [3]. The authors include a medical doctor and two computer scientists who have been using generative AI for a few years. To whet your appetite for the kind of breakthrough we're talking about, on page 100 of *The AI Revolution in Healthcare*, co-author Isaac Kohane (a paediatrician) describes how he was called to a newborn baby with ambiguous genitalia (a tiny penis with hypospadias – the urine

How to Read a Paper: The Basics of Evidence-Based Healthcare, Seventh Edition.
Trisha Greenhalgh and Paul Dijkstra.

hole was not right at the tip but some way down – and what looked like a scrotum but no palpable testes). Was this a chromosomal male with underdeveloped genitalia or a chromosomal female who had been androgenised in utero? And what to tell the parents? A fast decision was needed for both medical and social reasons.

Kohane put this clinical query into the newly developed GPT-4, an AI digital assistant, which you can now access through an application on your smartphone. Within seconds, he got a response listing several possible diagnoses: congenital adrenal hyperplasia, androgen insensitivity syndrome, gonadal dysgenesis and pituitary or hypothalamic dysfunction. Some of these conditions were feminised boys; others were androgenised girls; some had rare subtypes as well as more common variants. For each option, the digital assistant had suggested some further tests to rule the condition in or out and identify subtypes. To cut a long story short, the suggestions from the digital assistant allowed Kohane to run a focused search of the literature (informed by many of the principles set out in other chapters in this book), send a panel of specialised tests on the infant, and establish a firm (and treatable) diagnosis in the space of a few days.

Having whet your appetite with this dramatic but, importantly, anecdotal example of what AI can *already* contribute to healthcare, we should also introduce some downsides. Lee and colleagues' book includes some salutary examples of advanced AI's tendency to 'hallucinate'; for example, cite papers that don't exist (which is why you should check any sources!).

More generally, AI can be like the clever kid in the class who is not actually as clever as they seem. In a recent paper, anthropologist Lisa Messeri and cognitive scientist Molly Crockett discuss four visions of AI ('AI as oracle', 'AI as arbiter', 'AI as quant' and 'AI as surrogate') for researchers to consider before they embed AI tools in their research [4]. They warn that these visions of AI, or cognitive 'traps', could amplify incorrect beliefs about the nature of one's understanding (so called 'epistemic risk'), highlighting the *illusion of explanatory depth* (assuming that the explanation produced by AI is more profound than it actually is), the *illusion of exploratory breadth* (assuming that the AI model has covered all possible hypotheses relevant to the question when it has actually covered only a limited number) and the *illusion of objectivity* (assuming that the AI model has produced an unbiased 'view from nowhere' when in reality it reflects, and may even magnify, the various biases inherent in the published literature on a topic) [4]. You have been warned!

In summary, the paper you are reading could be about AI, written by AI, or AI could have read (and summarised) the paper for you. Recently, several papers have been published with random AI-written phrases embedded in the text, like 'Certainly, here is a possible introduction for your topic' or 'In summary, the management of bilateral iatrogenic I'm very sorry, but I don't have access to real-time information or patient-specific data, as I am an AI language model.' Obviously, a huge embarrassment – and warning – for authors, peer reviewers and journal editors!

Now let's wind back and take a broader overview of all the different kinds of AI you might come across in a healthcare setting.

Artificial intelligence

Let's start with a definition of AI (Table 17.1). AI is intelligence demonstrated by machines. It is also an interdisciplinary field of research that spans, among other disciplines, computer science, psychology, linguistics and philosophy [5]. Professor Nick Bostrom from the University of Oxford (have a listen

Table 17.1 Terminology and definitions

Artificial Intelligence (AI)	Intelligence demonstrated by machines
AI system	A decision support system that incorporates AI (consists of the AI : algorithm and its supporting software and hardware platforms
Big data	Data characterized by very high volume, velocity and variety requiring special technology and analytical methods to transform it into value. Only a 'volume' definition has also been proposed: '. . .a dataset could be qualified as "big dataset" only if Log(n*p) is superior or equal to 7.' [10]. The authors list eight properties of big data: great variety, high velocity, challenge on veracity, challenge on all aspects of the workflow, challenge on computational methods, challenge on extracting meaningful information, challenge on sharing data, challenge on finding human experts [10].
ChatGPT	Chat Generative Pre-trained Transformer, a commercial digital assistant (accessible via a smartphone app, for example). Includes a free basic version and a more sophisticated version for a monthly fee.
Cloud computing	The on-demand availability of computing resources (such as storage and infrastructure) over the internet.
Computer processing power	The ability of a computer to process information or the speed at which it can process information
Conversational AI	An AI system which engages in an intelligent conversation with a human user
Data leakage	When information about the test data is 'leaked' into the model during training
Deep learning	A type of machine learning that uses a layered structure of artificial neural networks

(*Continued*)

Table 17.1 (Continued)

Artificial Intelligence (AI)	Intelligence demonstrated by machines
Generative AI	A subset of AI technologies that generate new content such as text, images, music, speech, video, or code by learning patterns and structure of large amounts training data
Intended AI use	The use for which an AI system is intended (e.g. targeted medical condition, patient and user populations and use environment)
Machine learning	A field of computer science involving models/ algorithms which learn patterns from data, rather than being programmed with rules.
Large language models (LLMs)	AI models that use computational AI algorithms with text data as input to generate language that resembles that produced by humans
Large multi-modal models (LMMs)	AI models that have the ability to accept one or more type of data inputs (e.g. text, videos, and images) and generate diverse outputs that are not limited to the type of data inputted
Reinforcement learning	A type of machine learning where an agent learns to interact with an environment by trial and error, based on the idea of rewarding desired behaviors and penalizing undesirable ones. It is a powerful technique for training AI agents to make decisions in complex environments by learning from experience. Examples include optimizing treatment plans (e.g. insulin dosing in diabetes).
Supervised learning	A type of machine learning where the algorithm is trained on a dataset with labeled examples using (e.g.) linear or logistic regression. These labels provide the correct output or target variable for each input. Examples include spam filtering, image recognition and medical diagnosis.
Unsupervised learning	A type of machine learning where the algorithm is trained on a dataset without any labels. The algorithm discovers patterns, structures, or relationships in the data using (e.g.) clustering or dimensionality reduction. Examples include disease clustering (e.g. for subtypes of breast cancer), early detection and drug discovery.

to his fascinating TED® talk *What happens when our computers get smarter than we are?* [6]) described three major levels of AI [7]:

1. Artificial narrow intelligence (ANI) refers to algorithms with excellent pattern recognising abilities in huge data sets. It is useful for solving text, voice or image-based classification and clustering problems. ANI excels at a precisely defined single task (like playing chess).

2. Artificial general intelligence refers to AI applications that can reason, argue, memorise and solve problems. This is what Bostrom calls 'human level' AI, in the sense that it displays a cognitive capacity which approximates to that of a human being.
3. Artificial super intelligence refers to AI applications which could theoretically have humanity's combined cognitive capacity and more!

In this chapter, we focus on direct medical uses, which include risk prediction, interactive note taking, patient chatbots, clinical decision support, drug discovery, image interpretation, diagnosis and prognosis of disease, identification of treatments and patient–doctor communication (see the systematic review by Kedia et al. [8] for more examples). One major category of AI in healthcare, which we don't address in this book, is its many administrative functions (for example, speech recognition products which allow you to dictate a letter and see it typed as you speak).

From a computational perspective, the diverse medical and healthcare uses of AI can be classified into four broad categories:

1. *prediction* (using historical data to predict the likelihood of future events)
2. *classification* (e.g. of images into normal or abnormal)
3. *association* (enhancing prediction by incorporating new knowledge; e.g. identifying new symptoms of disease)
4. *optimisation* (mostly, administrative tasks) [9].

Table 17.1 lists some key terminology and definitions.

Big data

'Big data' (see Table 17.1 for defintion) refers to large or complex datasets which it would be impossible to analyse without advanced computer power [11]. As the sheer size of cohort studies and the number of variables to be analysed has increased, calculations can no longer be done on a desktop spreadsheet but require vast computer power. This is why cloud computing and the rapid growth in the ability of computers to process information (computer processing power) are *the* key drivers of the AI revolution.

One example of such a big data platform is OpenSAFELY (https://www.opensafely.org/), a secure analytics platform for NHS electronic health records in the UK. You can read more about it in Nab et al. [12]. A big-data cohort study by the OpenSAFELY collaborative [13] investigated the impact of vaccination on the association of COVID-19 with cardiovascular disease. Defining a 'prevaccination' cohort of more than 18,000,000 people, and 'vaccinated' and 'unvaccinated' cohorts (of 13,572,399 and 3,161,485, respectively), they concluded that COVID-19 vaccination significantly reduces the risk of cardiovascular events after COVID-19 infection.

For an accessible introduction to big data more generally, see the paper by Car and Sheikh [14].

Machine learning

Artificial intelligence works through machine learning, a field of computer science involving models/algorithms which learn patterns from data, rather than being programmed with rules (Table 17.1). You should be able to identify the type of machine learning used in the paper you are reading: supervised learning, unsupervised learning, reinforcement learning and deep learning. Be sceptical if the authors did not describe the subtype of machine learning or deep learning in detail (see question four below). A comprehensive overview of machine learning is beyond the scope of this chapter. However, you should be aware of the problem of 'data leakage' (Table 17.1), which has been long recognised as an important cause of errors in machine learning applications. It leads to inflated model performance and decreased reproducibility. You can read more about it in Kapoor and Narayanan's paper [15]. If you want to read more, the paper by Meskó and Görög provides an excellent overview of AI for healthcare professionals [5].

Generative artificial intelligence: large language and multimodal models

Generative AI, which we can only cover briefly in this book but which is covered in more detail elsewhere [16], includes large language models (LLMs) [17] and large multimodal models (LMMs) [17,18]; these are all defined in Table 17.1. LLM AI systems use algorithms 'trained on billions of words derived from articles, books and other [text-based] internet-based content' [17] to generate language (talk) like humans [17,18]; LMMs do the same but accept many types of data input, including text, images, audio and video (and sometimes other data types such as sensory data). LMMs generate diverse outputs that are not necessarily related to the type of data fed to the algorithm (you could, for example, feed images in and get text back or vice versa) [19,28]. LLMs and LMMs are increasingly used in medicine to retrieve knowledge, support clinical decision-making, summarise key findings, triage patients and so on.

If you are interested in *how* LLMs encode clinical knowledge, including their limitations and suggestions for future research, see the paper by Singhal et al. in *Nature* [20]. Our PubMed search for the term 'ChatGPT' on 16 January 2024 revealed 2167 papers (2060 published in 2023 and 189 in the first 16 days of 2024!). ChatGPT has passed the US Medical License Exam [21], and is used to answer common patient questions about colonoscopy, for example [22]. LLM-driven chatbots are increasingly used in healthcare, including in medical education, in the resource constrained neuro-ophthalmic field, for example [23]. Chatbots are also used to provide clinical advice to patients. Because they operate in a *conversational* format (you ask a question, the LLM replies, you explain why the response isn't quite what you wanted and so on), LLMs and LMMs can *feel* like you're interacting with a human or human-like agent. And because they are designed to find and take account of context rather than focusing only on the inputted text, these models can potentially adapt what they say (and how they say it) to accommodate different patient personalities and levels of health literacy. They can also, potentially, respond in the patient's preferred language. All this is very exciting: generative AI could potentially overcome some of the brittleness of previous-generation digital health applications and produce fewer punch-the-screen moments. But, at the time of writing, we're talking mostly about *potential* rather than *actual* benefits for patients.

Ethical principles for the use of artificial intelligence for health

What comes out of an AI system depends on how it is built ('garbage in, garbage out'). If, for example, the designers incorporate (consciously or unconsciously) stereotypical or incorrect assumptions about patients or other users, the responses generated by the models will themselves be biased or misleading. Furthermore, whatever its data processing ability, a machine is still a machine; there are aspects of medicine and healthcare (compassion, comfort, care) which still, arguably, require human input. AI applications are, for the most part, designed to be used by a human who has professional training, not to *substitute* for that human. For this reason, ethical considerations and human rights must be central to their design, development and implementation. The World Health Organization (WHO) endorsed six key ethical principles for the use of AI for health [24]:

1. *Protecting human autonomy*. Humans should remain in control of medical decisions and people should understand how AI is used in their care (including how their privacy and confidentiality are protected).
2. *Promoting human wellbeing and safety and the public interest*. AI should not harm people: the designers of AI technology should comply with regulatory requirements for safety, accuracy and efficacy.
3. *Ensuring transparency, explainability and intelligibility*. AI technology should be understandable to developers, healthcare professionals, patients, users and regulators 'according to the capacity of those to whom they are explained'.

4. *Fostering responsibility and accountability.* Patients and clinicians should evaluate the development and deployment of AI technologies. This should include mechanisms for questioning and for redress for individuals and groups that are adversely affected by decisions based on algorithms.
5. *Ensuring inclusiveness and equity.* AI for health should be designed 'to encourage the widest possible appropriate, equitable use and access, irrespective of age, sex, gender, income, race, ethnicity, sexual orientation, ability or other characteristics protected under human rights codes'. AI technologies should not encode biases to the disadvantage of identifiable groups (especially already minoritised groups).
6. *Promoting AI that is responsive and sustainable.* All AI role players (designers, developers and users) should 'continuously, systematically and transparently' assess AI applications during actual use. Two aspects are important for sustainable AI systems. First, their environmental consequences should be minimal. Second, their impact on the workplace, including workplace disruptions, training of healthcare workers and potential job losses, should be addressed by governments and companies.

Guidance on the ethics and governance of LMMs is a complex and expanding topic; see the WHO's new review if you are interested [19].

Appraising artificial intelligence papers: a plethora of checklists

When can you trust a paper describing an AI intervention, and when can't you? The APPRAISE-AI tool was developed to evaluate the methodological and reporting quality of 28 clinical AI studies using a quantitative approach [25]. However, it is only one of several such tools in the literature (indeed, a 2022 literature review identified 14 frameworks including 8 providing reporting checklists for medical applications of AI) [26]. We summarise some of the current frameworks in Table 17.2.

You should select the specific reporting guideline relevant to the study design of the paper you are appraising; for example, TRIPOD-AI for prediction model studies, STARD-AI for diagnostic accuracy studies and SPIRIT/CONSORT-AI for randomised controlled trials. These AI extensions to current reporting guidelines include additional items to, for example, address potential sources of bias specific to AI systems [27]. Reporting guidelines, although a good starting point when evaluating a paper, should not be used uncritically as quality checklists.

As we write this chapter, no reporting standards yet exist for studies that evaluate the performance of LLM-linked chatbots when providing clinical advice. To bridge this gap, a group of researchers are currently developing CHART (chatbot assessment reporting tool) to guide researchers interested

Table 17.2 Artificial intelligence reporting guidelines

Name	Stage	Study design	Comment
TRIPOD-AI	Preclinical development	Prediction model evaluation[a]	Extension of TRIPOD and used to report development, validation and updates of diagnostic and prognostic prediction models (diagnostic or prognostic)
STARD-AI	Preclinical development, offline validation	Diagnostic accuracy studies[a]	Extension of STARD and used to report diagnostic accuracy studies
DECIDE-AI	Early live clinical evaluation	Various (prospective cohort studies, non-RCTs, etc.)	Stand-alone guideline which is used to report the early evaluation of AI systems as an intervention in live clinical settings (guideline used for all study designs and any AI system modality, e.g. diagnostic, prognostic, therapeutic). This guideline focuses on clinical utility, safety, and human factors
SPIRIT-AI	Comparative prospective evaluation	RCTs (protocol)	Extension of SPIRIT. Used to report the protocols of randomised controlled trials evaluating AI systems as interventions
CONSORT-AI	Comparative prospective evaluation	RCTs[a]	Extension of CONSORT and used to report large-scale RCTs evaluating AI systems as interventions (for any AI system modality, e.g. diagnostic, prognostic, therapeutic). This guideline focuses on effectiveness and safety
CLAIM	All AI in medical imaging studies	Studies reporting medical imaging[a]	A checklist to guide reporting of AI in medical imaging
CHART	All studies assessing the use of chatbots in healthcare	Chatbot assessment studies[a]	Chatbot assessment reporting tool (CHART) currently being developed

[a] Primary target of the guidelines (either specific stage or a specific design).
RCT, randomised controlled trial.
Source: [28] / BMJ Publishing Group Ltd.

Chapter 17

in evaluating the performance of LLM-linked chatbots that summarise health evidence and provide clinical advice [29]. You might want to track that publication in Google Scholar.

A further challenge of AI studies is that even when your critical appraisal confirms that the AI study was done rigorously and its findings can be trusted, there is a further question: does the AI technology or intervention work in (clinical) practice? The patients in your clinic may not be comparable to the patient sample on which the algorithm was trained.

We can't reproduce or summarise all the checklists in this chapter, so we have chosen the DECIDE-AI checklist (see Table 17.3) for evaluating AI-based decision support systems. This field poses some methodological challenges (Box 17.1 and Table 17.3) [25]. Most of these challenges are also applicable to other AI studies; for example, how humans and machines 'collaborate' while protecting the important ethical principle of human autonomy, and how AI systems could harm (e.g. algorithm bias and data breaches).

Box 17.1 Issues to consider in AI-based decision support systems

- AI-based decision support systems represent complex interventions. We need to account for the associated complexities and evaluate how these systems integrate within existing healthcare ecosystems.
- People who use AI-based decision support systems vary a lot; this could add biases. We need to account for user variability and the added biases.
- Two forms of intelligence (human and AI system) are collaborating. We therefore need to evaluate human factors.
- AI-based decision support systems involve both physical patients and their data representations. We therefore need to account for patients and their data when evaluating these AI systems.
- AI-based decision support systems represent a interventions that continuously change (either due to early prototyping, version updates, or continuous learning design). We need to account for this complexity and analyse related performance changes.
- AI-based decision support systems could embed and reproduce existing health inequality and systemic biases. We need to evaluate and address these challenges.
- Findings of AI-based decision support system studies might not be relevant for different settings to those studies. We need to estimate the generalisability of findings across different sites and populations.
- AI-based decision support systems represent a field of dynamic innovation and intellectual property protection. We need to evaluate (and enable) reproducibility of the findings in the context of these challenges.

Source: adapted from Vasey et al. [28].

Table 17.3 Simplified DECIDE-AI checklist

Theme	Recommendation
Title	Include mention of AI in the title
Abstract	Provide a structured summary.
Introduction	
Intended use	Describe what condition(s) the AI is being used for, the intended patient population, and current standard practice Describe who will use the AI system, how it will fit into the care pathway, and what the anticipated impact will be
Objectives	State the study objectives
Ethics and governance	Link to the study protocol and give details of ethics approval
Methods	
Participants	Describe how patient participants *and* users of the AI system were recruited, including what inclusion and exclusion criteria were used (for patients, at both patient and data level), and justify the sample sizes; Describe how users were taught to use the AI system.
AI system	Describe the AI system (include version and type of underlying algorithm). Describe/ reference the characteristics of the patient population on which the algorithm was trained (and its performance in preclinical development and validation studies) Identify and describe input data. (including how data were acquired and entered, for example) Describe the AI system outputs and how they were presented to users (add image if possible)
Implementation	Describe the settings in which the AI system was evaluated, including details of clincal workflow, who made actual clinical decisions and how
Outcomes	Specify primary and any secondary outcomes measured
Safety and errors	Describe how errors or malfunctions were defined and identified, and how risks to patient safety were identified, analysed and minimised
Human factors	Describe the human factors tools, methods or frameworks used, the used cases considered, and the users involved
Analysis	Describe and justify how data were analysed including statistical tests
AI ethics	Give details of any specific methodologies used to ensure algorithmic fairness or other ethical goal
Patient involvement	Say how patients were involved in any aspect of the study
Results	
Participants	Give details of both the patient population and users of the AI system
Implementation	Report on how much the AI system was used, whether users adhered to the protocol, and any changes to workflow or care pathway

(*Continued*)

Table 17.3 (Continued)

Theme	Recommendation
Main findings	Report on the primary and secondary outcomes, with subgroup analyses if appropriate
Modifications	Report on any changes made to the AI platform or its hardware throughout the study
Human-computer agreement	Report on how closely the human user agreed with the AI system's recommendations and explain and comment on instances of disagreement
Safety and errors	List and comment on significant errors or malfunctions, including how common they were, whether they could be corrected and impacts on patient care. Report on any risks or harms to patients, including indirect harm.
Human factors	Report on the usability evaluation (perhaps using a recognised framework for this)
Discussion	
Conclusions about intended use	Discuss whether the study results support the intended use of the AI system in clinical settings
Safety and errors	Discuss the implications of the safety profile of the AI system, including the extent to which limitations might be mitigated
Strengths and limitations	Discuss the strengths and limitations of the study
Statements	
Data availability	Say what data are available (including code) to others
Disclosures	Disclose any conflicts of interest (e.g. commercial interests)

Source: simplified and adapted from Vasey et al. [28].

Ten questions to ask about a paper that reports AI studies in healthcare

In preparing these ten questions, we have drawn on several AI quality tools and reporting guidelines—mostly the CONSORT-AI [30] and DECIDE-AI [28] extensions. The questions focus on studies on decision support systems driven by AI.

Question one: What is the intended use of the AI system, and who are the intended users? Based on this, is the AI system relevant to your patients and practice?
As we mentioned in Chapter 8, this is the 'so what' question, or the *clinical utility* of the AI system. What are the targeted medical condition(s) (e.g. breast cancer) and associated problem(s) (e.g. reducing false-positive screens and increase breast cancer detection rates), current standard practice, and the intended patient population? Who are the intended users of the AI system and how could it be integrated in their care pathways? For example, radiologists are the intended users of an AI system developed to improve accuracy of

breast cancer screening programmes [31]. How might the AI system improve on current standard practice? If so, would you or your patient(s) use it in preference to existing solutions/systems?

Question two: Is it clear what type of AI study is reported in the paper?
Does the paper, for example, report a clinical trial, diagnostic accuracy study or prediction model study? As mentioned above, the applications of AI (in general and in healthcare) are broadly grouped into one or a combination of four capabilities: prediction (e.g. the risk of a person developing a specific health outcome), classification (e.g. presence of absence of a disease), association (e.g. drug discovery or new risk factors for a specific health condition) and optimisation (e.g. administrative tasks).

Question three: Who participated in the study (patients and users)?
Here, you should consider three important aspects: the patients on which the AI algorithm was trained, the users of the AI system and how users were familiarised with the AI system. First, considering patients, it should be clear from the manuscript who the patients were on which the AI algorithm was trained: how patients were recruited, including sample size and inclusion and exclusion criteria at both patient and data level. For example, at patient level a participant could meet all inclusion criteria but still be excluded from the study due to incomplete or poor quality of the data. Second, as AI systems are complex interventions, it is important to consider how the interaction between users and the AI system influenced overall AI system performance and study results. This is similar to surgical innovation studies where both patient and operator characteristics are important and should be reported [32]. Finally, how users were familiarised with the AI system should help you to anticipate how much time and work might be required for the AI system to be used reliably and with confidence in your own practice. Look for a training protocol, the type and number of training and practice sessions delivered, and training materials (as supplementary information). Finally, look for the baseline characteristics of the patients included in the AI system dataset and the users of the AI system in the study.

Question four: What AI system was used in this study?
First, look for a concise description of the AI system, especially its version, the underlying algorithm, supporting hardware, and software (if relevant). You can usually find this in the methods section of the paper. Do not expect a full description of the AI algorithm or mathematical model in the paper, it could be complicated! Rather, if you are mathematically inclined, look for references (either published or in an open science repository or as supplementary material) to the development and validation studies of the algorithm. Here, you should find information on the components of the algorithm (e.g. neural network architecture), the patient populations used in

the development/validation studies, the performance metrics used and the study results. A description of the supporting hardware might give you an indication of the benefits and limitations of the platform in your own clinical setting. Also look for specific algorithmic thresholds used in the study (e.g. cut-off set to not exceed a specific false positive rate).

Second, identify the data used as inputs for the AI system. How did the research team acquire the data? What method was used to input the data into the AI system? What preprocessing was applied and how were missing or low-quality data handled? Finally, look for a description of the AI system outputs and how they were presented to the users. The human-computer interface (specifically how information is displayed) is important for how users will interact with the AI system [33].

Question five: What are the clinical setting(s) and clinical workflow/pathway in which the AI system was evaluated?
You need to know whether the settings and conditions of the study are representative of the AI system's intended use. How the AI system has been integrated in the clinical workflow/care pathway (including the clinical decisions made using the AI system) is important. Anchoring bias, a form of cognitive bias [34], is possible when users see the AI system recommendations at the same time as they receive other information on which clinical decision-making is based (so called 'concurrent reading mode'). In second reading mode, users see the AI system recommendations after they have made the decision about a case, and re-evaluate their initial decision based on the new AI system information. Authors should report any significant changes to the clinical workflow or care pathways caused by the AI system.

Question six: Were possible errors, including algorithm and use errors (and malfunctions of the supporting software/hardware) defined, described and reported? Did the authors describe their approach to mitigate safety concerns or patient harm? Did the authors report and discuss any safety concerns or instances of harm?
Errors and malfunctions impact patient safety and could harm patients. Three main categories of errors and malfunctions should be considered (look for this in the methods section of the paper) and reported in the results section (e.g. rate, causes and impact on patient care of AI system errors/malfunctions):

1. algorithm errors (e.g. the AI system did not detect all cancers in women's digital mammograms [35])
2. malfunction of the supporting software or hardware (e.g. the AI system failed to produce a recommendation due to data extraction issue)
3. errors involving users (e.g. clinician input inaccurate patient details or applied the AI system to a medical indication its not been designed for).

Safety assessment is a continuous process which occurs before, during and after a clinical study as new risks or harms might be uncovered after AI system implementation in clinical settings. AI system researchers should describe their risk management process in the methods section of the paper and report and discuss any observed risks to patient safety or instances of harm in the results and discussion sections of the paper. Authors should report any changes made to the AI system during the study.

Question seven: How did the authors deal with human factors?
Human factors (also called ergonomics) can make or break AI systems in healthcare. Here, the aim is to describe and understand the interactions among humans and the AI system, including factors like situation awareness, workload and automation bias. Authors should consider AI system evaluation (preclinical and ongoing while used in clinical settings), the clinical context and specific AI system, and usability (using validated tools to evaluate, for example, workload, display interface or user satisfaction). You can read more about human factors and ergonomics principles for healthcare AI in this paper [36].

Question eight: What is the approach to ethical use of the AI system?
This question relates to the key ethical principles discussed earlier in this chapter (and to question six above). Did the authors report and describe how they worked to detect, quantify and mitigate bias in the AI system's algorithmic outputs (e.g. through algorithmic fairness: adjustments in an attempt to correct for bias). Therefore, algorithmic bias in AI systems could harm groups that are already underrepresented and marginalised [37].

Question nine: Did the authors share the code and data used to train and validate their AI system?
As noted above, explainability of any AI system is very important. The authors should share the code and data used to train and validate their AI system. Bonus points to the authors if they annotated their code to explain what each bit does to allow the reader to follow regardless of their background. Ideally, you should be able to easily generate plots, charts and matrices that tell you all about the data's metrics, by running the algorithm. Good papers that are transparent about their code and data will let you do this.

Question ten: What kind of collaborative model between authors was used to build the AI system?
Who performed the research? Was it a diverse team of AI scientists, clinicians and patient partners, for example, to counteract the risk of 'monocultures of knowing and knowers' referred to earlier in this chapter [4]? While this could be difficult to tell, by looking at the author list as well as data sources you could

form an idea: were clinicians involved in building the AI tool if it's aimed at clinical care (not just testing it, but building it! Here, Yosra Mekki argues that clinicians should build their own AI models [38]). Do the authors explain to what extent clinicians and patient partners, for example, were involved in the project? (And not just a tokenistic checklist tick of the 'collaboration' box). Did the authors discuss how they supported clear communication between team members of different backgrounds? This reflects on model quality.

Summary

In summary, before we use an AI system to inform our clinical decisions, we should ask two over-arching questions. First, 'What is the accuracy, reliability, and validity of the AI system in diagnosing or making a recommendation for my patient's specific condition and context?' And second, 'How well has the AI system been tested against diverse patient populations and various clinical scenarios?' We should understand the limitations and potential biases of an AI system – AI systems can only supplement but not replace a healthcare professional's expertise and contextual praxis. A well-informed clinician would consider the results from such technologies within the context of the science, and the individual patient's personal circumstances.

Exercises based on this chapter

1. Listen to the *NEJM-AI* podcast by Dr Ziad Obermeyer [39]. Discuss the complex issues of bias, safety and generalisability of medical AI. How do siloed and inaccessible data amplify these AI challenges? Why should clinicians and AI researchers collaborate to develop AI systems for healthcare?
2. Take a look at the paper by Wong et al. [40], who used a big-data 'deep learning' approach to discover a new class of antibiotic. Why do you think this innovation was not possible before the advent of advanced computer power? To what extent do you think AI can help us keep ahead of antimicrobial resistance?
3. According to this paper, machine learning may outperform conventional statistical methods to predict next-season athlete injuries [41]. What are the challenges of applying machine learning to predict a future health condition? Is machine learning always better than conventional statistical models such as logistic regression?
4. A US-based classification algorithm for melanoma diagnosis [42] was trained on images of skin lesions in mainly light-skinned patients and then used on images of lesions among African-American patients [43]. How did the system perform? Referring to the WHO's six key ethical principles for the use of AI for health [24], what would you do to ensure ethical and safe AI in your own (clinical or research) setting?

5. Review the paper 'The role of artificial intelligence in early cancer diagnosis' [44]. Now, search PubMed and find an artificial intelligence paper on a topic of your choice. What was the health condition that the AI system targeted? What type of AI algorithm did the researchers use in the paper? (artificial neural network, deep neural network, convolutional neural network, recurrent neural network etc.). Could you describe the problem-solving approach that the AI algorithm followed (classification, regression etc.)? What was the source of data used to develop the AI algorithm? Was the data source representative or could the AI algorithm be biased?
6. Read this paper on the use of AI to predict whether a person is at risk of ventricular arrhythmia [45]. What type of machine learning did the researchers use? Could you use such an AI system in your practice?

References

1. Johnson. Our word of the year for 2023. *The Economist* 7 December 2023. https://www.economist.com/culture/2023/12/07/our-word-of-the-year-for-2023 (accessed 9 December 2023).
2. Zhang J, Whebell S, Gallifant J, et al. An interactive dashboard to track themes, development maturity, and global equity in clinical artificial intelligence research. *Lancet Digital Health*. 2022; **4**: e212–3.
3. Lee P, Goldberg C, Kohane I. *The AI Revolution in Medicine: GPT-4 and beyond.* Hoboken, NJ: Pearson; 2023.
4. Messeri L, Crockett MJ. Artificial intelligence and illusions of understanding in scientific research. *Nature* 2024; **627**: 49–58.
5. Meskó B, Görög M. A short guide for medical professionals in the era of artificial intelligence. *npj Digital Medicine* 2020; **3**: 126.
6. Bostrom N. What happens when our computers get smarter than we are? *TED* March 2015. https://www.ted.com/talks/nick_bostrom_what_happens_when_our_computers_get_smarter_than_we_are (accessed 8 March 2024).
7. Bostrom N. *Superintelligence: Paths, dangers, strategies.* New York, NY: Oxford University Press; 2014.
8. Kedia N, Sanjeev S, Ong J, et al. ChatGPT and Beyond: An overview of the growing field of large language models and their use in ophthalmology. *Eye* 2024; **38**: 1252–61.
9. De Silva D, Alahakoon D. An artificial intelligence life cycle: from conception to production. *Patterns* 2022; **3**: 100489.
10. Baro E, Degoul S, Beuscart R, et al. Toward a literature-driven definition of big data in healthcare. *BioMed Research International* 2015; **2015**: 639021.
11. Dhindsa K, Bhandari M, Sonnadara RR. What's holding up the big data revolution in healthcare? *BMJ* 2018; **363**: k5357.
12. Nab L, Schaffer A, Hulme W, et al. OpenSAFELY: a platform for analysing electronic health records designed for reproducible research [preprint]. 3 February 2024 https://doi.org/10.31219/osf.io/hj2sg.
13. Cezard GI, Denholm RE, Knight R, et al. Impact of vaccination on the association of COVID-19 with cardiovascular diseases: An OpenSAFELY cohort study. *Nature Communication* 2024; **15**: 2173.

14. Car J, Sheikh A, Wicks P, et al. Beyond the hype of big data and artificial intelligence: building foundations for knowledge and wisdom. *BMC Medicine* 2019; **17**: 143.
15. Kapoor S, Narayanan A. Leakage and the reproducibility crisis in machine-learning-based science. *Patterns (NY)* 2023; **4**: 100804.
16. Yu P, Xu H, Hu X, et al. Leveraging generative AI and large language models: a comprehensive roadmap for healthcare integration. *Healthcare (Basel)* 2023; **11**: 2776.
17. Thirunavukarasu AJ, Ting DSJ, Elangovan K, et al. Large language models in medicine. *Nature Medicine* 2023; **29**: 1930–40.
18. Clusmann J, Kolbinger FR, Muti HS, et al. The future landscape of large language models in medicine. *Communications Medicine* 2023; **3** :141.
19. World Health Organization. WHO releases AI ethics and governance guidance for large multi-modal models. https://www.who.int/news/item/18-01-2024-who-releases-ai-ethics-and-governance-guidance-for-large-multi-modal-models (accessed 21 January 2024).
20. Singhal K, Azizi S, Tu T, et al. Large language models encode clinical knowledge. *Nature* 2023; **620**: 172–80.
21. Kung TH, Cheatham M, Medenilla A, et al. Performance of ChatGPT on USMLE: potential for AI-assisted medical education using large language models. *PLOS Digital Health*. 2023; **2**: e0000198.
22. Lee T-C, Staller K, Botoman V, et al. ChatGPT Answers common patient questions about colonoscopy. *Gastroenterology* 2023; **165**: 509-511.e7.
23. Waisberg E, Ong J, Masalkhi M, et al. Large language model (LLM)-driven chatbots for neuro-ophthalmic medical education. *Eye* 2024; **38**: 639–41.
24. World Health Organization. *Ethics and Governance of Artificial Intelligence for Health*. WHO Guidance. Geneva: WHO; 2021.
25. Kwong JCC, Khondker A, Lajkosz K, et al. APPRAISE-AI Tool for quantitative evaluation of ai studies for clinical decision support. *JAMA Network Open* 2023; **6**: e2335377.
26. Crossnohere NL, Elsaid M, Paskett J, et al. Guidelines for artificial intelligence in medicine: literature review and content analysis of frameworks. *Journal of Medical Internet Research* 2022; **24**: e36823.
27. Nagendran M, Chen Y, Lovejoy CA, et al. Artificial intelligence versus clinicians: systematic review of design, reporting standards, and claims of deep learning studies. *BMJ* 2020; **368**: m689.
28. Vasey B, Nagendran M, Campbell B, et al. Reporting guideline for the early stage clinical evaluation of decision support systems driven by artificial intelligence: DECIDE-AI. *BMJ* 2022; **377**: e070904.
29. Huo B, Cacciamani GE, Collins GS, et al. Reporting standards for the use of large language model-linked chatbots for health advice. *Nature Medicine* 2023; **29**: 2988–2988.
30. Liu X, Rivera SC, Moher D, et al. Reporting guidelines for clinical trial reports for interventions involving artificial intelligence: the CONSORT-AI Extension. *BMJ* 2020; **370**: m3164.

31. Marinovich ML, Wylie E, Lotter W, et al. Artificial intelligence (AI) for breast cancer screening: BreastScreen population-based cohort study of cancer detection. *eBioMedicine* 2023; **90**: 104498.
32. Hirst A, Philippou Y, Blazeby J, et al. No surgical innovation without evaluation: evolution and further development of the IDEAL framework and recommendations. *Annals of Surgery* 2019; **269**: 211–20.
33. Dudley JJ, Kristensson PO. A review of user interface design for interactive machine learning. *ACM Transactions on Interactive Intelligent Systems* 2018; **8**(2): 1–37.
34. Furnham A, Boo HC. A literature review of the anchoring effect. *Journal of Socio-Economics* 2011; **40**: 35–42.
35. Freeman K, Geppert J, Stinton C, et al. Use of artificial intelligence for image analysis in breast cancer screening programmes: systematic review of test accuracy. *BMJ* 2021; **374**: n1872.
36. Sujan M, Pool R, Salmon P. Eight human factors and ergonomics principles for healthcare artificial intelligence. *BMJ Health and Care Informatics* 2022; **29**: bmjhci-2021-100516.
37. Aquino YSJ, Carter SM, Houssami N, et al. Practical, epistemic and normative implications of algorithmic bias in healthcare artificial intelligence: a qualitative study of multidisciplinary expert perspectives [published online ahead of print 23 February 2023]. *Journal of Medical Ethics* 2023. https://doi.org/10.1136/jme-2022-108850
38. Mekki YM. Physicians should build their own machine-learning models. *Patterns* 2024; **5**:100948.
39. Development P. Manrai A, Beam A, hosts. The double-edged sword of AI, with Dr. Ziad Obermeyer [podcast]. *NEJM AI Grand Rounds* 27 July 2023. https://ai-podcast.nejm.org/e/the-double-edged-sword-of-ai-with-dr-ziad-obermeyer (accessed 1 January 2024).
40. Wong F, Zheng EJ, Valeri JA, et al. Discovery of a structural class of antibiotics with explainable deep learning. *Nature* 2024; **626**: 177–85.
41. Karnuta JM, Luu BC, Haeberle HS, et al. Machine learning outperforms regression analysis to predict next-season major league baseball player injuries: epidemiology and validation of 13,982 player-years from performance and injury profile trends, 2000–2017. *Orthopaedic Journal of Sports Medicine* 2020; **8**: 2325967120963046.
42. Brinker TJ, Hekler A, Enk AH, et al. Deep neural networks are superior to dermatologists in melanoma image classification. *European Journal of Cancer* 2019; **119**: 11–17.
43. Norori N, Hu Q, Aellen FM, *et al.* Addressing bias in big data and AI for health care: a call for open science. *Patterns* 2021; **2**: 100347.
44. Hunter B, Hindocha S, Lee RW. the role of artificial intelligence in early cancer diagnosis. *Cancers (Basel)* 2022; **14**: 1524.
45. Barker J, Li X, Kotb A, et al. Artificial intelligence for ventricular arrhythmia capability using ambulatory electrocardiograms. *European Heart Journal Digital Health* 2024; 2024: ztae004.

Chapter 18 EBM+: the importance of mechanistic evidence

What is mechanistic evidence? An example

Mechanistic evidence means evidence about the causal mechanism through which an intervention achieves an effect. A few years ago, Trisha participated in a Cochrane review of school feeding programmes for disadvantaged children [1]. To her surprise, there were some randomised controlled trials (RCTs) on this topic, although many studies were done as before-and-after designs for ethical and practical reasons (it is hard to assign starving children to a 'control group', even temporarily). It came as no surprise that, generally but not always, feeding children at school when they weren't getting enough food at home led to improvements in nutritional status, growth, school performance and other key outcome measures [1]. But *how* did providing a meal at school produce these outcomes? And in the studies where the intervention had no effect, *why* did it fail?

To answer these questions, the review team needed to produce mechanistic evidence. In the school feeding studies, which were a *complex social intervention* (see Chapter 7), the review looked at qualitative studies, including process evaluations of the RCTs, for information on who exactly did what and how this affected the outcomes [2]. It found that, in some studies, the improvements were very short-term: children who hadn't eaten breakfast were sleepy and unattentive in class; a good meal on arrival perked them up, so they did better in class. In other studies, the gains were more long term: correction of protein-calorie malnutrition, anaemia and vitamin deficiency. These children were taller and heavier 6 months later as well as doing better in class. In one study of disadvantaged teenagers in a deprived part of the United States, the teacher cooked the class a hearty breakfast before giving a lesson. The teens said they felt valued and cared for, and became less disaffected with school in general.

How to Read a Paper: The Basics of Evidence-Based Healthcare, Seventh Edition.
Trisha Greenhalgh and Paul Dijkstra.

In studies where school feeding produced no effect, the mechanistic evidence was even more interesting. In one study, where the intervention was a daily carton of chocolate milk, it turned out that children couldn't digest the milk because lactose intolerance was widespread in that region. More prosaically, some meals (which were nutritionally balanced by the world's top food scientists, packaged in carefully measured portions in plastic wrappers and shipped in from abroad) were alien and unpalatable to the children, so only a fraction of the supplement was actually consumed.

These mechanistic findings led to an important general conclusion: if you're going to feed starving children, leave your fancy supplements out of the equation. Just give them what their parents would give them if they could afford it. Some of the most successful school feeding studies got local women (and maybe men too) to help prepare the meals from local ingredients; a measure which had the happy side effect of educating some parents in what and how to cook.

Finally, in one or two studies, whenever a child in abject poverty was fed at school, the family withheld a meal from the child at home. This was not because they didn't love the child, but because there was, perhaps, a starving grandparent who had been sacrificing their own meal for the younger generation. Maybe we need to address poverty in general, rather than just give undernourished children the occasional plate of food at school?

Hopefully, this example has illustrated why scholars within the evidence-based medicine (EBM) movement have been calling for 'EBM+' [3, 4]; that is, use an approach which systematically considers mechanistic evidence (defined as *studies which aim to explain which factors and interactions are responsible for a phenomenon* [5]) on a par with the probabilistic evidence from clinical trials and observational cohort studies.

The many types of mechanistic evidence and a preliminary hierarchy

In a paper called 'Adapt or die', Trisha and colleagues argued that the evidence-based healthcare (EBHC) movement needs to embrace mechanistic evidence or it will die as a paradigm [5]. In that paper, many examples of mechanistic evidence were given, including in vitro experiments, biomedical imaging, autopsy, established theory, animal experiments, aerosol science, engineering research and simulations [5].

As these examples show, mechanistic evidence can be of many different types and can operate at multiple levels. A mechanism, for example, might involve molecules, genes, drugs, receptors, immune responses (antibodies, cells), people's thought processes or emotional reactions, cultural movements, laws, policies or the entire economy (recessions, for example, tend to have effects on people's health).

Table 18.1 A preliminary hierarchy of evidence for mechanistic evidence

Level	Criteria and standard
1	Necessary and sufficient conditions for causality (e.g. multiple features of the causal chain) supported by multiple independent studies, confirmed by multiple independent research groups using accepted best research methods. No high-quality disconfirming studies found
2	Indicators of causality (e.g. more than one feature of the causal chain) supported, especially if by more than one method and confirmed by independent studies. No high-quality disconfirming studies found
3	Suggestion of causality (e.g. one feature of the causal chain) supported by multiple independent studies. No high-quality disconfirming studies found
4	Sparse evidence supporting feature(s) of the causal chain. Disconfirming studies found but these are not definitive
5	No supporting studies. High-quality disconfirming studies found

Source: reproduced from Greenhalgh et al. [5] with permission of BMJ Publishing Group Ltd.

Like all evidence, mechanistic studies can be of variable quality, and you may decide that a piece of mechanistic evidence is *definitive* (i.e. so solid that you don't need to do, or look for, more empirical research studies) or that it is not.

Table 18.1 shows some preliminary criteria for grading mechanistic evidence, based partly on previous work by others [6–8], which would benefit from further elaboration. This 'hierarchy' should be interpreted cautiously, however. While a lot of good evidence is always better than a meagre supply of weak evidence, you can't judge the totality of mechanistic evidence on a topic just by counting the number of publications or adding up the smiley faces on a checklist.

EBM+ means 'both and', not 'either or'

No one kind of evidence stands alone. We need *both* controlled experiments (and where these are impossible or unethical, non-randomised comparative and observational studies as in the school feeding studies example above) *and* explanations for why each study produced the findings it did [7]. Sir Austin Bradford Hill, who led the first modern RCT (of streptomycin in tuberculosis) proposed a set of indicators (Table 18.2) for assessing whether an association is causal [9]. The table also draws on some more recent work by philosophers of science [10,11]. The presence of high-quality and consistent mechanistic evidence greatly increases the external validity of an RCT finding; absence of such evidence, and especially mechanistic evidence that goes *against* what a RCT appears to be

Table 18.2 Bradford Hill indicators of causality, showing the importance of both probabilistic evidence (e.g. from RCTs) and mechanistic evidence (e.g. from laboratory studies or qualitative process evaluations)

Indicator	Explanation	Probabilistic or mechanistic	Preferred types of evidence
Strength of association	A strong association is more likely to be causal than a weak one	Both	RCTs or high-quality observational studies (e.g. longitudinal cohort) which allow calculation of a measure of association such as relative risk or odds ratio, and adjustment for confounding
Consistency	Multiple observations made by different observers with different instruments mean the association is more likely to be causal	Both	Systematic review. Exploration of heterogeneity via tools such as meta-regression may help identify and quantify inconsistency in effects across studies
Specificity	If an outcome is best predicted by one primary factor, the causal claim is more credible	Neither	A problematic indicator, as it is common for a single exposure to be causally associated with multiple outcomes (e.g. tobacco smoking and heart disease, stroke, cancer)
Temporality	A cause must precede an effect	Both	Any longitudinal design (e.g. clinical trial, non-cross-sectional observational study)
Biological gradient	There should be a direct 'dose–response' relationship between the independent variable (e.g. a risk factor) and the dependent one (e.g. people's status on the disease variable)	Both	Basic science (e.g. toxicology-based risk analysis), varying-dose RCTs, unbiased observational studies with adjustment for confounding
Plausibility	An association is more likely to be causal if there is a rational and theoretical basis for it	Mechanistic	Basic science

(*Continued*)

Chapter 18

Table 18.2 (Continued)

Indicator	Explanation	Probabilistic or mechanistic	Preferred types of evidence
Coherence	An association is more likely to be causal if it coheres with other knowledge (i.e. does not conflict with what is known about the variables under study and there are no plausible competing theories or rival hypotheses)	Both	Systematic review; integration of both mechanistic AND probabilistic evidence is key here
Experimental manipulation	Any related research that is based on experiments will make a causal inference more plausible	Both	Basic science or RCT (which may be considered 'epidemiological experiments' as exposure is defined by the investigator)
Analogy	Sometimes a commonly accepted phenomenon in one area can be applied to another area	Both	Requires a broad understanding of all relevant fields; potentially subject to logical fallacy

showing, should make us question RCT findings [12]. As we pointed out in Chapter 15, the same goes for other probabilistic study designs such as genome-wide association studies (GWAS). If GWAS findings are affirmed by laboratory studies, we can trust those findings more than if no mechanistic evidence existed.

Mechanistic evidence in the COVID-19 pandemic

If you are interested in how mechanistic evidence takes EBM or EBHC to a new level, you might like to look out some of Trisha's work on the controversial topic of mask wearing to reduce transmission of respiratory infections [5,13].

As many of us know from bitter experience during COVID-19, pandemics are very difficult contexts for generating and appraising evidence. Things happen fast and people are busy. Many aspects of the pandemic were characterised by a combination of complexity (multiple variables interacting dynamically with a high degree of uncertainty), urgency (decisions needed in days not years) and impending peril (the consequences of not acting could be catastrophic). In such circumstances, RCTs of community interventions such as universal masking can be difficult or impossible. Mechanistic evidence may be particularly crucial here.

Whether and to what extent masks work became a hotly contested topic during the pandemic, not least because it became associated with certain political and ideological viewpoints. The body of evidence on masks comes from multiple sources and represents many different levels of causality, both probabilistic and mechanistic. In its entirety, this evidence amounts to a lengthy monograph with hundreds of references [13]. Here, we summarise some key points.

There is extensive evidence from laboratory and other mechanistic studies that the SARS-CoV-2 virus spreads significantly (and almost certainly *predominantly*) through the air. One classic piece of mechanistic research, for example, studied the cross-infection of ferrets who were kept in different cages. Sick ferrets in one cage transmitted COVID-19 to previously healthy ferrets in another cage when the cages were connected with air pipes that contained a series of 90-degree bends [14]. Droplets can't make the journey round corners and against gravity, but particles suspended in the air can!

Some sceptics say that the ferret study is low-level evidence because the findings of animal studies don't necessarily apply to humans. But this is a misreading of the hierarchy of evidence. Testing a drug in an animal and claiming that the drug therefore works in humans would be bad science. But demonstrating the airborne nature of a virus using an animal model means that that virus *must* be airborne for every creature. If you are interested in other mechanistic studies on the airborne nature of SARS-CoV-2, see Trisha and colleagues' summary paper in the *Lancet* [15] or their more recent 'state of the science' review on masks [13].

Right from the earliest months of the COVID-19 pandemic, precautions were designed around a 'droplet' mode of transmission. For example, hand-washing and scrubbing of surfaces were strongly encouraged, and people were asked to 'socially distance' by staying 1.5 or 2 metres apart on the assumption that a droplet emitted by one person would fall to the ground under the influence of gravity within that distance. But the actual mode of transmission is *airborne*: the virus gets into the depths of our lungs when we breathe in air that others (who may be asymptomatic or presymptomatic) have exhaled [16]. Because airborne particles spread in the air, they are like cigarette smoke – they eventually spread to fill an entire room. This means that while you are more likely to catch COVID-19 from an infected person if you're sitting or standing close to them, you might still catch it if you share indoor air at *any* distance.

The mechanism of transmission matters hugely here. Standard medical or surgical masks have a waterproof backing and a not-particularly-close-fitting design. This is because they are designed to stop droplets, *not* filter out pathogens from the air. Contrast this with *respirator* masks – the ones that form part of high-grade personal protective equipment and which need to be 'fit tested' to make sure they don't leave any gaps. If someone is wearing a standard medical or surgical mask, *some* of the air they breathe in and out bypasses the actual mask material. The standard mask is still better than no mask at all, but the level of protection is relatively low.

This mechanistic evidence *should* have influenced the design of all RCTs of masks and respirators in preventing respiratory disease transmission, but sadly it did not. Some triallists did design their RCTs to reflect airborne transmission. For example, when studying the efficacy of respirators in protecting healthcare workers, these authors made sure that staff in the intervention arm wore their respirators *all the time* when at work. But other researchers assumed that significant airborne transmission didn't happen and designed their RCTs around the prevention of *droplet* transmission. For example, they required the respirators to be worn only when working within 2 metres of a patient with known or suspected COVID-19 or when doing a so-called 'aerosol-generating procedure'. Here's the interesting part: the former studies demonstrated that respirators are significantly better than medical masks in preventing workplace-acquired COVID-19, whereas the latter studies found no difference between respirators and medical masks. You can read the detail in Greenhalgh et al. [13].

Another way that mechanistic evidence should have influenced trial design, especially in trials of masking in the community, was taking account of both egress and ingress. Masks and respirators may, theoretically, reduce transmission of pathogens in two ways. First, to the extent that they filter effectively, they reduce *egress* (outward movement) of pathogens *from* an infected person into the environment. Wearing a mask to prevent egress is known as *source control*. Second, to the extent that they filter effectively, masks reduce *ingress* of pathogens from the environment into an uninfected person. This is known as *protecting the wearer*. An RCT that is designed *only* to detect if the wearer is protected will underestimate the overall effect of masking on the wider community because it won't capture the impact of source control. For this reason, the ideal design for community masking studies is randomising whole communities (e.g. villages), as Jason Abaluk and his team did, impressively, in Bangladesh [17].

Mechanistic evidence should have informed systematic reviews of mask trials, for example by weighting the trials by how far the intervention design was informed by evidence of mechanism of transmission, and also by whether trials took account of the extent to which the masks were actually worn. You probably know that RCTs should be designed on an intention-to-treat basis (see Chapter 6), but it is surely common sense that if a person does not wear the mask they are advised to wear, a 'negative' trial result does not mean that the *mask* doesn't work, it means that the *advice* to mask didn't work. Not all RCTs of advice to mask measured compliance, but a systematic review of mask trials which did measure compliance demonstrated a 'dose–response' effect; that is, the more the trial participants actually wore masks, the less likely they were to become infected [18].

In short, RCTs of masks in the control of respiratory infections include some that were well designed and reflected what is known about mechanism of transmission and some whose authors ignored mechanistic evidence *both* when they designed the intervention *and* when they interpreted their findings.

Thousands of lives were probably lost as a result of what was incorrectly claimed to be an 'evidence-based' approach, dismissing or downgrading mechanistic evidence, over-valuing findings from poorly designed or irrelevant RCTs and advocating for inaction where RCT evidence was lacking. As we argued in 'Adapt or die' [5], the mask example put EBM/EBHC in a poor light. This and other examples from the COVID-19 pandemic should be seen as an epistemic opportunity for the EBHC movement to come to better understand, debate and embrace EBM+.

One final word of warning. Mechanistic evidence comes in many forms, and you may or may not be an expert in the kind of research presented in a paper which purports to demonstrate causality. The critical appraisal of mechanistic evidence is beyond the scope of this book, but before you accept a published mechanistic study as evidence of causality, do ask an expert in the relevant scientific subfield to help you interpret it.

Exercises based on this chapter

1. Take a look at Beaulé and colleagues' paper on mechanistic evidence on the significance of cam morphology in the development of hip osteoarthritis [19]. They apply the Bradford Hill criteria to examine whether cam morphology (a bony bump at the head-neck junction of the hip on x-ray or scan), which is relatively common in adolescent athletes and often asymptomatic, is *causally* linked to the development of hip arthritis at an early age. On the basis of the evidence they present, do you believe that cam morphology *causes* arthritis?
2. Consider the question of whether repetitive head trauma in sport leads to brain damage (chronic traumatic encephalopathy). Some sports involve this kind of trauma, and ex-athletes may develop premature dementia, but did the repetitive head trauma *cause* the condition? Read the paper by Nowinski et al. [20], then make a list of arguments for and against a causal link.

References

1. Kristjansson EA, Robinson V, Petticrew M, *et al*. School feeding for improving the physical and psychosocial health of disadvantaged elementary school children. *Cochrane Database of Systematic Reviews* 2007; **(1)**: CD004676.
2. Greenhalgh T, Kristjansson E, Robinson V. Realist review to understand the efficacy of school feeding programmes. *BMJ* 2007; **335**: 858–61.
3. Tresker S. Treatment effectiveness and the Russo–Williamson thesis, EBM+, and Bradford Hill's viewpoints. *International Studies in the Philosophy of Science* 2021; **34**: 131–58.
4. Aronson JK, Auker-Howlett D, Ghiara V, et al. The use of mechanistic reasoning in assessing coronavirus interventions. *Journal of Evaluation in Clinical Practice* 2021; **27**: 684–93.
5. Greenhalgh T, Fisman D, Cane DJ, et al. Adapt or die: how the pandemic made the shift from EBM to EBM+ more urgent. *BMJ Evididence-Based Medicine* 2022; **27**: 253–60.
6. Clarke B, Gillies D, Illari P, et al. Mechanisms and the evidence hierarchy. *Topoi* 2014; **33**: 339–60.
7. Williamson J. Establishing causal claims in medicine. *International Studies in the Philosophy of Science* 2019; **32**: 33–61.
8. Williamson J. Establishing the teratogenicity of Zika and evaluating causal criteria. *Synthese* 2021; **198**: 2505–18.
9. Bradford Hill A. The environment and disease: association or causation? *Proceedings of the Royal Society of Medicine* 1965; **58**: 295–300.
10. Fedak KM, Bernal A, Capshaw ZA, Gross S. Applying the Bradford Hill criteria in the 21st century: how data integration has changed causal inference in molecular epidemiology. *Emerging Themes in Epidemiology* 2015; **12**:14.
11. Russo F, Williamson J. Interpreting causality in the health sciences. *International Studies in the Philosophy of Science* 2007; **21**: 157–70.
12. Parkkinen V-P, Wallmann C, Wilde M, et al. *Evaluating Evidence of Mechanisms in Medicine: Principles and procedures*. Berlin: Springer Nature; 2018.
13. Greenhalgh T, MacIntyre CR, Baker MG, et al. Masks and respirators for prevention of respiratory infections: a state of the science review. *Clinical Microbiology Reviews* 2024; **37**:e00124-23. doi: 10.1128/cmr.00124-23.
14. Kutter JS, de Meulder D, Bestebroer TM, et al. SARS-CoV and SARS-CoV-2 are transmitted through the air between ferrets over more than one meter distance. *Nature Communications* 2021; **12**: 1653.
15. Greenhalgh T, Jimenez JL, Prather KA, et al. Ten scientific reasons in support of airborne transmission of SARS-CoV-2. *Lancet* 2021; **397**: 1603–5.
16. Greenhalgh T, Ozbilgin M, Tomlinson D. How covid-19 spreads: narratives, counter narratives, and social dramas. *BMJ* 2022; **378**: e069940.
17. Abaluck J, Kwong LH, Styczynski A, et al. Impact of community masking on COVID-19: a cluster-randomized trial in Bangladesh. *Science* 2022; **375**: eabi9069.
18. Kollepara PK, Siegenfeld AF, Taleb NN, Bar-Yam Y. Unmasking the mask studies: why the effectiveness of surgical masks in preventing respiratory infections has been underestimated. *Journal of Travel Medicine* 2021; **28**: taab144.

19. Beaulé PE, Grammatopoulos G, Speirs A, et al. Unravelling the hip pistol grip/cam deformity: origins to joint degeneration. *Journal of Orthopaedic Research* 2018; **36**: 3125–35.
20. Nowinski CJ, Bureau SC, Buckland ME, et al. Applying the Bradford Hill criteria for causation to repetitive head impacts and chronic traumatic encephalopathy. *Frontiers in Neurology* 2022; **13**: 938163.

Chapter 19 Papers that report consensus exercises

Think about the last time you and fellow students or colleagues discussed a contentious healthcare topic – say a journal club on the benefits and possible harms of intermittent fasting, or the appropriate level of medical intervention during pregnancy and labour. Why was this topic important enough to be discussed? Did everyone in the room have a good grasp of the current evidence? How did you and your colleague-friends *interpret* the evidence? Did everyone agree? When sharing their views, were some people more passionate than others? Did you appreciate how different priorities, different professional or cultural backgrounds, different experiences, and maybe different ages and genders shaped opinions? Did one or two people perhaps dominate the discussion? Who *facilitated* the discussion and how did they do? How were differences of opinion reconciled? Did you reach consensus? And, importantly, were you still good colleagues at the end of the discussion?

Consensus in healthcare is difficult. Even when good evidence on a topic exists, 'experts' often disagree on, for example, how to *interpret* and *apply* evidence (in clinical practice, research agendas, policy etc). Opinions matter, especially in the absence of good or high-quality evidence. Even high-quality evidence is contextual; do you and your colleagues always agree how to apply the evidence in your *specific context*? Probably not! A consensus exercise on a controversial healthcare topic is therefore often necessary to define the *level of agreement* and, importantly, surface areas of tension, dissent and disagreement. Here, *power* matters – who (individual or group) in a consensus discussion could potentially dominate – and how can we ensure that all voices are heard?

When consensus researchers neglect to specifically address power dynamics in their expert panels, marginalised and minoritised individuals and groups will be even more sidelined. And the consensus exercise will dismally fail in its objective to represent the views of a *group* of experts on a topic. A detailed discussion of power (and its influence on consensus discussions) is

How to Read a Paper: The Basics of Evidence-Based Healthcare, Seventh Edition.
Trisha Greenhalgh and Paul Dijkstra.

beyond the scope of this chapter. If you are interested in this topic, you might want to read social science studies of the links between power, status and knowledge in science (one example is a paper by Trisha and co-authors [1]).

This chapter orients you to think critically when reading a consensus method paper and equips you with a basic appraisal framework: ten questions to ask about such a paper.

Why are consensus method papers important?

Uncertainty fuels anxiety, especially in healthcare. Clinician and patient uncertainty breed decision-making anxiety that could lead to medical errors and resource overuse. On the other hand, when clinicians struggle to embrace uncertainty, their overconfidence could inevitably lead to medical reversal (when well-designed trials prove popular health practices, like arthroscopy for knee osteoarthritis, wrong [2]). The quest for more certainty in healthcare is therefore one of the main drivers of consensus exercises. During a consensus exercise, a group of 'experts', ideally using consensus methods, come together to agree on (or rate the importance of) several items (e.g. actions or statements) to bridge the gap between empirical evidence on a specific topic and what to do. Such consensus from a group of experts using formal methods is generally more reliable than individual opinions or experiences.

Consensus methods are used in different areas of healthcare, especially when 'experts' need to agree on definitions, taxonomy (e.g. classification of disease), patient-reported outcome measures, clinical practice guidelines, diagnostic guidelines, research priority setting, forecasting, healthcare rationing, policy and research reporting guidelines and so on. The International Olympic Committee (IOC), for example, has published 29 consensus statements on topics like relative energy deficiency in sport (REDs), concussion and mental health in elite athletes (https://olympics.com/ioc/medical-scientific).

How do experts choose and reach consensus on a specific topic?

A consensus exercise is hard work. It always involve differences of opinion, emotions and tension (and, as mentioned above, power!) that must be grappled with for it to be a true 'consensus exercise'. This is important. We often see haphazard GOBSATs ('good old boys sat around a table'; see Chapter 1) reported as a 'consensus agreement'. While we might read: 'Experts agreed on…', it is obvious that a small group of 'expert friends' (often predominantly white, medically qualified men) reached consensus without any mention of grappling with disagreement and tension! Minoritised groups or less powerful individuals (e.g. patient) were either not present or not heard…

Before discussing the most-used consensus methods and ten questions to ask when appraising a consensus method paper, a few words on our own research and the influence of the COVID-19 pandemic on consensus research. The COVID-19 pandemic disrupted not only clinical services but also research, including consensus method research. Largely driven by lockdowns and governments banning group meetings in early 2020, consensus researchers (like us!) were forced to explore alternatives, including online consensus methods. During this time, Paul, as part of his doctoral studies (with Trisha supervising), led the Oxford consensus studies on primary cam morphology (a bony bump that develops, due to high-load sporting activity, at the head–neck junction of the femur in the hip joint of many young athletes) and femoroacetabular impingement syndrome [3,4].

Why was this topic important enough for a consensus exercise? Apart from the fact that primary cam morphology is highly prevalent among some athletes (such as competitive football players) and could lead to early hip osteoarthritis in an unfortunate few, the clinical and research community at the time had to agree on five key aspects, including: a new conceptual definition for primary cam morphology; best terminology to use; taxonomy distinguishing between primary and secondary cam morphology; how to operationalise primary cam morphology using radiographs and more advanced imaging; and a prioritised research agenda for the field. What was originally planned as a relatively small in-person consensus meeting of 15–20 experts changed into a much larger (and more rigorous) online Delphi method consensus involving 65 experts and six different stakeholder groups, including patient partners.

Following the two-round Delphi panel, steering group members and patient partners, co-led online discussions to grapple with areas of tension, dissent and disagreement. These discussions, reported separately in the consensus paper, captured the views of potentially marginalised groups like athlete coaches and people from the Global South. The Oxford consensus highlights three key aspects of any consensus exercise: the topic (why was the specific topic chosen?), the experts (who were the experts and why them?) and, the process (what formal consensus method was used and how were dissenting views captured?).

Figure 19.1 represents eight steps of an example consensus exercise:

Step 1: Choose the consensus topic (an important, or rare, healthcare topic with emergent, inconsistent or limited evidence, for example).

Step 2: Consider research methodology (the philosophy that guides how and when to apply specific research methods).

Step 3: Design the study (including the formal consensus method, e.g. Delphi; consider publishing a protocol).

Step 4: Prepare for the study (confirm methods; recruit experts; synthesis of current evidence, e.g. scoping or systematic review(s); prepare

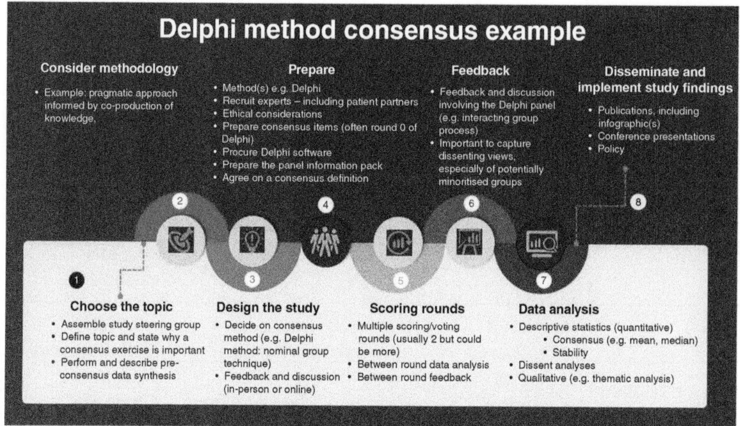

Figure 19.1 Example of an eight-step consensus exercise.

consensus items/statements – this could be round 0 of a Delphi panel; procure software; prepare panel information pack; agree on a consensus definition).

Step 5: Execute the study (e.g. a Delphi panel: two to four formal scoring or voting rounds with between round data analysis and individual panellist feedback).

Step 6: Feedback and discussion (following the formal Delphi rounds, for example; important to capture and document dissenting views, especially of potentially minoritised groups).

Step 7: Analyse data (quantitative and qualitative; could include a formal dissent analysis).

Step 8: Disseminate and implement study findings (data visualisation; peer-reviewed publications, including infographic(s); conference presentations; policy).

Consensus methods

Since the late 1940s, RAND Corporation (it started as 'Project RAND' in the aftermath of World War II when key military and industry leaders in the United States realised the importance of connecting military planning with research and development decisions: www.rand.org) has played a key role in shaping how 'experts' work towards consensus (while also surfacing areas of tension, dissent or disagreement).

By now, you should appreciate that research teams planning a consensus exercise should use formal consensus methods; group interaction *methods* can have a significant influence on the results and output of a consensus exercise. Applying best consensus methods, however, is easier said than done. In what follows, we briefly describe the most common consensus methods used in health studies: Delphi method (including modified Delphi), nominal group technique (NGT), and consensus meetings (Table 19.1).

Table 19.1 Some consensus methods in healthcare

Method	What is it?	Key characteristics	Comments examples
Delphi	A series of structured rounds in which panelists rank a set of statements for their importance and relevance; statements may be modified in subsequent rounds	Anonymity: panellists provide rankings and give their opinions anonymously. Iteration: iteration takes place over multiple rounds of voting. Feedback: formal individual feedback after each voting round (each panelist is told how their own ranking compares to others'). Analysis: analysis of group responses (statistical and qualitative)	See *RAND Methodological Guidance for Conducting and Critically Appraising Delphi Panels* [5]
Modified Delphi, e.g. RAND/ UCLA appropriateness method (RAM)	A shorter and more formalised version of a Delphi exercise, using fewer panelists	RAM introduced five important changes to classical Delphi [5]: number of rounds was specified and limited; review of evidence shared with experts before the first Delphi round (replacing the open-ended round of the classical Delphi); in-person discussion round added between two Delphi rounds; number of panelists limited number of panelists to 9-18 experts, with emphasis on complimentary expertise; 9-point Likert scales with formal measure of consensus	*Consensus-Based Guidance on Opioid Management in Individuals With Advanced Cancer-Related Pain and Opioid Misuse or Use Disorder* [6]

Chapter 19

Table 19.1 (Continued)

Method	What is it?	Key characteristics	Comments examples
Nominal group technique (NGT) [7,8]	A structured brainstorming exercise in which a large group is divided into smaller groups (or into individuals); after an idea-generating stage, each person (or small group) in turn offers one suggestion, continuing until all suggestions have been shared and discussed	Silent writing exercise. Good for generating new ideas, information and for fact-finding. Outspoken individuals cannot dominate the process. Modified NGT include four stages: silent and solo idea generation; round robin idea feedback (one idea per person per round); clarification through discussion; voting (ranking or rating)	Note the difference originally described between NGT and Interacting Group Process [7]: group of individuals interacting; individuals considering other dimensions of a problem; help synthesising and evaluating alternative solutions; good process to elaborate, modify, and work toward a consensus when implementing solutions to problems
Consensus meetings (or conference/ workshop)	Real-time (traditionally in-person) meeting to discuss evidence and its implications for practice	Face-to-face (or online) meetings, with some form of pre-meeting evidence synthesis by experts in the field (e.g. reviews – narrative, scoping of systematic), with semi-structured discussion and voting	International Olympic Committee consensus statements, e.g. *How much is too much? (Part 1) International Olympic Committee consensus statement on load in sport and risk of injury* [9]

Delphi method

The Delphi method is an iterative and anonymous group-based exercise to elicit and aggregate experts' opinions on a topic with the goal to explore (and work towards) consensus and, importantly, surface areas of tension, dissent or disagreement [10,11]. It has four key characteristics (Table 19.1): anonymity, iteration, feedback and statistical analysis of responses. The Delphi method remains one of the most popular consensus methods in healthcare; two-thirds of all Delphi method peer-reviewed articles (since the first peer-reviewed article on the Delphi method was published in 1963 [12]) have been in health journals [11]. The *classical Delphi* usually begins with a series of open-ended questions to panellists (round 0), asking them to nominate statements or issues to be considered for future rounds.

Following this open round, the study steering group aggregate and synthesise panellists' statements and craft final statements for panellists to judge (and explain their responses) in at least two more rounds. Between rounds, the study steering group collate responses and provide an anonymised group summary to each panellist (including each panellist's original responses). After the final round, individual judgements are aggregated and summarised as one or more measures of central tendency (e.g. median) and dispersion (e.g. interquartile range). Statistical consensus is determined by calculating the percent responses above and below a certain point (for the Oxford consensus studies discussed earlier, for example, consensus was defined as 70% or more of responses 7 to 9, and less than 15% of responses 1–3 on a 1–9 Likert scale). Panellists' qualitative feedback is also analysed (e.g. thematic analysis) and reported.

A recently published manual by Rand Corporation provides a very comprehensive overview for conducting and appraising Delphi panels [5]. In addition to the classical Delphi, the authors describe four more Delphi types: policy Delphi, modified Delphi, E-Delphi and real-time Delphi.

Nominal group technique

The NGT is a highly structured face-to-face group interaction [8] and, therefore, when described in the majority of consensus studies, most likely not 'nominal' (as originally described) but 'interacting' or a combination of the two. The word 'nominal' refers to something that exists in name only (a nominal ruler in a constitutional monarchy like the UK, for example). Therefore, purists might argue an NGT is not a *real* group technique; it was described as a silent group process, with the emphasis on writing, *not* talking. This is how Delbecq and Ven de Ven described NGT in their seminal 1971 paper: 'nominal groups' refer to groups in which individuals work in the presence of one another (nowadays online too!) but *do not interact* [7]. They argued that NGT is good for fact-finding and 'generating' information, while *interacting* group processes is preferred when the focus is information synthesis, evaluation or group consensus [7,13]. Interestingly, when group members don't interact (nominal technique) when they create key problem variables, their views on problems are richer (more multidimensional), they produce more high-quality suggestions and they craft a greater number of possible solutions to the problem [13]. NGT has evolved into a group process with four key stages (Table 19.1): silent generation, round robin, clarification and voting [8].

Consensus meetings, workshops or conferences

Commonly used in health research, consensus meetings or conferences are organised meetings of experts in a given field. Usually face to face (but, increasingly, online since the COVID-19 pandemic), these meetings of 10–15 panel members are flexible, interactive and foster dialogue, debate and discussion. For 37 years (1977–2013), the US National Institutes of Health (NIH) produced more than 160 consensus statements on important and controversial topics in medicine - all based on their consensus development conference method [14]. Several other organisations have adopted and adapted this method for in-person or online consensus meetings, workshops or conferences; for example, the National Academies (e.g. *Improving Representation in Clinical Trials and Research – Building research equity for women and underrepresented groups* [15]) and the IOC's consensus statements mentioned earlier in this chapter (https://olympics.com/ioc/documents/athletes/medical-and-scientific-consensus-statements).

Ten questions to ask about a paper that reports a consensus statement

The questions you should ask about a specific consensus methods paper obviously depend on the specific consensus method. For a Delphi method paper, for example, it is important to ask if the consensus process was truly anonymous and how between-round feedback was given.

The ten questions below apply to any consensus method paper. In preparing these questions, we have drawn on the ACCORD (ACcurate COnsensus Reporting Document) reporting guideline for consensus methods in biomedicine [16]. The 35 ACCORD items relate to the article title (1 item), introduction (3 items), methods (21 items), results (5 items), discussion (2 items) and other information (3 items).

Question one: What is the consensus topic? Is this topic potentially important to my patients and my practice?
This question is about relevance. Consensus statements are often detailed, pernickety and time-consuming to read. They matter greatly to frontline practitioners and policymakers in a particular topic area, but unless you specialise in that area yourself you may not need this level of detail and nuance. You might be a family physician or physiotherapist providing care to players from a local rugby club. A consensus statement on concussion in sport might therefore be relevant to you; see Patricios et al. [17]. You might be working for a large organisation planning the delivery of care during pandemics. The recommendations of this multinational Delphi consensus on the COVID-19 public health threat might therefore be of interest [18].

Question two: Why is a consensus on the topic needed?
Not every topic needs a consensus exercise. If the evidence is strong, definitive and with unambiguous implications for practice, there may be little need to discuss it. On the other hand, if the evidence is ambiguous or if there is wide dissent among experts about what it means for practice or policy, a consensus exercise may provide a way forward. You should check whether the consensus exercise was preceded by a thorough review of the literature (either scoping, narrative or systematic review etc.) and whether the points of tension and disagreement were clearly highlighted in the briefing materials. The Oxford consensus on primary cam morphology and related conditions, built on recommendations from previous consensus research in the field and the results of a systematic review-informed concept analysis [19].

Question three: Who directed the consensus exercise and were all [conflicts of] interest declared?
Was the consensus exercise led by a chairperson, co-chairs and/or a steering group? If so, who were they and how were they chosen? Look for a paragraph or table describing the steering group's demographics and their relevant expertise and experience. Some papers might also include a steering group positionality statement. Another important aspect is consensus researchers' conflict of interest; were they declared for all members of the steering group and panellists? It is important to note that there is no 'view from nowhere'; in other words, everyone on a steering group or panel is likely to have some 'skin in the game'. Some may have had paid consultancies to a drug company which makes a treatment for the condition; others may have written a previous article questioning whether the condition exists at all. We need to know, so we can take these perspectives into account.

Question four: Who was in the room and what kind of expertise did they have? Were patients included (if not, why not)?
As you will be aware, there are many kinds of expert, including experts in research or systematic reviewing, experts in clinical practice and experts in lived experience. Different clinical experts bring contrasting perspectives (it is sometimes said, for example, that midwives bring expertise in normal births and obstetricians bring expertise in abnormal births). You need to consider what kinds of expertise would enrich your chosen topic and whether that expertise was represented among the consensus experts (the panellists who would score the statements, for example). It is also useful to consider how these experts were identified and recruited. A key – and often neglected – expert group are patients (people who know the condition from having lived it) and the public (people who bring a commonsense perspective). For the Oxford consensus studies, the steering group applied the 'closeness continuum' to recruit panellists. The closeness continuum represents a more inclusive approach to identifying experts, including people with: (i) *subjective* closeness (people with deep experiential knowledge or real-life experiences, e.g. patients); (ii) *mandated* closeness (people with professional and/or legal/ethical responsibility, e.g. clinicians managing patients with the specific health condition being discussed), and (iii) *objective* closeness (people who study the topic, exploring and inquiring without preconceived bias, e.g. researchers) to the topic of interest (see figure 2 and table 1 of the Oxford consensus paper) [3].

Question five: How did the consensus authors address equity, diversity and inclusion?
Equity, a multidimensional concept, is about treating people with fairness and recognising and addressing systemic barriers for marginalised individuals and groups. For example, people from low-income countries and people with a disability are often excluded from consensus panels. This may not be direct or planned exclusion, but when an in-person consensus conference is hosted in an expensive high-income country, panellists from low-income countries may not be able to afford to travel or may have their visa applications rejected! Diversity is complex and includes people's and groups' unique experiences and perspectives relevant to the consensus topic. Here, individual characteristics (such as personality) and identity (race, ethnicity, sex/gender etc.) matter; diverse perspectives and experiences are key for rich consensus discussions. If consensus panels are dominated by white men from the Global North, their deliberations, however well-informed by evidence and good intentions, will be less rich. Finally, inclusion includes efforts to enable members of the consensus group (or panel) to feel valued, supported and respected. For this, consensus authors should pay special attention to

those with support needs (e.g. the patient on a panel may value a mentor, a 'buddy' or a named member of staff as a point of contact).

Question six: How did the experts work towards consensus? (The method)
Based on the consensus methods discussed earlier in this chapter, did the authors describe their consensus method in detail? Did they use a modified Delphi method or NGT, or a combination, for example? Importantly, did the authors *justify* why they chose the specific consensus method or combination of methods? After reading their justification, are you convinced that the authors chose the most appropriate consensus method? Is there evidence that all the key steps in the method were followed? You might have access to a protocol in the form of a peer-reviewed paper (like this one [20]), as a supplementary file to the published consensus paper (e.g. data supplement 1 of the Oxford Consensus study [3]) or preregistered online (e.g. Open Science Framework). If the authors, for example, described a modified Delphi method consensus, did they clarify how their Delphi method was different from the classical Delphi method?

Question seven: Was a definition of consensus set before the start of the consensus exercise?
It is important for consensus researchers to agree on a consensus definition prior to the consensus rounds or meeting. For the Oxford consensus on primary cam morphology and femoroacetabular impingement syndrome [3], for example, we defined consensus prior to the Delphi rounds (see table 2 of the open access paper). Panellists scored statements using a 9-point Likert scale ranging from 1 ('not important/disagree') to 9 ('critical/agree'). For 'consensus in' or 'high agreement', 70% or more panel members must have scored 7–9 *and* less than 15% of panel members scored 1–3. Several other consensus measures, using either descriptive statistics or qualitative analysis, have been used [21].

Question eight: Did the researchers perform an appropriate analysis of all the panellist responses (quantitative and qualitative) and was this made available?
Usually, data analyses include simple descriptive statistics to communicate quantitative results: how panellists on average scored each statement. In the data analysis section of the Oxford consensus [3], for example, we described the quantitative analyses, including, for each statement, the overall median and interquartile range (IQR), reported for each of the two Delphi rounds in table 4 of the published paper. In addition to medians and IQRs, we visually reported (using histograms) how stakeholder groups scored statements in each Delphi round. Panellists had access to this report and their individual scores after the first Delphi round. Based on this between-round individual

feedback, they could then reconsider their scores in the next Delphi round (see data supplement 5: https://bjsm.bmj.com/content/bjsports/suppl/2022/12/06/bjsports-2022-106085.DC1/bjsports-2022-106085supp005_data_supplement.pdf).

Another important construct is the stability of responses for each statement between rounds, relevant to the Delphi method. Stability of experts' responses is an indication of whether agreement (or dissensus or disagreement) is present throughout and whether it develops between rounds. Stable disagreement across rounds, for example, could highlight differences in experts' opinions and stimulate discussion about future research. Some Delphi methodologists advocate for group stability as a good criterion for stopping a Delphi study (in other words, the study is topped when members agree to disagree).

Did the authors conduct a qualitative analysis of panellists' answers to any open-ended questions or explanations of their numeric responses? Consensus authors should therefore integrate qualitative and quantitative analyses to inform a rich discussion of the consensus exercise results. In a Delphi exercise on assessing the severely unwell patient with acute COVID-19, for example, Trisha identified high agreement among an online panel on two items (the cut-off for 'red flag' levels of pulse and respiratory rate), but there was a single 'outlier' who was sure the cut-off values should be different. This individual declared themselves as an experienced first responder who had attended hundreds of respiratory emergencies (and, in retrospect, probably had more accumulated experience in assessing vital signs in this context than most of the rest of the panel put together). The first responder had used the free-text box to write a detailed justification of their ranking (including references to peer-reviewed publications) and explain that this issue was often misunderstood by clinicians. When their argument was circulated to the wider panel, almost everyone changed their rankings in line with the 'outlier' [22].

Finally, did the authors specify their plan for handling missing data? This is important as panellist attrition is common over Delphi rounds. Authors should also explore any patterns (e.g. demographic) of panellists who did not complete all rounds.

Question nine: How did the researchers deal with dissent? Did they report it? Did they perform a proper dissent analysis?

Dissent and disagreement are important constructs in any consensus exercise. Note the subtle but important difference between these two words. Dissent refers to strong opposition (and refusal to conform). In 2022, for example, three liberal justices (Breyer, Kagan and Sotomayor) wrote a strong dissenting opinion when the majority US Supreme Court justices voted to overturn *Roe v. Wade* and remove the constitutional right to receive an abortion. The basis of this dissent was that the majority opinion had assumed XXX but the liberal judges were firmly of the view that this was NOT the case; rather, they took the opposite position YYY. Disagreement is a more neutral and versatile term indicating a difference of opinion; natural (and inevitable) for any consensus exercise involving people with different perspectives, experiences and backgrounds, for example. Example of disagreement in clinical consensus include when to start investigating (or screening), where to draw the line between normal and abnormal in a continuously varying biomarker, and when to start actively treating a condition. For the Oxford consensus [3], we performed a formal dissent analysis, including *outlier analysis, bipolarity analysis* and *stakeholder group analysis*. Following the two-round Delphi exercise, we organised online mixed stakeholder group meetings co-led by steering group members and patient partners (we called it the 'interacting group process' part of our consensus exercise). During these meetings, experts discussed topics of dissent and disagreement (we reported summaries of these discussions in boxes one to four in the published paper [3]).

Question ten: Did the researchers produce a clear bottom line for decision-makers?
Even small consensus exercise studies generate a lot of data. Did the authors discuss their results in the context of existing literature and clinical application? And, importantly, did they *present* the results (often a long list of statements!) in a way that makes it easy for the reader to understand and apply? Did the authors discuss the 'so what?' and 'what now?' questions? Did the authors address the limitations of their consensus exercise and how these might have influenced their conclusions? In short, are you able to read the consensus paper and feel more informed about your own practice or policy decision?

In sum, we hope that this chapter will help you to think critically when reading a consensus method paper and that you feel more equipped to perform a basic consensus method paper appraisal. The three exercises based on this chapter will help to further cement some of the key aspects relevant to most consensus method papers.

Exercises based on this chapter

1. Read and apply the ten appraisal questions to Nurek et al.'s paper on long COVID [23]:
   a. Why was the specific topic important?
   b. Who were the experts and how was the consensus exercise facilitated (methods)?
   c. Did the authors capture marginalised and dissenting views (focusing on the processes outside the formal group process)?

2. Find a consensus method paper in your clinical or research area of interest. Use the ten questions above to appraise this paper. After your appraisal, could you trust the consensus paper's results? Were all the different views on the topic considered and reported?
3. Compare the consensus methods used by the ACCORD [16] and REFORMS [24] reporting guideline research teams. Would you have approached the consensus exercise differently?

References

1. Greenhalgh T, Ozbilgin M, Contandriopoulos D. Orthodoxy, *illusio*, and playing the scientific game: a Bourdieusian analysis of infection control science in the COVID-19 pandemic. *Wellcome Open Research* 2021; **6**: 126.
2. Haslam A, Livingston C, Prasad V. Medical reversals in family practice: a review. *Current Therapeutic Research* 2020; **92**: 100579.
3. Dijkstra HP, McAuliffe S, Ardern CL, et al. Oxford consensus on primary cam morphology and femoroacetabular impingement syndrome. Part 1: definitions, terminology, taxonomy and imaging outcomes. *British Journal of Sports Medicine* 2022; **57**: 325–41.
4. Dijkstra HP, McAuliffe S, Ardern CL, et al. Oxford consensus on primary cam morphology and femoroacetabular impingement syndrome. Part 2: research priorities on conditions affecting the young person's hip. *British Journal of Sports Medicine* 2022; **57**: 342–58.
5. Khodyakov D, Grant S, Kroger J, et al. *RAND Methodological Guidance for Conducting and Critically Appraising Delphi Panels*. Santa Monica, CA: RAND Corporation; 2023. https://doi.org/10.7249/TLA3082-1.
6. Fitzgerald Jones K, Khodyakov D, Arnold R, et al. Consensus-based guidance on opioid management in individuals with advanced cancer-related pain and opioid misuse or use disorder. *JAMA Oncology* 2022; **8**: 1107–14.
7. Van de Ven A, Delbecq AL. Nominal versus Interacting Group Processes for Committee Decision-Making Effectiveness. *Academy of Management Journal* 1971; **14**: 203–12.
8. McMillan SS, King M, Tully MP. How to use the nominal group and Delphi techniques. *International Journal of Clinical Pharmacology* 2016; **38**: 655–62.
9. Soligard T, Schwellnus M, Alonso J-M, et al. How much is too much? (Part 1) International Olympic Committee consensus statement on load in sport and risk of injury. *British Journal of Sports Medicine* 2016; **50**: 1030–41.
10. Helmer-Hirschberg O. *Systematic Use of Expert Opinions. Document no. P-3721*. Santa Monica, CA: RAND Corporation; 1967. https://www.rand.org/pubs/papers/P3721.html (accessed 25 March 2024).
11. Khodyakov D, Grant S, Kroger J, et al. Disciplinary trends in the use of the Delphi method: a bibliometric analysis. *PLoS One* 2023; **18**: e0289009.
12. Dalkey N, Helmer O. An experimental application of the delphi method to the use of experts. *Management Science* 1963; **9**: 458.

13. Delbecq AL, Van de Ven AH. A group process model for problem identification and program planning. *Journal of Applied Behavioral Science*. 1971; **7**: 466–92.
14. Ferguson JH. The NIH Consensus Development Program: the evolution of guidelines. *International Journal of Technology Assessment in Health Care* 1996; **12**: 460–74.
15. Bibbins-Domingo K, Helman A (eds). *Improving Representation in Clinical Trials and Research: Building research equity for women and underrepresented groups*. Washington DC: National Academies Press; 2022. https://doi.org/10.17226/26479.
16. Gattrell WT, Logullo P, Zuuren EJ van, et al. ACCORD (ACcurate COnsensus Reporting Document): A reporting guideline for consensus methods in biomedicine developed via a modified Delphi. *PLoS Medicine* 2024; **21**: e1004326.
17. Patricios JS, Schneider KJ, Dvorak J, et al. Consensus statement on concussion in sport: the 6th International Conference on Concussion in Sport–Amsterdam, October 2022. *British Journal of Sports Medicine* 2023; **57**: 695–711.
18. Lazarus JV, Romero D, Kopka CJ, et al. A multinational Delphi consensus to end the COVID-19 public health threat. *Nature* 2022; **611**: 332–45.
19. Dijkstra HP, Ardern CL, Serner A, et al. Primary cam morphology; bump, burden or bog-standard? A concept analysis. *British Journal of Sports Medicine* 2021; **55**: 1212–21.
20. Santaguida P, Dolovich L, Oliver D, et al. Protocol for a Delphi consensus exercise to identify a core set of criteria for selecting health related outcome measures (HROM) to be used in primary health care. *BMC Family Practice* 2018; **19**: 152.
21. von der Gracht HA. Consensus measurement in Delphi studies: review and implications for future quality assurance. *Technological Forecasting and Social Change* 2012; **79**: 1525–36.
22. Greenhalgh T, Thompson P, Weiringa S, et al. What items should be included in an early warning score for remote assessment of suspected COVID-19? Qualitative and Delphi study. *BMJ Open* 2020; **10**: e042626.
23. Nurek M, Rayner C, Freyer A, et al. Recommendations for the recognition, diagnosis, and management of long COVID: a Delphi study. *British Journal of General Practice* 2021; **71**: e815–25.
24. Kapoor S, Cantrell E, Peng K, et al. REFORMS: consensus-based recommendations for machine-learning-based science. *Science Advances* 2024; **10**(18): https://doi.org/10.1126/sciadv.adk3452.

Chapter 20 **Criticisms of evidence-based healthcare**

What's wrong with evidence-based healthcare when it's done badly?

There is, quite appropriately, a growing body of scholarship that offers legitimate criticisms of evidence-based healthcare (EBHC)'s assumptions and core approaches. There is also a somewhat larger body of misinformed critique, and a grey zone of 'anti-EBHC' writing that contains more than a grain of truth but is itself one-sided and poorly argued. This chapter seeks to set out the criticisms that are fair and reasonable, and point the interested reader towards more in-depth arguments.

This chapter draws on a number of sources, including a book by Timmermans and Berg [1] called *The Gold Standard: The challenge of evidence-based medicine and standardization in health care*; a paper by Timmermans and Mauck [2] on the promises and pitfalls of EBM; Ben Goldacre's book *Bad Pharma* [3] and a paper written by Trisha and colleagues, called 'Evidence based medicine – a movement in crisis?' [4]. That paper was published in the *BMJ* in 2014 and has so far been cited almost 2000 times, which suggests that a lot of people are interested in the flaws of EBHC as well as its benefits. However, it is also worth pointing out that soon after Trisha published the paper examining some of the flaws of EBHC, she developed a potentially life-threatening cancer and was treated (with surgery, chemotherapy and something called molecular targeted therapy) in accordance with the results of randomised controlled trials (RCTs), meta-analyses and clinical practice guidelines. She's now approaching 10 years from being declared cancer free. So while EBHC isn't perfect, Trisha's the first to admit that she owes her life to it.

The first thing we need to get clear is the distinction between EBHC when it is practised badly (this section) and EBHC when it is practised well (next

How to Read a Paper: The Basics of Evidence-Based Healthcare, Seventh Edition.
Trisha Greenhalgh and Paul Dijkstra.

section). As a starter for this section, we reproduce two paragraphs from the preface to this book, written for the first edition way back in 1995 and still more or less unchanged in this seventh edition:

> *Many of the descriptions given by cynics of what evidence-based medicine is (the glorification of things that can be measured without regard for the usefulness or accuracy of what is measured, the uncritical acceptance of published numerical data, the preparation of all-encompassing guidelines by self-appointed 'experts' who are out of touch with real medicine, the debasement of clinical freedom through the imposition of rigid and dogmatic clinical protocols, and the over-reliance on simplistic, inappropriate, and often incorrect economic analyses) are actually criticisms of what the evidence-based medicine movement is fighting against, rather than of what it represents.*
>
> *Do not, however, think of me as an evangelist for the gospel according to evidence-based medicine. I believe that the science of finding, evaluating and implementing the results of medical research can, and often does, make patient care more objective, more logical, and more cost-effective. If I didn't believe that, I wouldn't spend so much of my time teaching it and trying, as a general practitioner, to practise it. Nevertheless, I believe that when applied in a vacuum (that is, in the absence of common sense and without regard to the individual circumstances and priorities of the person being offered treatment or to the complex nature of clinical practice and policymaking), 'evidence-based' decision-making is a reductionist process with a real potential for harm.*

Let's unpack these issues further. What does 'EBHC practised badly' look like? Trisha once gave a lecture called 'Is evidence-based medicine broken?' on the difference between 'real' and 'rubbish' EBHC (you can see it on YouTube if you're interested: https://www.youtube.com/watch?v=qYvdhA697jI&t=203s). 'Rubbish EBHC' is EBHC practised badly. What do we mean by that?

First, rubbish EBHC cites numbers derived from population studies but asks no upstream questions about where those numbers (or studies) came from. If you have spent time on the wards or in general practice, you will know the type of person who tends to do this: a fast-talking, technically adept individual who appears to know the literature and how to access it (perhaps via applications on their state-of-the-art tablet computer) and who always seems to have a number needed to treat or odds ratio at their fingertips. But the fast talker is less skilled at justifying why *this* set of 'evidence-based' figures should be privileged over some other set of figures. Their evidence, for example, may come from a single trial rather than a high-quality and recent meta-analysis of all available trials. Self-appointed EBHC 'experts' tend to be unreflective (i.e. they don't spend much time thinking deeply about things) and they rarely engage *critically* with the numbers they are citing. They may not, for example, have engaged with the arguments about surrogate endpoints we set out in Chapter 6.

Rubbish EBHC considers the world of published evidence to equate to the world of patient need. Hence, it commits two fallacies: it assumes that if (say) an RCT exists that tested a treatment for a 'disease', that disease is necessarily a real medical problem requiring treatment; and it also assumes that if 'methodologically robust' evidence does not exist on a topic, that topic is unimportant. This leads to a significant bias. The evidence base will accumulate in conditions that offer the promise of profit to the pharmaceutical and medical device industries, such as the detection, monitoring and management of cholesterol level (a risk factor for cardiovascular disease) [6], the development and testing of new drug entities for diabetes [7] or the creation and treatment of non-diseases such as 'female hypoactive sexual desire' [8]). Evidence will also accumulate in conditions that government chooses to recognise and prioritise for publicly funded research, but it will fail to accumulate (or will accumulate much more slowly) in Cinderella conditions that industry and/or government deem unimportant, hard to classify or 'non-medical'. One example is the paucity of trials which addressed the question 'What is the impact of giving disadvantaged children a free meal at school?' [9]. On the one hand, perhaps we don't need too many studies asking whether it's a good idea to feed starving children. But on the other hand, some governments have been slow to support school feeding programmes because of an alleged lack of evidence!

Rubbish EBHC has little regard for the patient perspective and fails to acknowledge the significance of clinical judgement. As we pointed out in Chapter 16, the 'best' treatment is not necessarily the one shown to be most efficacious in RCTs but the one that fits a particular set of individual circumstances and aligns with the patient's preferences and priorities.

Finally, rubbish EBHC draws on rubbish research; for example, research that has used weak sampling strategies, unjustified sample sizes, inappropriate comparators, statistical trick-cycling and so on. Chapter 6 set out some specific ways in which research (and the way it is presented) can mislead. While people behaving in this way will often claim to be members of the EBHC community (e.g. their papers may have 'evidence-based' in the title), the more scholarly members of that community would strongly dispute such claims. Indeed, in our 'movement in crisis' paper, we gave examples of how the pharmaceutical industry has learnt to 'game' the quality standards and risk-of-bias tools beloved of the EBHC movement [5].

What's wrong with evidence-based healthcare when it's done well?

While we worry as clinicians about EBHC done badly, EBHC also has some important limitations *even when done well.* This is because there are good philosophical reasons why EBHC will never be the fount of all knowledge.

A significant criticism of EBHC, highlighted by Timmermans and colleagues [2,3], is the extent to which EBHC is a formalised method for imposing an unjustifiable degree of standardisation and control over clinical practice. These authors argue that in the modern clinical world, EBHC can be more or less equated with the production and implementation of clinical practice guidelines. 'Yet', argue Timmermans and Berg [2, p. 3]:

> *such evidence is only rarely available to cover all the decision moments of a guideline. To fill in the blanks and to interpret conflicting statements that might exist in the literature, additional, less objective steps [such as consensus methods] are necessary to create a guideline [2].*

It is for this reason that we have included a new chapter on consensus methods in this edition of the book (Chapter 19).

Because of these (sometimes subtle) gaps in the research base, Timmermans and Berg contend that an 'evidence-based' guideline is usually not nearly as evidence-based as it appears to be. But the *formalisation* of the evidence into guidelines, which may then become ossified in protocols or computerised decision support programmes, lends an unjustified level of significance – and sometimes coercion – to the guideline. The rough edges are sanded down, the holes are filled in and the resulting recommendations start to acquire biblical significance!

One nasty side effect of this ossification is that *yesterday's* best evidence drags down *today's* guidelines and clinical pathways. An example is the lowering of blood glucose in type 2 diabetes. For many years, the 'evidence-based' assumption was that the more intensively a person's blood glucose was controlled, the better the outcomes would be. But more recently, a large meta-analysis showed that intensive glucose control had no benefit over moderate control but was associated with a two-fold increase in the incidence of severe hypoglycaemia [10]. Yet for some years after it was published, UK general practitioners were still being performance managed through a scheme called the *Quality and Outcomes Framework* (QOF) to strive for intensive glucose control *after* the publication of that meta-analysis had shown an adverse benefit–harm ratio [11]. This is because it takes time for practice and policy to catch up with the evidence, but the existence of the QOF, introduced to make care more evidence-based, actually had the effect of making it *less* evidence-based!

Perhaps the most powerful criticism of EBHC is that, if over-assiduously applied, it dismisses the patient's own perspective on the illness in favour of an average effect on a population sample or a column of quality-adjusted life-years (see Chapter 11) calculated by a medical statistician. Some writers on EBHC are enthusiastic about using a decision-tree approach to incorporate the patient's perspective into an evidence-based treatment choice. In practice, this often proves impossible because, as we pointed out in Chapter 16, patients' experiences are complex stories that refuse to be reduced to a tree of yes/no (or 'therapy on, therapy off') decisions.

The (effective) imposition of standardised care reduces the clinician's ability to respond to the idiosyncratic, here-and-now issues emerging in a particular consultation. The very core of the EBHC approach is to use a population average (or more accurately, an average from a sample that is hopefully representative of the population) to inform decision-making for that patient. But as many others before me have pointed out, a patient is not a mean or a median but an individual, whose illness inevitably has unique and unclassifiable features. Not only does over-standardisation make the care offered less aligned to individual needs, it also de-skills practitioners so that they lose the ability to customise and personalise care (or, in the case of recently trained clinicians, fails to gain that ability in the first place).

As Spence [12] put it:

> *Evidence engenders a sense of absolutism, but absolutism is to be feared absolutely. "I can't go against the evidence" has produced our reductionist flowchart medicine, with thoughtless polypharmacy, especially in populations with comorbidity. Many thousands of people die directly from adverse drug reactions as a result.*

Here is another example. Trisha recently undertook some research that required her to spend a long period of time watching junior doctors in an emergency department. She discovered that whenever a child was seen with an injury, the junior doctor completed a set of questions on the electronic patient's record. These questions were based on an evidence-based guideline to rule out non-accidental injury. But because the young doctors filled these boxes for every child, it seemed to her that the 'hunch' that they might have had in the case of any *particular* child was absent. This standardised approach contrasted to Trisha's own junior doctor days 30 years ago, when there were no guidelines but doctors spent quite a bit of time playing and honing their hunches.

Another concern about 'EBHC done well' is the sheer volume of evidence-based guidance and advice that now exists. As we describe in Chapter 10, even 20 years ago, the guidelines needed to manage the handful of patients seen on a typical 24-hour acute take ran to over 3000 pages and would have required over a week of reading by a clinician [13]. And that doesn't include point-of-care prompting for other evidence-based interventions (e.g. risk factor management) in patients seen in a non-acute setting. For a time, whenever a general practitioner saw a patient of between 16 and 25 years, a pop-up prompt would remind them to 'offer chlamydia screening'. Such advice may, on one level, be 'evidence based', but it takes no account of the interactional dynamics of abruptly introducing the possibility of a sexually transmitted infection when the patient has attended for something else. Qualitative research has shown how disruptive such electronic prompts are to the dynamic of the clinician–patient consultation, whatever the clinical indication [14].

A more philosophical criticism of EBHC is that it is predicated on a simplistic and naïve version of what knowledge is. The assumption is that knowledge can be equated with 'facts' derived from research studies that can be formalised into guidelines and 'translated' (i.e. implemented by practitioners and policymakers). But as Trisha has argued elsewhere, knowledge is a complex and uncertain beast [15]. For one thing, only some knowledge can be thought of as something an individual can know as a 'fact'; there is another level of knowledge that is *collective* – that is, socially shared and organisationally embedded [16]. As Tsoukas and Vladimirou [17] put it:

> *Knowledge is a flux mix of framed experiences, values, contextual information and expert insight that provides a framework for evaluating and incorporating new experiences and information. It originates and is applied in the minds of knowers. In organizations, it often becomes embedded not only in documents or repositories but also in organizational routines, processes, practices, and norms.*

Gabbay and May [18] illustrated this collective element of knowledge in their study of clinical mindlines. While these researchers, who watched GPs in action for several months, never observed the doctors consulting guidelines directly, they did observe them discussing and negotiating these guidelines among themselves and also acting in a way that showed they had somehow absorbed and come to embody the key components of many evidence-based guidelines 'by osmosis'. These collectively embodied, socially shared elements of guidelines are what Gabbay and May called *mindlines*.

Facts held by individuals (e.g. a research finding that one person has discovered on a thorough literature search) may become collectivised through a variety of mechanisms, including efforts to make it relevant to colleagues (timely, salient, actionable), legitimate (credible, authoritative, reasonable) and accessible (available, understandable, assimilable) and to take account of the points of departure (assumptions, world views, priorities) of a particular audience.

These mechanisms reflect a body of research on the philosophy of knowledge – a major topic that is beyond the scope of this book. The key point here is that to present EBHC purely as the sequence of individual tasks set out in earlier chapters is over-simplistic. If you are comfortable with the basics of EBHC, you may wish to pursue the literature on these wider dimensions of knowledge [15–21].

Why is 'evidence-based policymaking' so hard to achieve?

For some people, the main criticism of EBHC is that it fails to get evidence simply and logically into policy. And the reason why policies don't flow simply and logically from research evidence is that there are so many other factors involved.

Take the question of publicly funded treatments for infertility, for example. You can produce a stack of evidence as high as a house to demonstrate that intervention X leads to a take-home baby rate of Y% in women with characteristics (such as age or comorbidity) Z, but that won't take the heat out of the decision to sanction infertility treatment from a limited health care budget. To use a real example from a few years ago, local policymakers operating with a finite budget had to balance this decision against competing options (outreach support for first episode of psychosis, for example, or a community-based diabetes specialist nurse for epilepsy). It wasn't that the members of the policy forum ignored the evidence – they had plenty – it was that values, rather than evidence, were what the final decision hung on. And as many have pointed out, policymaking is as much about the struggle to resolve conflicts of values in particular local or national contexts as it is about getting evidence into practice [22].

In other words, the policymaking process cannot be considered as a 'macro' version of the sequence depicted in section 1.1 ('convert our information needs into answerable questions . . .' etc.). Like other processes that fall under the heading 'politics' (with a small 'p'), policymaking is fundamentally about persuading one's fellow decision-makers of the superiority of one course of action over another. This model of the policymaking process is strongly supported by research studies, which suggest that at its heart lies unpredictability, ambiguity, and the possibility of alternative interpretations of the 'evidence' [22–24].

The quest to make policymaking 'fully evidence based' may actually not be a desirable goal, as this benchmark arguably devalues democratic debate about the ethical and moral issues faced in policy choices. A mantra used in many political manifestos claims that 'what matters is what works'. But what matters, surely, is not just what 'works', but what is appropriate in the circumstances, and what is agreed by society to be the overall desirable goal. Deborah Stone, in her book *Policy Paradox*, argues that much of the policy process involves debates about values masquerading as debates about facts and data. In her words:

> *The essence of policymaking in political communities [is] the struggle over ideas. Ideas are at the centre of all political conflict . . . Each idea is an argument, or more accurately, a collection of arguments in favour of different ways of seeing the world [23].*

One of the most useful theoretical papers on the use of evidence in healthcare policymaking is by Dobrow and colleagues [24]. They distinguish the philosophical–normative orientation (that there is an objective reality to be discovered and that a piece of 'evidence' can be deemed 'valid' and 'reliable' independent of the context in which it is to be used) from the practical–operational orientation, in which evidence is defined in relation to a specific decision-making context, is never static, and is characterised by emergence, ambiguity and incompleteness. From a practical–operational standpoint, research evidence is based on designs (such as randomised trials) that explicitly strip the study of contextual 'contaminants' and which therefore ignore the multiple, complex and interacting determinants of health. It follows that a complex intervention that 'works' in one setting at one time will not necessarily 'work' in a different setting at a different time, and one that proves 'cost-effective' in one setting will not necessarily provide value for money in a different setting. Many of the arguments raised about EBHC in recent years have addressed precisely this controversy about the nature of knowledge.

Questioning the nature of evidence – and indeed, questioning evidential knowledge itself – is a somewhat scary place to end a basic introductory textbook on EBHC, because most of the previous chapters in this book assume what Dobrow would call a philosophical–normative orientation. Here's some advice: if you are a humble student or clinician trying to pass your exams or do a better job at the bedside of individual patients, and if you feel thrown by the uncertainties we've raised in this final section, you can probably safely ignore them until you're actively involved in policymaking yourself. But if your career is at the stage when you're already sitting on decision-making bodies and trying to work out the answer to the question posed in the title to this section, we suggest you explore some of the papers and books referenced below. Do watch for the next generation of EBHC research, which increasingly addresses the fuzzier and more contestable aspects of this important topic.

Exercises based on this chapter

1. Take a look at these papers arguing that evidence-based medicine/healthcare is 'too simplistic': Fernandez et al. [25], 'too utilitarian' Anjum et al. [26] and 'doesn't answer the question about the individual patient' Horwitz et al. [27].
2. Read the paper by Te Meerman et al. [28] on how the disease of attention deficit hyperactivity disorder is 'constructed' differently by different scholars and clinicians. What are the implications for the evidence base on this condition?
3. Now look at this paper published by two of the founding fathers (sic) of evidence-based medicine: Djulbegovic and Guyatt [29], and this one, Ioannidis [30], published by a epidemiologist scholar who likes to play devil's advocate. Both are arguing that the advantages of EBHC outweigh the downsides. To what extent do you think these writers have engaged with the *philosophical* criticisms of EBHC rather than simply reiterating its well-rehearsed strengths?

References

1. Timmermans S, Berg M. *The Gold Standard: The challenge of evidence-based medicine and standardization in health care.* Philadelphia, PA: Temple University Press; 2003.
2. Timmermans S, Mauck A. The promises and pitfalls of evidence-based medicine. *Health Affairs* 2005; **24)**: 18–28.
3. Goldacre B. *Bad Pharma: How drug companies mislead doctors and harm patients.* London: Fourth Estate; 2013.
4. Greenhalgh T, Howick J, Maskrey N. Evidence based medicine: a movement in crisis? *BMJ* 2014; **348**: g3725.
5. Jauho M. Patients-in-waiting or chronically healthy individuals? People with elevated cholesterol talk about risk. *Sociology of Health and Illness* 2019; **41**: 867–81.
6. Hunt LM, Arndt EA, Bell HS, Howard HA. Are corporations re-defining illness and health? The diabetes epidemic, goal numbers, and blockbuster drugs. *Journal of Bioethical Inquiry* 2021; **18**: 477–97.
7. Kleinplatz PJ. History of the treatment of female sexual dysfunction (s). *Annual Review of Clinical Psychology* 2018; **14**: 29–54.
8. Lugtenberg M, Burgers JS, Clancy C, et al. Current guidelines have limited applicability to patients with comorbid conditions: a systematic analysis of evidence-based guidelines. *PloS One* 2011; **6**: e25987.
9. Kristjansson E, Osman M, Dignam M, et al. School feeding programs for improving the physical and psychological health of school children experiencing socioeconomic disadvantage. *Cochrane Database of Systematic Reviews* 2022; **2022**(8): CD014794.

10. Boussageon R, Bejan-Angoulvant T, Saadatian-Elahi M, et al. Effect of intensive glucose lowering treatment on all cause mortality, cardiovascular death, and microvascular events in type 2 diabetes: meta-analysis of randomised controlled trials. *BMJ* 2011; **343**: d4169.
11. Calvert M, Shankar A, McManus RJ, et al. Effect of the quality and outcomes framework on diabetes care in the United Kingdom: retrospective cohort study. *BMJ* 2009; **338**: b1870.
12. Spence D. Why evidence is bad for your health. *BMJ* 2010; **341**: c6368.
13. Allen D, Harkins K. Too much guidance? *Lancet* 2005; **365**: 1768.
14. Swinglehurst D, Greenhalgh T, Roberts C. Computer templates in chronic disease management: ethnographic case study in general practice. *BMJ Open* 2012; **2**: e001754.
15. Greenhalgh T. What is this knowledge that we seek to 'exchange'? *Milbank Quarterly* 2010; **88**: 492–9.
16. Contandriopoulos D, Lemire M, DENIS JL, et al. Knowledge exchange processes in organizations and policy arenas: a narrative systematic review of the literature. *Milbank Quarterly* 2010; **88**: 444–83.
17. Tsoukas H, Vladimirou E. What is organizational knowledge? *Journal of Management Studies* 2001; **38**: 973–3.
18. Gabbay J, May Al. Evidence based guidelines or collectively constructed "mindlines?" Ethnographic study of knowledge management in primary care. *BMJ* 2004; **329**: 1013.
19. Greenhalgh T, Wieringa S. Is it time to drop the 'knowledge translation' metaphor? A critical literature review. *Journal of the Royal Society of Medicine* 2011; **104**: 501–9.
20. Wieringa S, Engebretsen E, Heggen K, Greenhalgh T. Has evidence-based medicine ever been modern? A Latour-inspired understanding of a changing EBM. *Journal of Evaluation in Clinical Practice* 2017; **23**: 964–70.
21. Wieringa S, Engebretsen E, Heggen K, Greenhalgh T. Rethinking bias and truth in evidence-based health care. *Journal of Evaluation in Clinical Practice* 2018; **24**: 930–8.
22. Greenhalgh T, Russell J. Evidence-based policymaking: a critique. *Perspectives in Biology and Medicine* 2009; **52**: 304–18.
23. Stone DA. *Policy Paradox:The art of political decision making*. New York:, NY: Norton; 1997.
24. Dobrow MJ, Goel V, Upshur R. Evidence-based health policy: context and utilisation. *Social Science and Medicine* 2004; **58**: 207–17.
25. Fernandez A, Sturmberg J, Lukersmith S, et al. Evidence-based medicine: is it a bridge too far? *Health Research Policy and Systems* 2015; **13**: 66.
26. Anjum RL, Mumford SD. A philosophical argument against evidence-based policy. *Journal of Evaluation in Clinical Practice* 2017; **23**: 1045–50.
27. Horwitz RI, Hayes-Conroy A, Caricchio R, Singer BH. From evidence based medicine to medicine based evidence. *American Journal of Medicine* 2017; **130**: 1246–50.

28. Te Meerman S, Freedman JE, Batstra L. ADHD and reification: Four ways a psychiatric construct is portrayed as a disease. *Frontiers in Psychiatry* 2022; **13**: 2713.
29. Djulbegovic B, Guyatt GH. Progress in evidence-based medicine: a quarter century on. *Lancet* 2017; **390**: 415–23.
30. Ioannidis JP. Hijacked evidence-based medicine: stay the course and throw the pirates overboard. *Journal of Clinical Epidemiology* 2017; **84**: 11–13.

Appendix 1 Checklists for finding, appraising and implementing evidence

Unless otherwise stated, these checklists can be applied to randomised controlled trials, other controlled clinical trials, cohort studies, case–control studies or any other research evidence.

Is my practice evidence-based? A context-sensitive checklist for individual clinical encounters (see Chapter 1)

1. Have I identified and prioritised the clinical, psychological, social and other factor(s) taking into account the patient's perspective?
2. Have I performed a sufficiently competent and complete examination to establish the likelihood of competing diagnoses?
3. Have I considered additional issues and risk factors that may need opportunistic attention?
4. Have I, where necessary, sought evidence (from systematic reviews, guidelines, clinical trials and other sources) pertaining to the problems?
5. Have I assessed and taken into account the completeness, quality and strength of the evidence?
6. Have I applied valid and relevant evidence to this particular set of problems in a way that is both scientifically justified and intuitively sensible?
7. Have I presented the pros and cons of different options to the patient in a way they can understand, and incorporated the patient's preferences into the final recommendation?
8. Have I arranged review, recall, referral or other further care as necessary?

How to Read a Paper: The Basics of Evidence-Based Healthcare, Seventh Edition.
Trisha Greenhalgh and Paul Dijkstra.

Checklist for searching (see Chapter 2)

1. Decide on the purpose of your search: browsing, seeking an answer to a clinical question or a comprehensive review (e.g. prior to undertaking a piece of research) and design your search strategy accordingly (see section 'What are you looking for?').
2. Go for the highest level of evidence you can (see section 'Levels upon levels of evidence'). For example, high-quality synthesised sources (e.g. systematic reviews and evidence-based summaries and syntheses such as Clinical Evidence or NICE guidelines; see section 'Synthesised sources: systems, summaries and syntheses') represent a very high level of evidence.
3. For keeping abreast of new developments, use synopses such as POEMS ('patient-oriented evidence that matters'), *ACP Journal Club* or *Evidence-Based Medicine* journal (see section 'Pre-appraised sources: synopses of systematic reviews and primary studies').
4. Make yourself familiar with the specialised resources in your own field and use these routinely (see section 'Specialised resources').
5. When searching the PubMed database for primary research, you will greatly increase the efficiency of your search if you do two broad searches and then combine them, or if you use tools such as the 'limit set' or 'clinical queries' function (see section 'Primary studies: tackling the jungle').
6. A very powerful way of identifying recent publications on a topic is to 'citation chain' an older paper (i.e. use a special electronic database to find which later papers have cited the older paper; see section 'Primary studies: tackling the jungle').
7. Federated search engines such as TRIP search multiple resources simultaneously and are free (see section 'One-stop shopping: federated search engines').
8. Experiment with artificial intelligence search tools such as Scite, but check the findings carefully (see section 'Using artificial intelligence to search the literature').
9. Human sources (expert librarians, experts in the field) are an important component of a thorough search (see section 'Asking for help and asking around').
10. To improve your skill and confidence in searching, try an online self-study course (see section 'Online tutorials for effective searching').

Checklist to determine what a paper is about (see Chapter 3)

1. Why was the study performed (what clinical question did it address)?
2. What type of study was performed?

- Primary research (experiment, randomised controlled trial, other controlled clinical trial, cohort study, case–control study, cross-sectional survey, longitudinal survey, case report or case series)?
- Secondary research (simple overview, systematic review, meta-analysis, decision analysis, guideline development, economic analysis)?

3. Was the study design appropriate to the broad field of research addressed (therapy, diagnosis, screening, prognosis, causation)?
4. Did the study meet expected standards of ethics and governance?

Checklist for the methods section of a paper (see Chapter 4)

1. Was the study original?
2. Who is the study about?
   - How were participants recruited?
   - Who was included in, and who was excluded from, the study?
   - Were the participants studied in 'real-life' circumstances?
3. Was the design of the study sensible?
   - What intervention or other manoeuvre was being considered?
   - What outcome(s) were measured, and how?
4. Was the study adequately controlled?
   - If a randomised controlled trial, was randomisation truly random?
   - If a cohort, case–control or other non-randomised comparative study, were the controls appropriate?
   - Were the groups comparable in all important aspects except for the variable being studied?
   - Was assessment of outcome (or, in a case–control study, allocation of caseness) 'blind'?
5. Was the study large enough, and continued for long enough, and was follow-up complete enough, to make the results credible?

Checklist for the statistical aspects of a paper (see Chapter 5)

1. Have the authors set the scene correctly?
   - Have they determined whether the study arms are comparable and, if necessary, adjusted for baseline differences?
   - What sort of data have they produced and have they used appropriate statistical tests?
   - If the statistical tests in the paper are obscure, why have the authors chosen to use them?
   - Have the data been analysed according to the original study protocol?

2. Paired data, tails and outliers:
   - Were paired tests performed on paired data?
   - Was a two-tailed test performed whenever the effect of an intervention could conceivably be a negative one?
   - Were outliers analysed with both common sense and appropriate statistical adjustments?
3. Correlation, regression and causation:
   - Has correlation been distinguished from regression and has the correlation coefficient ('*r*-value') been calculated and interpreted correctly?
   - Have assumptions been made about the nature and direction of causality?
4. Probability and confidence:
   - Have '*p*-values' been calculated and interpreted appropriately?
   - Have confidence intervals been calculated and do the authors' conclusions reflect them?
5. Have the authors expressed their results in terms of the likely harm or benefit that an individual patient can expect, such as:
   - relative risk reduction?
   - absolute risk reduction?
   - number needed to treat?

Checklist for material provided by a pharmaceutical company representative (see Chapter 6)

See particularly Table 6.1 for questions on randomised trials based on the CONSORT statement.

1. Does this material cover a subject that is clinically important in my practice?
2. Has this material been published in independent peer-reviewed journals? Has any significant evidence been omitted from this presentation or withheld from publication?
3. Does the material include high-level evidence such as systematic reviews, meta-analyses or double-blind randomised controlled trials against the drug's closest competitor given at optimal dosage?
4. Have the trials or reviews addressed a clearly focused, important and answerable clinical question that reflects a problem of relevance to patients? Do they provide evidence on safety, tolerability, efficacy and price?
5. Has each trial or meta-analysis defined the condition to be treated, the patients to be included, the interventions to be compared and the outcomes to be examined?

6. Does the material provide direct evidence that the drug will help my patients live a longer, healthier, more productive and symptom-free life?
7. If a surrogate outcome measure has been used, what is the evidence that it is reliable, reproducible, sensitive, specific, a true predictor of disease and rapidly reflects the response to therapy?
8. Do trial results indicate whether (and how) the effectiveness of the treatments differed and whether there was a difference in the type or frequency of adverse reactions? Are the results expressed in terms of numbers needed to treat, and are they clinically as well as statistically significant?
9. If large amounts of material have been provided by the representative, which three papers provide the strongest evidence for the company's claims?

Checklist for a paper describing a study of a complex intervention (see Chapter 7)

1. What is the problem for which this complex intervention is seen as a possible solution?
2. What was done in the developmental phase of the research to inform the design of the complex intervention?
3. What were the core and non-core components of the intervention?
4. What was the theoretical mechanism of action of the intervention?
5. What outcome measures were used and were they sensible?
6. What were the findings?
7. What process evaluation was performed and what were the key findings from it?
8. If the findings were negative, to what extent can this be explained by implementation failure and/or inadequate optimisation of the intervention?
9. If the findings varied across different subgroups, to what extent have the authors explained this by refining their theory of change?
10. What further research do the authors believe is needed and is this justified?

Checklist for a paper that claims to validate a diagnostic or screening test (see Chapter 8)

1. Is this test potentially relevant to my practice?
2. Has the test been compared with a true gold standard?
3. Did this validation study include an appropriate spectrum of participants?
4. Has workup bias been avoided?

5. Has observer bias been avoided?
6. Was the test shown to be reproducible both within and between observers?
7. What are the features of the test as derived from this validation study?
8. Were confidence intervals given for sensitivity, specificity and other features of the test?
9. Has a sensible 'normal range' been derived from these results?
10. Has this test been placed in the context of other potential tests in the diagnostic sequence for the condition?

Checklist for a systematic review or meta-analysis (see Chapter 9)

1. Did the review address an important clinical question?
2. Was a thorough search carried out of the appropriate database(s) and were other potentially important sources explored?
3. Was methodological quality (especially factors that might predispose to bias) assessed and the trials weighted accordingly?
4. How sensitive are the results to the way the review has been performed?
5. Have the numerical results been interpreted with common sense and due regard to the broader aspects of the problem?

Checklist for a set of clinical guidelines (see Chapter 10)

1. Did the preparation and publication of these guidelines involve a significant conflict of interest?
2. Are the guidelines concerned with an appropriate topic and do they state clearly the goal of ideal treatment in terms of health and/or cost outcome?
3. Was a specialist in the methodology of secondary research (e.g. meta-analyst) involved?
4. Have all the relevant data been scrutinised and are guidelines' conclusions in keeping with the data?
5. Are the guidelines valid and reliable?
6. Are they clinically relevant, comprehensive and flexible?
7. Do they take into account what is acceptable to, affordable by, and practically possible for patients?
8. Do they take account of the realities of clinical practice in a particular locality (e.g. availability of particular services or drugs, affordability of interventions, presence of trained staff)?
9. Do they include recommendations for their own dissemination, implementation and periodic review?

Checklist for an economic analysis (see Chapter 11)

1. Is the analysis based on a study that answers a clearly defined clinical question about an economically important issue?
2. From whose viewpoint are costs and benefits being considered?
3. Have the interventions being compared been shown to be clinically effective?
4. Are the interventions sensible and workable in the settings where they are likely to be applied?
5. Which method of economic analysis was used, and was this appropriate?
   - if the interventions produced identical outcomes ⇒ cost-minimisation analysis
   - if the important outcome is unidimensional ⇒ cost-effectiveness analysis
   - if the important outcome is multidimensional ⇒ cost-utility analysis
   - if the cost–benefit equation for this condition needs to be compared with cost–benefit equations for different conditions ⇒ cost-benefit analysis
   - if a cost–benefit analysis would otherwise be appropriate but the preference values given to different health states are disputed or likely to change ⇒ cost-consequences analysis.
6. How were costs and benefits measured?
7. Were incremental, rather than absolute, benefits compared?
8. Was health status in the 'here and now' given precedence over health status in the distant future?
9. Was a sensitivity analysis performed?
10. Were 'bottom-line' aggregate scores overused?

Checklist for a qualitative research paper (see Chapter 12)

1. Did the article describe an important clinical issue addressed via a clearly formulated question?
2. Was a qualitative approach appropriate?
3. How were: (i) the setting, and (ii) the participants selected?
4. What was the researcher's perspective and has this been taken into account?
5. What methods did the researcher use for collecting data and are these described in enough detail?
6. What methods did the researcher use to analyse the data and what quality control measures were implemented?
7. Are the results credible and, if so, are they clinically important?
8. What conclusions were drawn and are they justified by the results?
9. Are the findings of the study transferable to other clinical settings?

Checklist for a paper describing questionnaire research (see Chapter 13)

1. What did the researchers want to find out and was a questionnaire the most appropriate research design?
2. If an 'off the peg' questionnaire (i.e. a previously published and validated one) was available, did the researchers use it (and if not, why not)?
3. What claims have the researchers made about the validity of the questionnaire (its ability to measure what they want it to measure) and reliability (its ability to give consistent results across time and within/between researchers)? Are these claims justified?
4. Was the questionnaire appropriately structured and presented, and were the items worded appropriately for the sensitivity of the subject area and the health literacy of the respondents?
5. Were adequate instructions and explanations included?
6. Was the questionnaire adequately piloted and was the definitive version amended in the light of pilot results?
7. Was the sample of potential participants appropriately selected, large enough and representative enough?
8. How was the questionnaire distributed (e.g. by post, email, telephone) and administered (self-completion, researcher-assisted completion) and were these approaches appropriate?
9. Were the needs of particular subgroups taken into account in the design and administration of the questionnaire? For example, what was done to capture the perspective of illiterate respondents or those speaking a different language from the researcher?
10. What was the response rate and why? If the response rate was low (< 70%), have the researchers shown that no systematic differences existed between responders and non-responders?
11. What sort of analysis was carried out on the questionnaire data and was this appropriate? Is there any evidence of 'data dredging' (i.e. analyses that were not hypothesis driven)?
12. What were the results? Were they definitive (statistically significant), and were important negative and non-significant results also reported?
13. Have qualitative data (e.g. free-text responses) been adequately interpreted (e.g. using an explicit theoretical framework)? Have quotes been used judiciously to illustrate more general findings rather than to add drama?
14. What do the results mean and have the researchers drawn an appropriate link between the data and their conclusions?

Checklist for a paper describing a quality improvement study (see Chapter 14)

1. What was the context?
2. What was the aim of the study?
3. What was the mechanism by which the authors hoped to improve quality?
4. Was the intended quality improvement initiative evidence based?
5. How did the authors measure success and was this method reasonable?
6. How much detail was given on the change process and what insights can be gleaned from it?
7. What were the main findings?
8. What was the explanation for the success, failure or mixed fortunes of the initiative and was this reasonable?
9. In the light of the findings, what do the authors feel are the next steps in the quality improvement cycle locally?
10. What did the authors claim to be the generalisable lessons for other teams and was this assessment reasonable?

Checklist for a paper describing a genetic association study (see Chapter 15)

1. What was the research question (and to what extent was it hypothesis driven)?
2. What was the population studied and was this appropriate? (Consider especially ethnic mix.)
3. Did the study follow established methodological quality criteria for an observational study (cohort or case–control)?
4. Were the alleles of interest distributed as expected in the population (i.e. can you reasonably assume that inbreeding and migration had not biased the genetic sample)?
5. Were phenotypes defined precisely and using standardised criteria?
6. How technically robust was the genetic analysis?
7. Are the findings consistent with other studies?
8. How large and how precise are the associations?
9. Are the conclusions justified by the findings?
10. What (if any) are the implications for patient care in my practice?

Checklist for involving patients in clinical decision-making (see Chapter 16)

1. Am I familiar with patient-reported outcome measures in my patient's condition?
2. Am I familiar with relevant shared decision-making tools (e.g. applications, option grids) for this condition?

3. When selecting a shared decision-making tool, have I taken account of quality features (e.g. does the tool take adequate account of):
   - the condition the patient wants treating
   - likely prognosis with and without treatment
   - all relevant treatment and self-management options (including doing nothing) and the outcome probabilities of each
   - degree of uncertainty of the evidence
   - diagrams and other visuals to help communicate
   - a means of helping the patient clarify their preferences
   - references and sources of further information
   - possible conflicts of interest (e.g. offered by a drug manufacturer).
4. Do I have a good, democratic clinical relationship with this patient so they feel able to converse (and disagree with me if they wish to)?
5. Have I created the time, privacy and permissive atmosphere for shared decision-making?
6. Have I portrayed equipoise where appropriate (e.g. when discussing active intervention versus non-interventional options)?
7. Have I ascertained and taken account of how much the patient wants to be involved in this decision (and/or whether they would like a relative to help decide on their behalf)?
8. Have I adapted the information and/or the tool to suit the patient's cultural background, educational level, health literacy and so on?
9. Have I explored the patient's concerns and attitudes about potential outcomes?
10. Have I offered the option of going away to think about it and having another appointment?

Checklist for a paper describing an artificial intelligence study (see Chapter 17)

1. What is the intended use of the artificial intelligence (AI) system and who are the intended users? Based on this, is the AI system relevant to your patients and practice?
2. Is it clear what type of AI study is reported in the paper?
3. Who participated in the study (patients and users)?
4. What AI system was used in this study?
5. What are the clinical setting(s) and clinical workflow/pathway in which the AI system was evaluated?
6. Were possible errors, including algorithm and use errors, and malfunctions of the supporting software/hardware) defined, described and reported? Did the authors describe their approach to mitigate safety concerns or

patient harm? Did the authors report and discuss any safety concerns or instances of harm?

7. How did the authors deal with human factors?
8. What is the approach to ethical use of the AI system?
9. Did the authors share the code and data used to train and validate their AI system?
10. What kind of collaborative model between authors was used to build the AI system?

Checklist for a paper on mechanistic evidence (see Chapter 18)

1. Have I understood what the term 'mechanistic evidence' means?
2. What kind of mechanistic evidence is relevant to my chosen topic? This might be at any level from molecular to societal, including molecules, genes, drugs, receptors, immune responses (antibodies, cells), people's thought processes or emotional reactions, cultural movements, laws, policies or the entire economy.
3. What is the quality and consistency of evidence supporting a causal mechanism?
4. What is the quality and consistency of evidence *refuting* a causal mechanism?
5. Overall, what is the level of mechanistic evidence (see Table 19.1)?
6. How does the mechanistic evidence align with the randomised controlled trial evidence (if any exists)?
7. What further studies, of what kind, are needed to strengthen the evidence base on causality in this topic?

Checklist for a paper describing a consensus study (see Chapter 19)

1. What is the consensus topic? Is this topic potentially important to my patients and my practice?
2. Why is a consensus on the topic needed?
3. Who directed the consensus exercise and were all [conflicts of] interest declared?
4. Who was in the room and what kind of expertise did they have? Were patients included (if not, why not)?
5. How did the consensus authors address equity, diversity and inclusion?
6. How did the experts work towards consensus (i.e. the method)?
7. Was a definition of consensus set before the start of the consensus exercise?

8. Did the researchers perform an appropriate analysis of all the panelist responses (quantitative and qualitative) and was this made available?
9. How did the researchers deal with dissent? Did they report it? Did they perform a proper dissent analysis?
10. Did the researchers produce a clear bottom line for decision-makers and, if so, what was it?

Appendix 2 **Assessing the effects of an intervention**

Group	Outcome event		Total
	Yes	No	
Control	*a*	*b*	*a* + *b*
Experimental	*c*	*d*	*c* + *d*

If outcome event is undesirable (e.g. death)
Control event rate (CER) = risk of undesirable outcome in control group = $a/(a+b)$
Experimental event rate (EER) = risk of undesirable outcome in experimental group = $c/(c+d)$
Relative risk of undesirable event in experimental versus control group = EER/CER
Absolute risk reduction in treated group (ARR) = CER − EER
Number needed to treat = 1/ARR = 1/(CER − EER)

If outcome event is desirable (e.g. cure)
CER = risk of desirable outcome in control group = a/(a + b)
EER = risk of desirable outcome in experimental group = c/(c + d)
Relative benefit increase in treated versus control group = EER/CER
Absolute benefit increase in treated versus control group = EER − CER
Number needed to treat = 1/ARR = 1/(EER − CER)

Acknowledgement

Thanks to Paul Glasziou from the Oxford Centre for Evidence-Based Medicine for clarification on these concepts.

How to Read a Paper: The Basics of Evidence-Based Healthcare, Seventh Edition.
Trisha Greenhalgh and Paul Dijkstra.

Index

How to Read a Paper: The Basics of Evidence-Based Healthcare, Seventh Edition.
Trisha Greenhalgh and Paul Dijkstra.